Melanocortins: Multiple Actions and Therapeutic Potential

ADVANCES IN EXPERIMENTAL MEDICINE AND BIOLOGY

Melanocortins:

Multiple Actions and Therapeutic Potential

Edited by

Anna Catania, MD
Center for Preclinical Investigation
Fondazione IRCCS ,Ca' Granda, Ospedale Maggiore Policlinico
Milano, Italy

Springer Science+Business Media, LLC

Landes Bioscience

Springer Science+Business Media, LLC
Landes Bioscience

Copyright ©2010 Landes Bioscience and Springer Science+Business Media, LLC

Printed in the USA.

Springer Science+Business Media, LLC, 233 Spring Street, New York, New York 10013, USA
http://www.springer.com

Please address all inquiries to the publishers:
Landes Bioscience, 1002 West Avenue, Austin, Texas 78701, USA
Phone: 512/ 637 6050; FAX: 512/ 637 6079
http://www.landesbioscience.com

The chapters in this book are available in the Madame Curie Bioscience Database.
http://www.landesbioscience.com/curie

Melanocortins: Multiple Actions and Therapeutic Potential, edited by Anna Catania. Landes Bioscience / Springer Science+Business Media, LLC dual imprint / Springer series: Advances in Experimental Medicine and Biology.

ISBN: 978-1-4419-6353-6

Library of Congress Cataloging-in-Publication Data

A C.I.P. catalog record for this book is available from the Library of Congress.

DEDICATION

To the many scientists who contributed to expand knowledge of the melanocortin system.

FOREWORD

It is clear that the melanocortins are of immense academic interest. Further, these molecules have remarkable potential as pharmaceutical agents for treatment of multiple human and veterinary disorders and diseases. The evidence to support academic interest and clinical applications lies in significant part within the chapters of this book, chapters written by noted experts in the field who have worked diligently to understand the molecules and to move them toward clinical applications. I personally believe that the α-MSH molecule and its derivatives will be used as routine therapeutics in the very near future. My belief is so strong that I left academia to form a company based on α-MSH analogs and have caused millions of dollars to be spent on melanocortin research. Now why would a sane professor pick up such a challenge and enter business, an essential step toward any clinical application? It is the α-MSH story that drove me. Consider that α-MSH occurs in exactly the same amino acid sequence in humans and in the sea lamprey, an organism unchanged since its appearance during the Pennsylvanian period of the Paleozoic era (about 300 million years ago—way before dinosaurs were to be considered). There is unpublished evidence that the stability of the molecule can be traced back a half billion years. Frankly, I believe that the molecule existed even when single cells began to live together. I speculate that the purpose of the molecule was then, as perhaps now, to modulate inflammation and infection, the earliest challenges to cells and cell colonies. We must await the motivation of cell physiologists to tell us if this is true but it is, in me, an unshakeable belief. I am an agrarian pragmatist and it seems that things must have been just this way, judging from what we know now.

Now, while Mother Nature was doing her work on α-MSH, we humans were simply oblivious to the events. We did not even know that such a molecule as α-MSH existed. That is, until Aaron Bunsen Lerner and his colleagues began to provide evidence for structure and function of the molecule in the early 1950s, not quite 60 years ago. As a slide from Dr. Catania's general presentation shows, by 1990 when she and I had begun working together, about 40 years after the reports from Lerner's lab, the annual production rate of α-MSH papers in the literature stood at 23. There was subsequently a dramatic and progressive rise in reports, with the total papers published from1990 to 2008 reaching over 5800. We need no further testament to the promise and excitement of melanocortin research.

As I have spent many years as editor and reviewer, always with an eye to the reader, I ask: What will readers get from this book? The answer after my personal review is: Quite a lot. The reader gets the latest perspectives on all aspects of the melanocortin molecules: from their amino acid sequences, their receptors, the mechanisms of their action, their roles in physiological and pathological processes, and the clinical significance of the molecules. Even the novice reader can see that it is likely that these ancient molecules operate in many different functions. They are said to be "pluripotential." From this perspective it is perhaps a pity that the major melanocortin molecule is called "α-melanocyte stimulating hormone" for we know it is much more than that. The term still leads students and novices to wrong conclusions and inaccurate theories concerning pigmentation. Still, no one would dare posit a more descriptive term because we all respect the name given to the molecule when it was discovered 60 years ago.

I can think of no other scientist I would recommend to edit this book. Dr. Catania is one of the most intelligent, knowledgeable and dedicated people I know and she takes our field very seriously. It was my pleasure to meet her some time ago at an international conference in Italy. I was immediately struck by her clinical background and avidity for science and the literature. It was immediately clear that she had an intense inherent interest and talent for science. At the time I told fellow faculty that her interests and capabilities were exceptional, truly unique. We arranged for her to travel to Southwestern Medical School at Dallas to collaborate with us on α-MSH research. My estimate of her abilities was proven correct and the collaboration was very fruitful... She calls me "mentor" but, in truth, I did little: just some basic ideas about scientific research and about writing research papers that I learned the hard way—through mistakes. She has become well-known based on her own self-generated projects, her high rate of research production, and on her many major summaries of where we are in the field, published as meritorious literature reviews.

James M. Lipton, PhD
Emeritus Professor of Physiology
University of Texas Southwestern Medical Center at Dallas
Dallas, Texas
USA

PREFACE

Melanocortin peptides and their receptors are key elements of ancient modulatory systems that appeared very early in evolution. Pro-opiomelanocortin (POMC) is a common precursor of melanocortins, the collective term for adrenocorticotropic hormone (ACTH), α-, β-, γ- melanocyte-stimulating hormone (α-, β-, γ-MSH), and endorphins. The pituitary of the lamprey, the most ancient of vertebrates, contains recognizable POMC sequences with structural similarity to those of teleosts and higher vertebrates. Melanocortin receptors are likewise very ancient.

The presence of melanocortins in primitive animals was paradoxically detrimental to research in higher organisms. It has not been long since melanocortins were considered an "evolutionary remnant" and the true potential of this system overlooked. Although adrenal, pigmentary, and behavioral effects of melanocortins have been known for over 50 years, the discovery that melanocortins have potent modulatory effects on host responses is much more recent. Significant progress stems from the signal contribution of my Mentor, Dr. James M. Lipton who discovered the antipyretic and anti-inflammatory actions of α-MSH. A major breakthrough in understanding melanocortin action came with the cloning of the melanocortin receptor (MCR) family by Dr. Kathleen Mountjoy, author of a chapter in this book. Characterization of receptors promoted substantial advances in understanding the nature and effects of melanocortins. The observation that melanocortinergic neurons exert a tonic inhibition of feeding behavior was a momentous discovery in melanocortin research. The multiple actions of natural peptides can be exploited therapeutically through design of synthetic analogues with specific effects.

This book represents the joint effort of an international group of scientists who are at the forefront of research in the field. The volume spans information on chemistry, pharmacology, distribution, and therapeutic potential of melanocortins. A recurrent theme in this volume is the role played by distinct melanocortin receptors in mediating melanocortin effects. Although these receptors have been identified and well-characterized, information in the book indicates that definite categorization of their expression and function in different conditions still needs major work. For example, it is clear that control of food intake mainly depends on central MC4R subtypes and pigmentation is regulated by MC1R in melanocytes. On the other hand, it appears that the anti-inflammatory effects of melanocortins are orchestrated by multiple receptors in the brain and in peripheral cells.

Several human disorders could benefit from melanocortin treatment. Obesity has become a major health problem in Western countries. Synthetic MC4R agonists are very promising candidates to treat this disorder; clinical trials are already in progress. The anti-cytokine action and the inhibitory effect on inflammatory cell migration make melanocortins potential new drugs for treatment of acute, chronic, and systemic inflammation. The neuroprotective action in vascular and inflammatory brain injury is likewise well established. Melanocortins could form a novel class of therapeutic agents for several disorders of the nervous system. Through activation of MC1R, α-MSH confers photoprotection to human melanocytes and reduces DNA damage caused by exposure to solar ultraviolet radiation. Based on these actions, MC1R agonists are promising agents for melanoma prevention strategies.

The severe disability caused by obesity, neurological, and inflammatory disorders has very high costs in terms of decrease in quality of life and ability to work. These conditions thus entail a heavy economic price for both the patients and the society. It is clear that effective treatments would be a beneficial response to significant needs. As research described in this book indicates, melanocortins have a remarkable potential for treatment of many dire conditions.

Anna Catania, MD
Center for Preclinical Investigation
Fondazione IRCCS, Ca' Granda, Ospedale Maggiore Policlinico
Milano
Italy

ABOUT THE EDITOR...

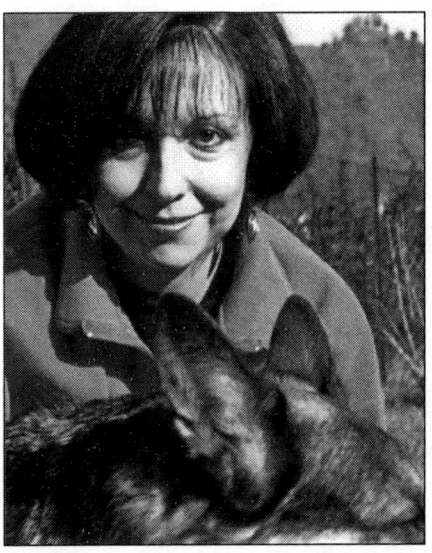

ANNA CATANIA, MD is the director of the Center for Preclinical Investigation at Fondazione Ca' Granda-Ospedale Maggiore Policlinico, Milano, Italy. She received her specialty degree in Medicine and Surgery at the University of Milan and postdoctoral degree in Endocrinology and Metabolism at the University of Genoa, Italy. For over a decade she has been visiting scientist at The University of Texas Southwestern Medical Center at Dallas, Texas.

During the past 20 years, her research activity has been focused on molecular biology and preclinical testing of melanocortins.

PARTICIPANTS

Zalfa A. Abdel-Malek
Department of Dermatology
University of Cincinnati
Cincinnati, Ohio
USA

Domenica Altavilla
 Department of Clinical
   and Experimental Medicine
   and Pharmacology
Section of Pharmacology
University of Messina
Messina
Italy

Jean-Philippe Bapst
Laboratory of Endocrinology
Department of Biomedicine
University Hospital Basel
   and University Children's Hospital
University of Basel
Basel
Switzerland

Carla Bazzani
Department of Biomedical Sciences
Section of Pharmacology
University of Modena
   and Reggio Emilia
Modena
Italy

Markus Böhm
Department of Dermatology
   and Ludwig Boltzmann
Institute for Cell Biology
   and Immunobiology of the Skin
University of Münster
Münster
Germany

Erin B. Bruce
Department of Pharmacodynamics
University of Florida
Gainesville, Florida
USA

Thomas Brzoska
Dr. Wolff Arzneimittel, GmbH
Bielefeld
Germany
and
Department of Dermatology
   and Ludwig Boltzmann
Institute for Cell Biology
   and Immunobiology of the Skin
University of Münster
Münster
Germany

Martine Calame
Laboratory of Endocrinology
Department of Biomedicine
University Hospital Basel
   and University Children's Hospital
University of Basel
Basel
Switzerland

Anna Catania
Center for Preclinical Investigation
Fondazione IRCCS Ca' Granda
Ospedale Maggiore Policlinico
Milano
Italy

Maija Dambrova
Latvian Institute of Organic Synthesis
Riga
Latvia

Alex N. Eberle
Laboratory of Endocrinology
Department of Biomedicine
University Hospital Basel
   and University Children's Hospital
University of Basel
Basel
Switzerland

Paula C. Eves
Department of Dental and Maxillofacial
   Medicine and Surgery
The School of Clinical Dentistry
The University of Sheffield
Claremont Crescent
Sheffield
UK

Sylvie Froidevaux
Actelion Pharmaceuticals, Ltd
Allschwil
Switzerland

Stefano Gatti
Center for Preclinical Investigation
Fondazione IRCCS Ca' Granda
Ospedale Maggiore Policlinico
Milano
Italy

Daniela Giuliani
Department of Biomedical Sciences
Section of Pharmacology
University of Modena and Reggio
   Emilia
Modena
Italy

Salvatore Guarini
Department of Biomedical Sciences
Section of Pharmacology
University of Modena
   and Reggio Emilia
Modena
Italy

Carrie Haskell-Luevano
Department of Pharmacodynamics
University of Florida
Gainesville, Florida
USA

Erica M. Haslach
Department of Pharmacodynamics
University of Florida
Gainesville, Florida
USA

John W. Haycock
Kroto Research Institute
Department of Engineering Materials
The University of Sheffield
Broad Lane
Sheffield
UK

Darren Lee
Schepens Eye Research Institute
Department of Ophthalmology
Harvard Medical School
Boston, Massachusetts
USA

Giovanna Leoni
The William Harvey Research Institute
Barts and the London School
   of Medicine
Queen Mary University of London
London
UK

James M. Lipton
University of Texas Southwestern
   Medical Center at Dallas
Dallas, Texas
USA

Caterina Lonati
Center for Preclinical Investigation
Fondazione IRCCS Ca' Granda
Ospedale Maggiore Policlinico
Milano
Italy

Karin Loser
Department of Dermatology
   and Ludwig Boltzmann
Institute for Cell Biology
   and Immunobiology of the Skin
University of Münster
Münster
Germany

Thomas A. Luger
Department of Dermatology
Ludwig Boltzmann Institute
   for Cell Biology and Immunobiology
   of the Skin
University of Münster
Münster
Germany

Andreas Lügering
Department of Internal Medicine
University of Münster
Münster
Germany

Trinidad Montero Melendez
The William Harvey Research Institute
Barts and the London School
   of Medicine
Queen Mary University of London
London
UK

Kathleen G. Mountjoy
Departments of Physiology
   and Molecular Medicine
   and Pathology
School of Medical Sciences
University of Auckland
Auckland
New Zealand

Ruta Muceniece
Faculty of Medicine
University of Latvia
Riga
Latvia

Alessandra Ottani
Department of Biomedical Sciences
Section of Pharmacology
University of Modena
   and Reggio Emilia
Modena
Italy

Hetal B. Patel
The William Harvey Research Institute
Barts and the London School
   of Medicine
Queen Mary University of London
London
UK

Mauro Perretti
Centre for Biochemical Pharmacology
The William Harvey Research Institute
Barts and The London School
   of Medicine
London
UK

André L.F. Sampaio
The William Harvey Research Institute
Barts and the London School
   of Medicine
Queen Mary University of London
London
UK
and
Department of Applied Pharmacology
Farmanguinhos
Fundação Oswaldo Cruz
Rio de Janeiro
Brazil

Jay W. Schaub
Department of Pharmacodynamics
University of Florida
Gainesville, Florida
USA

Anamika Singh
Department of Pharmacodynamics
University of Florida
Gainesville, Florida
USA

Andrea Sordi
Center for Preclinical Investigation
Fondazione IRCCS Ca' Granda
Ospedale Maggiore Policlinico
Milano
Italy

Francesco Squadrito
 Department of Clinical
   and Experimental Medicine
   and Pharmacology
 Section of Pharmacology
 University of Messina
 Messina
 Italy

Heidi Tanner
Laboratory of Endocrinology
Department of Biomedicine
University Hospital Basel
   and University Children's Hospital
University of Basel
Basel
Switzerland

Andrew W. Taylor
Schepens Eye Research Institute
Boston, Massachusetts
USA

CONTENTS

4. DRUGS, EXERCISE, AND THE MELANOCORTIN-4
RECEPTOR—DIFFERENT MEANS, SAME ENDS:
TREATING OBESITY 49

Jay W. Schaub, Erin B. Bruce, and Carrie Haskell-Luevano

5. MELANOCORTINS IN BRAIN INFLAMMATION:
THE ROLE OF MELANOCORTIN RECEPTOR SUBTYPES 61

Ruta Muceniece and Maija Dambrova

6. MELANOCORTINS AND THE CHOLINERGIC
ANTI-INFLAMMATORY PATHWAY 71

Daniela Giuliani, Alessandra Ottani, Domenica Altavilla, Carla Bazzani,
     Francesco Squadrito and Salvatore Guarini

7. MELANOCORTIN CONTROL OF CELL TRAFFICKING
IN VASCULAR INFLAMMATION.. 88

Hetal B. Patel, Giovanna Leoni, Trinidad Montero Melendez, André L.F. Sampaio
    and Mauro Perretti

8. TERMINAL SIGNAL: ANTI-INFLAMMATORY EFFECTS
OF α-MELANOCYTE-STIMULATING HORMONE
RELATED PEPTIDES BEYOND THE PHARMACOPHORE 107

Thomas Brzoska, Markus Böhm, Andreas Lügering, Karin Loser
    and Thomas A. Luger

9. PROTECTIVE EFFECTS OF MELANOCORTINS
IN SYSTEMIC HOST REACTIONS 117

Stefano Gatti, Caterina Lonati, Andrea Sordi and Anna Catania

10. DEVELOPMENT OF α-MELANOCORTIN ANALOGS FOR MELANOMA PREVENTION AND TARGETING 126

Zalfa A. Abdel-Malek

11. MSH RADIOPEPTIDES FOR TARGETING MELANOMA METASTASES 133

Alex N. Eberle, Jean-Philippe Bapst, Martine Calame, Heidi Tanner
    and Sylvie Froidevaux

12. APPLICATIONS OF THE ROLE OF α-MSH IN OCULAR IMMUNE PRIVILEGE.. 143

Andrew W. Taylor and Darren Lee

Structure-Activity Relationships (SAR) of Melanocortin and Agouti-Related (AGRP) Peptides

Anamika Singh, Erica M. Haslach and Carrie Haskell-Luevano*

Abstract

Structure-activity relationship (SAR) studies are a key feature of peptide and peptidomimetic research to improve the biological properties of native peptides and convert them into more drug-like compounds. Peptide SAR studies involve the systematic modification of a lead peptide to provide insight into the molecular determinants of the ligand-receptor interactions that result in either receptor stimulation or inhibition. This chapter will discuss structure-activity relationships of the endogenous and synthetic agonists and the antagonists of the melanocortin system.

Introduction

The melanocortin receptors (MCRs) belong to the family of seven transmamebrane (TM) spanning G-protein coupled receptors (GPCRs) that stimulate the cAMP signal transduction pathway. Five subtypes of melanocortin receptors have been identified to date MC1R-MC5R.[1-7] The endogenous melanocortin agonists peptides, α, β, γ-melanocyte stimulating hormones (MSH) and adrenocorticotropic hormone (ACTH) are derived by the posttranslational processing of the proopiomelanocortin (POMC) gene transcript (Fig. 1).[8] All MSH ligands contain a His-Phe-Arg-Trp core sequence (Fig. 1), which is important for melanocortin receptor stimulation.[9,10] The melanocortin receptor system is unique among GPCRs in terms of having both naturally occurring agonists and antagonists. The melanocortin antagonists, agouti and agouti-related protein (AGRP) are the only two endogenous antagonists of GPCRs identified to date.[11,12]

Cloning of melanocortin receptor subtypes rejuvenated the field in terms of research relating to SAR of MSH and ACTH peptides from the traditional studies dating back to the early 1960s utilizing frog and lizard skin bioassays. The MC1R is expressed in melanocytes and is involved in coat coloration and pigmentation. The MC2R only responds to stimulation by ACTH, is expressed in the adrenal cortex and adipocytes and is involved in steroidogenesis. The MC3R is expressed in the brain, placenta, heart and gut, whereas, the MC4R primarily expressed in the brain. Both the MC3R and MC4R are involved in the regulation of energy homeostatis, as related to the feeding behavior, satiety and obesity.[13-15] The MC5R is expressed in the muscle, liver, spleen, lung, brain, adipocytes and variety of other tissues where it is involved in the exocrine gland function.[16] Some of the known physiological functions and primary ligands for MCRs are summarized in the Table 1.

*Corresponding Author: Carrie Haskell-Luevano—Department of Pharmacodynamics, University of Florida, PO Box 100487, Gainesville Florida, 32610-0487 USA. Email: carrie@cop.ufl.edu

Melanocortins: Multiple Actions and Therapeutic Potential, edited by Anna Catania. ©2010 Landes Bioscience and Springer Science+Business Media.

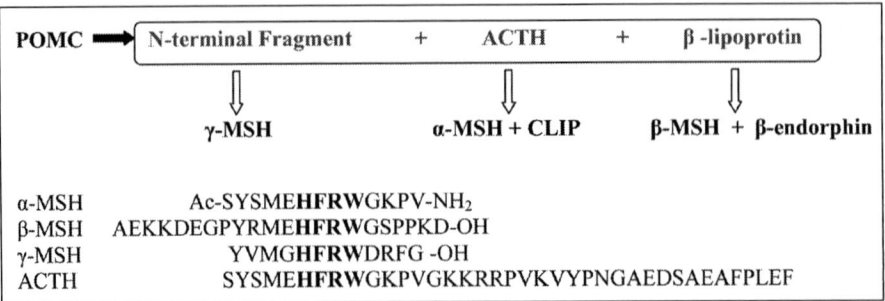

Figure 1. POMC processing of the melanocortins and primary sequence of the melanocortin peptides with core "His-Phe-Arg-Trp".

Table 1. Expression and function of melanocortin receptors

Receptor	Expression	Primary Ligand	Physiological Function
MC1R	Melanocytes, adipocytes, macrophages, sebocytes	α-MSH	Skin pigmentation, animal coat coloration, melanocyte function
MC2R	Adrenal cortex, adipocytes	ACTH	Steroidogenesis
MC3R	Brain, placenta, heart, gut	α, γ-MSH	Energy homeostasis
MC4R	Brain	α, β-MSH	Energy homeostasis, erectile function
MC5R	Muscle, liver, spleen, lung, brain, adipocytes,	α-MSH, ACTH	Sebaceous gland lipid secretion

Table 2. Amino acid sequence of different forms of γ-MSH

γ₁-MSH	Tyr-Val-Met-Gly-His-Phe-Arg-Trp-Asp-Arg-Phe-NH₂
γ₂-MSH	Tyr-Val-Met-Gly-His-Phe-Arg-Trp-Asp-Arg-Phe-Gly
γ₃-MSH	Tyr-Val-Met-Gly-His-Phe-Arg-Trp-Asp-Arg-Phe-Gly-Pro-Arg-Asn(glycosyl)-Ser-Ser-Ala-Gly-Gly-Ser-Ala-Gln

Structure and Chemistry of Melanocortin Peptides

α-MSH is the first thirteen N-terminal amino acid residues of ACTH and is identical in all mammals. It is acetylated at the N-terminus and amidated at the C-terminus. β-MSH is a 22 residue peptide and β-MSH(5-22), is found in the human hypothalamus with the C-terminal exists as the free acid.[17] γ-MSH peptides are endogenously present in three pharmacologically active forms, γ₃-MSH, γ₂-MSH and γ₁-MSH (Table 2). γ-MSH peptides have been detected in the pituitary and plasma, brain, vascular system, the bronchi and kidneys. ACTH is composed of 39 amino acids, having serine at the N-terminus and the phenylalanine residue at the C-terminus.

Structure-Activity Relationships (SAR)

Modification of biological activity or selectivity of the compound by altering its chemical structure is the primary goal of structure-activity relationship studies. The insight generated by SAR

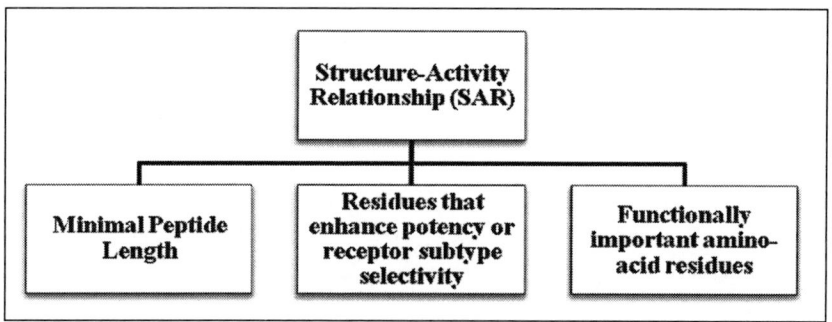

Figure 2. Summary of the "Classical" peptide structure-activity relationship (SAR) studies.

studies provide valuable information about the ligand, receptor binding pocket and ligand-receptor interactions which serve as a tool to the drug design process (Fig. 2).

Linear Melanocortin Peptides

The melanocortin ligands, both endogenous and synthetic, have been subjected to various structure-activity studies which led to valuable information about the receptor-ligand interactions. Receptor-ligand interactions are postulated to be responsible for molecular recognition, ligand binding and receptor stimulation. Structure-activity relationship (SAR) studies enable the identification of the chemical groups responsible for producing a target biological effect which aids in the design of ligands with more potency and selectivity. The SAR studies of melanocortin peptides are discussed herein. A summary of earlier findings precede more recent studies in each section.

α-MSH

Extensive SAR studies have been performed on melanotropin peptides, especially α-MSH and reviewed periodically.[9,18-20] α-MSH is a nonselective agonist at four melanocortin receptors, MC1 and MC3-MC5. Extensive structure-function studies of α-MSH eventually resulted in a more potent and enzyme-resistant analogue [Nle[4], DPhe[7]]-α-MSH (NDP-MSH), that contains the "active core" fragment of melanocortin peptides with Nle substitution at position 4 instead of Met which is prone to oxidation and DPhe at position 7 in place of Phe.[21] Radiolabeled derivatives of NDP-MSH are extensively used for melanocortin receptor studies. Truncation studies of α-MSH, which involves selective removal of N- and/or C-terminal residues, followed by evaluation of the truncated analogues for binding and/or functional activity revealed that residues 4, 10 and 12 contributes to the potency of the peptide. The minimum sequence identified for the biological activity was Ac-His-Phe-Arg-Trp-NH$_2$ (core message sequence) for α-MSH in classical frog (*Rana Pipiens*) and lizard (*Anolis carolinensis*) bioassays.[10,22,23] Moreover, it is hypothesized that a bioactive conformation involves a β-turn containing the core message sequence.[9,11,24,25,67,68] Using the lizard skin bioassay, residues 1-3, 5 and 13 were identified not to be important for agonist potency. The NDP-MSH truncation studies at the MC4R determined that the minimum sequence required for activity was Ac-DPhe-Arg-Trp-NH$_2$, with the addition of His, potency was significantly increased at mouse melanocortin receptors.[26]

An Alanine scan is a classical SAR method, which also complements the truncation studies in determining the residues responsible for, or contributing to, the biological properties of the native peptide important for molecular recognition and functional activity. Positional Ala scan of α-MSH revealed that positions 4, 6, 7, 8 and 9 (Table 3) are important for the receptor binding at MC1R.[27] Important points which were revealed after SAR studies of α-MSH are summarized in Table 4. More recent work on α-MSH includes cyclic analogues which will be discussed in a different section.

Table 3. Alanine substitution of core HFRW in α-MSH

AA	α-MSH at mMC1R (B16 melanoma cell assay)
His	100 fold ↓in binding; 6 fold ↓in activity
Phe	200 fold ↓in binding; 260 fold ↓in activity
Arg	2080 fold ↓in binding; 100 fold ↓in activity
Trp	2000 fold ↓in binding; 125 fold ↓in activity

Data taken from reference 8.

Tetrapeptide Ac-His-DPhe-Arg-Trp-NH$_2$

Several SAR studies of the core tetrapeptide sequence were carried out in search of more drug-like melanocortin ligands. Ala scan of the tetrapeptide Ac-His-DPhe-Arg-Trp-NH$_2$ showed that substitution of His with Ala resulted in greater reduction of potency, whereas, substitution of DPhe resulted in 1500-fold decreased potency at mMC1R and complete loss of activity at the mMC3R-mMC5R at concentrations up to 100 μM.[28] Replacement of Arg with Ala gave decreased potency ranging from 170-1,740 fold at the mouse MC1R and MC3-5R.[29] Complete loss of activity was seen for Trp replacement with Ala at mMC3R, however, 220-, 2540- and 9700-fold decreased potency was observed at mMC1R, mMC4R and mMC5R, respectively.[30] Holder et al have reported SAR studies of the Ac-His-DPhe-Arg-Trp-NH$_2$ tetrapeptide template using a positional scanning approach.[28-31] Several novel compounds with unique pharmacology were identified in these studies (Table 5). It was reported that introducing biphenylalanine (Bip) or tetrahydroisoquinoline (Tic) (peptides 2 and 3) instead of Trp in the Ac-His-DPhe-Arg-Trp-NH$_2$ template results in increased affinity for the MC1R and MC5R over the centrally expressed MC3 and MC4 receptors (Table 5). In a similar study corresponding to the alteration of the DPhe position, it was reported that Ac-His-(pI)DPhe-Arg-Trp-NH$_2$ (peptide 4, Table 5) possesses novel pharmacology as an antagonist and partial agonist at the mMC3R and a potent full agonist at the mMC4R (Table 5).[31,32] Substitution at the His position in the Ac-His-DPhe-Arg-Trp-NH$_2$ template revealed that various natural and unnatural amino acids can increase selectivity for the centrally expressed MC4R over the MC3R (Peptides 5 and 6; Table 5). Positional scanning of the Arg position has shown that the guanidine side chain of Arg is important for ligand receptor interactions in peptide ligands (peptides 7 and 8, Table 5).[33]

In a similar study, a series of pentapeptides, based on the hMC4R agonist (Ac-His⁶-DPhe⁷-Arg⁸-Trp⁹-Gly¹⁰-NH$_2$), were synthesized in which either DPhe⁷ or Trp⁹ residue systematically substituted.[34] A number of interesting DPhe surrogates [DThi, (3-CF$_3$) DPhe, 2- DNal and (3,4-diCl) DPhe)] as well as Trp surrogates (2-Nal and Bta) were identified in this study. Cheung et al have reported positional scanning approach on Bu-His-DPhe-Arg-Trp-Gly-NH$_2$ template and screened the compounds on human melanocortin receptors.[35] This study suggested that replacement of the His residue with the rigid, nonbasic Atc residue resulted in the selective hMC4R agonists without any stimulatory activity at the hMC3R. Substitution of the DPhe residue in the butanoyl-His-DPhe-Arg-Trp-Gly-NH$_2$ template with unusual amino acids resulted

Table 4. Summary of SAR studies for α-MSH

A. Ac-His-Phe-Arg-Trp-NH$_2$ (Core Sequence): important for biological activity.

B. Residues 4, 10 and 12 are important to retain equipotency to the parent peptide.

C. Residues 1-3, 5, 11 and 13 are not important and contribute minimally to the potency.

D. N-acetylation and C-amidation is necessary for enzymatic stability.

E. Reverse turn is proposed in the core sequence region.

Table 5. Functional activity of selected peptides at the mouse MC1, MC3-5 receptors

Peptide	Substitution				mMC1R EC$_{50}$ (nM)	mMC3R EC$_{50}$ (nM)	mMC4R EC$_{50}$ (nM)	mMC5R EC$_{50}$ (nM)	Ref.
1	His	DPhe	Arg	Trp	20.1 ± 0.57	156 ± 9.21	7.2 ± 2.78	3.96 ± 0.94	71
2	His	DPhe	Arg	**Bip**	51.9 ± 9.9	13400 ± 810	2700 ± 460	100 ± 20	71
3	His	DPhe	Arg	**Tic**	43.0 ± 12.5	23200 ± 2300	8500 ± 930	700 ± 99	71
4	His	**(pI)DPhe**	Arg	Trp	60.4 ± 13.4	Partial agonist pA$_2$ = 7.25 ± 0.18	25.0 ± 9.78	1.60 ± 0.35	73
5	**Anc**	DPhe	Arg	Trp	7900 ± 4200	pA$_2$ = 5.60 ± 0.11	21.1 ± 6.0	45.6 ± 6.9	72
6	**Phe**	DPhe	Arg	Trp	503 ± 100	11900 ± 1800	70.6 ± 13.8	143 ± 5	72
7	His	DPhe	**Ala**	Trp	3400 ± 1600	42000 ± 8900	23000 ± 4100	6900 ± 1500	70
8	His	DPhe	**Lys**	Trp	770 ± 500	25500 ± 1900	830 ± 140	320 ± 14	70

Slight agonist denotes that some stimulatory activity was observed but not enough to determine EC$_{50}$ values.

in some very potent agonists at the hMC1R and hMC4R.[34] The (pCl)DPhe and (pBr)DPhe pentapeptide analogues possessed low EC_{50} values at the hMC1R and hMC4R, similar to the (pI)DPhe analogue that was characterized at the mouse melanocortin receptor in the Table 5. However, no characterization was performed at the hMC3R and hMC5R. Substitution of the Trp residue in the butanoyl-His-DPhe-Arg-Trp-Gly-NH$_2$ template resulted in the identification of a potent agonist at the hMC1R and hMC4R without any increase of selectivity or potency than the parent compound.[34] Only a slight decrease in potency as compared to the reference compound was observed for the DTrp modified peptide. Positional scanning at the Arg position resulted in acylguanidine and cyanoguanidine derivatives (less basic surrogates) that retained melanocortin stimulatory activity of the parent at the hMC1R and hMC4R.[36] Introduction of other natural and unnatural amino acids in place of Arg resulted in decreased potency that was similar to the observations reported in the Ac-His-DPhe-Arg-Trp-NH$_2$ template which may suggest that positive charge of Arg[8] is not essential for efficient interaction of pentapeptides with both hMC1 and hMC4Rs.

Previous structure-activity relationship (SAR) studies, modifying the DPhe[7] of synthetic melanocortin ligands (α-MSH numbering) such as MTII,[37] SHU9119[38] (Table 7) and the tetrapeptide template Ac-His-DPhe-Arg-Trp-NH$_2$ led to the hypothesis that bulky substituent at the DPhe[7] position may be responsible for antagonism at the MC3 and MC4 receptors. Ac-His-DNal(2')-Arg-Trp-NH$_2$ was identified as an antagonist, similar to that of SHU9119, however, with decreased potency.[31] Unexpectantly, modification at the DPhe position with pI, resulted in the tetrapeptide Ac-His-DPhe(pI)-Arg-Trp-NH$_2$ that possessed "mixed pharmacology" as discussed earlier with antagonist/partial agonist activity at the mMC3R, while retaining full nanomolar agonist potency and efficacy at the mMC4R.[31] Recently, Proneth et al has published the study based on the hypothesis that the DPhe[7] position can be exploited for improvement of receptor selectivity for the mMC3R versus the mMC4R and for the differentiation of agonist versus antagonist activity at the mMC3R.[32] Several residues with diverse ranges of electronic, polar properties and size were chosen to replace the DPhe[7] at para and meta positions. Selected compounds pharmacology at the mouse melanocortin receptors (MC1R, MC3R-MC5R) are summarized in (Table 6).

The incorporation of the smaller fluorine, chlorine and bromine substituents at the para position of DPhe slightly improved ligand potency for mMC1R, mMC4R and mMC5R, whereas the larger p-I substituent in peptide 12 and the pCF$_3$ in peptide 13 or a Cl substituent in the meta position (Peptide 15, 16) slightly decreases ligand potency for these receptor subtypes. Peptides with fluorine or chlorine substituents at the para position of DPhe have slightly improved agonist potency for mMC3R, whereas the peptides with large halogens or -CF$_3$ at the para position or with chlorine in the meta position, function as partial agonist/antagonists or as very poor agonists. Comparison of the halogen-containing tetrapeptides revealed that peptide 9 with DPhe(pF) was the most potent tetrapeptide agonist for mMC3R (EC_{50} = 50 nM), whereas peptides 12 with DPhe(pI) and 15 with DPhe(3,4-diCl) were the most potent tetrapeptide antagonists for the mMC3R with Ki = 260 nM (Table 6). It was suggested that antagonism of bromo-, iodo-, dichloro- and trifluoromethyl-containing tetrapeptides at mMC3R may be attributed to a combination of hydrophobicity and van der Waals interactions with surrounding receptor atoms from the putative hydrophobic ligand binding pocket.[32]

N-Terminus Modifications

α-MSH contains a N-terminal acetyl group as a result of endogenous posttranslational processing. Modification of the N-terminus is another approach to generate SAR data. The addition of fatty acid conjugates,[39,40] biotin[41] and chlorotriazinylaminofluorescein[42] to the N-terminus of melanocortin peptides have been reported and resulted in enhanced or decreased potencies in the classical skin and tyrosinase melanocortin bioassays. In a more recent study, Bowen et al synthesized a branched flexible linker that incorporates a fluorescent dansyl moiety and used to connect two high affinity NDP-α-MSH ligands or two low affinity Ac-MSH ligands.[43] It was

Table 6. Agonist EC$_{50}$ (nM) pharmacology at the mouse melanocortin receptor

Peptide	His	DPhe	Substitution Arg	Trp	mMC1R EC$_{50}$ (nM)	mMC3R EC$_{50}$ (nM)	mMC4R EC$_{50}$ (nM)	mMC5R EC$_{50}$ (nM)
9	His	DPhe(pF)	Arg	Trp	53.7 ± 8.62	53.7 ± 5.30	0.45 ± 0.10	2.04 ± 0.27
10	His	DPhe(pCl)	Arg	Trp	38.2 ± 3.3	84.8 ± 21.0	0.40 ± 0.12	1.47 ± 0.44
11	His	DPhe(pBr)	Arg	Trp	40.8 ± 10.4	~50% at 100 µM pA$_2$ = 7.54 ± 0.12	1.07 ± 0.46	2.60 ± 1.52
12	His	DPhe(pI)	Arg	Trp	40.7 ± 2.73	~40% at 100 µM pA$_2$ = 7.41 ± 0.08	3.94 ± 1.32	7.41 ± 0.08
13	His	DPhe(pCF$_3$)	Arg	Trp	540 ± 120	~25% at 100 µM pA$_2$ = 6.79 ± 0.15	12.8 ± 1.94	8.03 ± 1.33
14	His	DNal(2')	Arg	Trp	92.8 ± 42.7	~25% at 100 µM pA$_2$ = 6.70 ± 0.12	pA$_2$ = 8.28 ± 0.13	22.4 ± 5.0
15	His	(3,4-diCl)	Arg	Trp	140 ± 30	~30% at 100 µM	3.40 ± 0.66	7.42 ± 0.26
16	His	(m-Cl)	Arg	Trp	320 ± 57.3	1240 ± 270	8.64 ± 1.73	30.0 ± 13.6

A percentage value indicates that some stimulatory agonist pharmacology resulted at upto 100 µM concentrations, but the maximal stimulation levels are less than the control level. The compounds not demonstrating full agonism were assayed for antagonism using Schild pA$_2$ analysis and the MTII peptide as agonist. Data taken from reference 78.

reported that binding to the hMC4R was not diminished for linker-ligand combinations relative to the corresponding ligand alone.

Additionally, the design and synthesis of N-terminally modified tri- and tetrapeptide ligands have been reported.[44-47] In these studies it was observed that the octanoyl-His-DPhe-Arg-Trp-NH$_2$ tetrapeptide is more potent at the mMC1R, mMC3-5R's than the reference peptide Ac-His-DPhe-Arg-Trp-NH$_2$. This compound exhibited approximately 80- to 100-fold difference in potency at the mMC1R, mMC3R, mMC4R and only about 8-fold difference in potency at the mMC5R.[44] In a similar study, it was reported that a 4-phenylbutanoyl derivative (C$_6$H$_5$ (CH$_2$)$_3$CO-His-DPhe-Arg-Trp-NH$_2$) is a 1440-fold more potent subnanomolar agonist at the hMC1R than the reference compound.[47] The increase in potency observed from addition of aliphatic chains to the tetrapeptides may be attributed to an increase in hydrophobic ligand—receptor interactions, since the melanocortin receptors putatively contain a hydrophobic binding pocket.[48,49] An alternative explanation may be that introduction of hydrophobic acyl groups to the N-terminus enhance peptide—lipid interactions along the membrane—liquid interface, thereby increasing availability of the ligand to the lipid bilayer.[40,50]

β-MSH

Yan et al have reported extensively on β-MSH as MC4R selective agonists and summarized their work in recent review.[51] Truncation of β-MSH has generated two more potent, but nonselective peptide agonists, β-MSH (7-22) and β-MSH(9-22). It was suggested that C-terminal amidation did not alter the ligand binding affinity or selectivity. Also the N-terminus was acetylated for increased enzymatic stability. Inversion of chirality at the Phe residue showed improved binding potency at melanocortin receptors, but no selectivity enhancement was observed. Introduction of a cyclic constraint resulted in a potent and selective ligand Ac-YR-c[CEHDPhe-RWC]-NH$_2$ with increased selectivity at MC4R over MC1R, MC3R and MC5R subtypes. In vivo studies showed reduction in food intake and body weight gain in rats treated with Ac-YR-c[CEHDPhe-RWC]-NH$_2$. Moreover, extensive SAR studies on Ac-YR-c[CEHDPhe-RWC]-NH$_2$ have resulted in a series of small, potent and selective MC4R agonists.[51] SAR studies designed to pharmacologically characterize α-MSH/β-MSH hybrid analogues have been presented.[52] In the same study, analogues were synthesized that contained the N-terminal residues 5-9 from α-MSH and the Pro-Pro-Lys-Asp sequence corresponding to the C-terminus of human β-MSH, connected by a disulfide bridge between the side chains of two cysteine residues. A series of compounds with different chiralities, but a similar disulfide template have been shown to significantly alter potency and selectivity at hMC3-5 receptors.

γ-MSH

Ala scan of γ$_2$-MSH revealed that when positions 5-8 (His-Phe-Arg-Trp) were substituted with Ala, analogues resulted with decreased potency at the hMC3-5Rs.[53] These data confirmed the postulated importance of the His-Phe-Arg-Trp sequence for stimulating potent agonist pharmacological responses at melanocortin receptors. A D-amino acid scan was also performed using the γ$_2$-template that discovered that changing the configuration of Trp-8 to DTrp increased the selectivity of the compound for the hMC3R versus the hMC4R (300-fold more selective), as compared to γ$_2$-MSH, which is only 17-fold selective in a cAMP functional bioassay.[54] Another important feature identified from this latter study was that when Phe^6 was replaced with DPhe, a loss of hMC3R versus hMC4R selectivity resulted. A cyclic scan was carried out to probe the receptor-active conformation of the His-Phe-Arg-Trp pharmacophore in γ-MSH.[55] Various cyclic analogues were designed and synthesized including 20-23 membered cyclic disulfides ring and 23-membered lactam rings. It was concluded that the 26-membered ring was important for selectivity, whereas, 23-membered analogues were desirable for alteration of potency. In the same study, replacement of His, Phe, or Trp with hydrophobic residues, converted agonist to antagonist in at least one of the melanocortin receptors, showing the role of these amino acids in structure-activity relationship.[98] In a different study, Asp-10 position in Lys-γ$_2$-MSH was found to be an important residue to get selectivity at MC3R over MC4R.[56]

ACTH

Truncation of ACTH in some studies increased the in vivo potency of the compound as compared to the ACTH (1-39).[57] SAR studies report that the [DSer^1, Lys^{17}, Lys^{18}]-ACTH(1-18)-NH$_2$ derivative is 5-fold more potent than the full length ACTH.[57] Other studies have revealed that the introduction of an extra amino acid at the N-terminus of ACTH(1-19)-NH$_2$ (i.e., alanine or proline) decreased steroidogenic activity by 40% and 65% respectively.[58] Replacement of Glu in ACTH(1-19) with Gln has been shown to reduce in vivo steroidogenic activity by two-thirds.[59] The His at the sixth position has been demonstrated to be important for proper steroidogenic activity of ACTH (1-19), as its replacement with Phe results in almost 90-fold decreased potency.[58] Several reports have been published in order to probe specific amino acid position in regards to the influence on adrenocorticotropic activity and the significance of an amide or acid at the C-terminal.[60,61] However, truncation and positional scanning studies data regarding the ACTH molecule is limited. Recently, it has been reported that truncated ACTH fragments such as ACTH(1-18) and ACTH(1-17) possess nM potency at the human MC2R.[61] Interestingly, N-terminally truncated ACTH(11-24) was reported to be a competitive antagonist of ACTH(1-24) in the isolated adrenal gland cell assay.[62]

NDP-MSH

It was observed during early studies that the heating of α-MSH in basic solution altered (increased) its biological properties as a result of partial amino acid racemization.[63] It was identified, using high-resolution gas chromatographic that the Phe-7 residue was the predominant racemized residue and speculated that this amino acid may be responsible for the enhanced properties observed for racemized α-MSH activity. These data resulted in the design and discovery of the highly potent and "prolonged" acting α-MSH analog, NDP-MSH.[21] Truncation studies of NDP-MSH have shown that the minimal sequence required to elicit a response in the μM range at the cloned mouse melanocortin receptors was Ac-DPhe-Arg-Trp-NH$_2$.[26] However, the introduction of the His residue at the N-terminus of the tripeptide results in an increase in potency (100-fold) for the ligand (Ac-His-DPhe-Arg-Trp-NH$_2$) at the four mouse melanocortin receptor subtypes examined. In two different studies from Bednarek et al, various analogues of NDP-MSH were synthesized and identified peptides selective for the hMC1R and hMC5R receptor subtypes.[64,65]

SAR of Cyclic Melanocortin Peptides

Many endogenous peptides are small and often conformationally flexible, making the correlation between conformation and pharmacological activity difficult.[66] Introduction of cyclic constraints can restrict conformation of the peptides and aid in structural analysis, as well as lead to more selective and potent ligands by stabilizing secondary structures, such as β-turns. Cyclic analogues of biologically active linear peptides have demonstrated the potential to: (1) increase agonist and antagonist potency; (2) withstand proteolytic degradation; (3) increase receptor selectivity; (4) enhance bioavailability; and (5) bioactive conformation of ligands.[67] There are four main ways to form constrained cyclic peptides. These cyclizations involve bridging between (i) two side chains; (ii) a side chain to N-terminus; (iii) a side chain to C-terminus; (iv) or two backbone residues either C-terminal or N-terminal. The most common cyclization is between two distant side-chains, for e.g., lactam or disulfide bridges. The effects of different cycles and their sizes on the melanocortin ligands, affinity to bind to the receptors, selectivity and their activity will be discussed. Both cyclic lactam and cyclic disulfide approaches were applied on α-MSH to give more potent and selective analogues on melanocortin receptors. The Ac-[Cys^4,Cys^{10}]-α-MSH,[68] which contains a disulfide bridge between Cys^4 and Cys^{10} amino acids and resulted in enhanced biological properties. This cyclic disulfide α-MSH analog was more potent in the frog skin bioassay, than α-MSH, but was not particularly potent in subsequent evaluations using mammalian bioassays. Sawyer et al suggested that cyclization constrains the analogue in a conformation favorable for peptide—receptor interactions, the "bioactive" conformation, which likely consisted of a reverse β-turn around the His-Phe-Arg-Trp sequence. Recently there has been renewed interest in using disulfide α-MSH analogs to help rigidify conformational flexibility that has led to the discovery of fairly potent and selective melanocortin ligands.[69-71] Schioth et al have reported potent and selective disulfide

Table 7. *Amino acid sequence of synthetic melanocortin peptides*

Ligand	Amino Acid Sequence	Ref.
NDP-MSH	Ac-Ser-Tyr-Ser-Nle-Glu-His-DPhe-Arg-Trp-Gly-Lys-Pro-Val-NH$_2$	59
MTII	Ac-Nle-c[Asp-His-DPhe-Arg-Trp-Lys]-NH$_2$	73
SHU9119	Ac-Nle-c[Asp-His-DNal(2′)-Arg-Trp-Lys]-NH$_2$	74
HS014	c[Cys-Glu-His-DNal(2′)-Arg-Trp-Gly-Cys]-Pro-Arg-Leu-Asp-NH$_2$	111

peptide antagonists for the MC4R that increase food intake following intracerebroventricularly (i.c.v.) as well as peripheral administration.[71] These compounds were more selective for the MC4R, however, the disulfides had decreased affinities than the lactam analogues with same 23-membered ring. Subsequently, by changing the ring size to 26-membered, a more MC4R selective compound HS014 was found and increasing the ring size to 29-memebered-MC3R selectivity was increased.[70,71] Three important observations led to the discovery of more potent cyclic analogues of α-MSH like MTII are discussed. (i) Both α-MSH and NDP-MSH adopted folded conformations that placed the aromatic His^6-Phe^7(or DPhe^7)-Trp^9 residues on the same face of the peptide in β-turn conformation; (ii) hydrophilic Glu^5, Arg^8 and Lys^{11} residues were oriented on the face of the peptide opposite the aromatic groups; (iii) although Glu^5 and Lys^{11} were in close proximity to one another, the charged groups were not close enough to form a strong ionic interaction. Later Al-Obeidi et al have demonstrated that the linear Ac-[Nle^4, DPhe^7, Lys^{10}]-α-MSH$_{(4-10)}$-NH$_2$ and the Ac-[Nle^4, Asp^5, DPhe^7, Lys^{10}]-α-MSH$_{(4-10)}$-NH$_2$ analogues, which contain Lys at position 10, adopt a folded configuration in which the side chain carboxyl group of either Asp or Glu and the side chain amino group of Lys were in close proximity and a putative reverse turn occurred around the His-DPhe-Arg-Trp residues.[72] Once this observation was made for the linear peptides, the corresponding lactam cyclized MTII and MTII-like peptides were synthesized and were found to be highly potent and exhibited prolonged activity.[37] MTII is a smaller peptide, the lactam derived from the (4-10)-fragment of NDP-MSH and more potent, but nonselective agonist at MC1 and MC3-5Rs. Subsequent structure-activity relationship studies of MTII modified with bulky aromatic amino acids led to the discovery of SHU9119 which is a high affinity antagonist for melanocortin MC3 and MC4Rs and an agonist for melanocortin MC1 and MC5Rs (Table 7).[38] I.C.V. administration of MTII reduced food intake and conversely administration of SHU9119 increased food intake and body weight.[73]

Backbone Cyclization and N-Methylation of Melanocortin Peptides

Backbone cyclization (BC) is one of the approaches that has been utilized to overcome the drawbacks of peptides being flexible. BC is formed by covalently connecting atoms in the backbone (N and/or C) of a target linear peptide via a linker to form a ring. BC has been shown to dramatically enhance the metabolic stability of peptides in serum and intestinal enzymes.[74] A library of backbone cyclic peptides with a basic parent peptide sequence with the same side chain pharmacophores and hence the same potential bioactivity, but they differ in their ring size and chemistry, conferring conformational diversity. Advantage of BC over other peptide cyclization methods is that it use the backbone atoms, leaving the side chain intact which are essential for biological activity at the receptor. This method has been shown to improve the metabolic stability of peptides in serum and also pharmacological selectivity of a given peptide. Utilizing this approach, Hess et al have synthesized a library of backbone cyclic analogues where the bridge was formed connecting the N-terminus to the Nα of the C-terminal Gly building unit by a dicarboxylic acid spacer.[74] All the peptides in the library bear the same parent sequence, but differ in ring size. From this study, they found the compound BL3020-1 which was selective for the MC4R and had favorable metabolic and pharmacokinetic properties. This peptide was detected in the brain (determined after 8h) following oral administration to rats.

N-methylation is another approach to improve the pharmacokinetic property of peptides and convert them into more drug-like candidates. Mono-N-methylation has been used for years to change pharmacological properties of peptides. However, multiple N-methylation is becoming more common in the field. In different study, Linde et al performed SAR studies on compound BL3020-1, utilizing both BC and N-methylation approaches.[75] Two libraries were synthesized, comprising 37 backbone cyclic (BL3020) and N-methylated backbone cyclic (N-Me) peptides with the same sequence as compound BL3020-1 (Phe^6-DPhe-Arg-Trp-Gly^{10}-NH$_2$) and a lactam bridge between the N-terminus and the backbone nitrogen of the C-terminal Gly. The peptides in the BL3020 library differed in ring size and ring chemistry, whereas the peptides in the N-Me libraries differed also in the number and position of the N-Me group. These libraries were screened to select peptide(s) with improved selectivity and activity towards the MC4R, while retaining resistance against intestinal enzymes. An N-Me and amide bond modification study has also been performed on the tetrapeptide Ac-His-DPhe-Arg-Trp-NH$_2$ sequence.[76]

Agouti-Related Protein (AGRP)

As mentioned previously, the melanocortin system is the only GPCR known to date to be regulated by endogenous antagonists. The agouti protein and agouti related protein (AGRP) modulate melanocortin receptor function with MCR subtype selectivity. They are paracrine signaling molecules exhibiting antagonistic activity at the MC1R, MC3R and MC4R.[11,12] Agouti protein is expressed in the skin and has been shown to antagonize the action of α-MSH at the MC1R, MC3R and MC4R.[11,77] AGRP was identified based upon its similarity in size and genomic structure to the agouti protein.[12,78] AGRP is a potent orexigenic (appetite stimulating) neuropeptide that has been shown to be expressed primarily in the arcuate nucleus of the hypothalamus and adrenal cortex, with slight expression in the lung and kidney. AGRP is a competitive antagonist and blocks the action of the melanocortin agonists at the MC3R and MC4R. In addition, studies have demonstrated AGRP to act as an inverse agonist at the MC4R.[79,80] It has been proposed that AGRP mediates obesity and hyperphagia through the MC4R due to the observation that an obese phenotype was exhibited by transgenic mice when the human AGRP gene was introduced into their genome. This phenotype is similar to that of the MC4R deficient mice.[12,78]

AGRP Structure

Within the 132 amino acid polypeptide chain of AGRP, there is a postulated signal peptide sequence, an asparate (glutamate)-rich acid region in the middle and a conserved C-terminal domain rich in cysteine residues. Both agouti and AGRP contain this conserved C-terminal cysteine rich domain (Fig. 3). This region contains ten cysteine residues that form five disulfide bonds which contribute to the stability of agouti.[77,95] AGRP,[81,87] their antagonistic effects, and has been shown to display similar pharmacology to that of the full protein.[81] McNulty et al used nuclear magnetic resonance (NMR) to determine the three-dimensional structure of the C-terminal of AGRP.[81] From NMR studies, it was observed that there are three loops that define the tertiary structure of hAGRP(87-132): the N-terminal loop amino acids LGQQ, hAGRP (95-98), the central loop containing the residues proposed to be responsible for antagonism of the C-terminal, hAGRP(111-116), and the C-terminal loop, hAGRP(121-128). Three hAGRP disulfide bonds (Cys87-Cys102, Cys94-Cys108, Cys101-Cys119) were identified to be involved in a mammalian inhibitor cysteine knot (ICK) motif in the C-terminal region that contributes to the conformation of the active loop. Within the ICK motif, a three-stranded anti-parallel β-sheet was identified. Two strands of this structural feature form a secondary structure known as a β-hairpin involving hAGRP residues (106-120), that has been observed to be important for the antagonistic activity of hAGRP (87-132).[81]

AGRP SAR

In 1999, Tota et al conducted the first structure-activity studies of hAGRP and it was found that that the N-terminal end of hAGRP is not necessary for it to bind to the MC3R and the MC4R, while the C-terminal was found to exhibit similar antagonistic pharmacology to that of the full

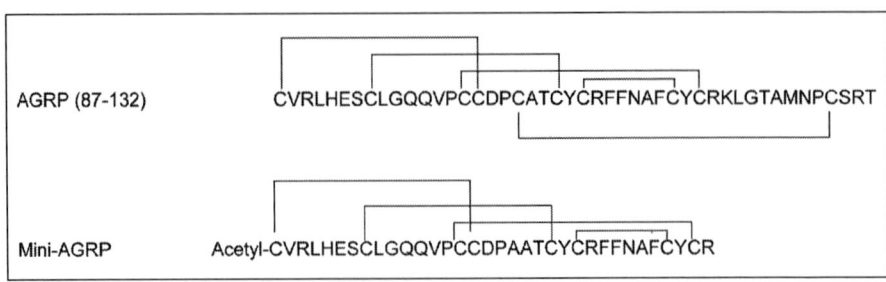

Figure 3. Structure of AGRP and mini-AGRP.

hormone.[82] Additional studies were then performed to identify which regions of the C-terminal domain contribute to antagonistic activity. Through SAR studies, it was found that the endogenous antagonists contain a conserved tripeptide motif, Arg-Phe-Phe, within the C-terminal domain that was postulated to mimic the binding of the core sequence of the melanocortin agonists. This triplet has been shown to be located in the active central loop CRFFNAFC, hAGRP (110-117). Only slight changes were observed for hAGRP(87-132) binding affinity when residues in the N-terminal loop and C-terminal loop were modified, adding further support that the central portion of hAGRP (87-132) is important for molecular recognition and stimulation. Tota et al synthesized monocyclic peptides based on the octapeptide loop, [Cys-Arg-Phe-Phe-Asn-Ala-Phe-Cys], containing the Arg-Phe-Phe triplet. All synthetic analogues displayed a lower affinity for the MC3R than the MC4R, however, were all still active. In the same study, linear analogues were synthesized in which Cys residues were replaced by Ser residues, however, these peptides were basically inactive. This study resulted in the reduction of a large ligand, hAGRP (87-132), to a ten residue analogue, Y-c[CRFFNAFC]-Y that retained a similar pharmacological profile to the C-terminal domain. This decapeptide was less potent at the MC4R, with an IC_{50} binding affinity of 57nM compared to the full length C-terminal peptide at the MC4R (3.5nM). Its shorter length may not have allowed it to achieve the ideal conformation modifying its IC_{50} value or it may lack additional pharmacophores found within AGRP that contribute to potent antagonistic activity.[82]

Although this monocyclic decapeptide was less potent at the MC3R and MC4R when compared to the C-terminal peptide, interestingly it was found to exhibit agonist activity at the mMC1R, which is not observed with the endogenous hAGRP protein.[83] Further studies were performed on this cyclic decapeptide due to the interesting activity observed at the mMC1R. A novel peripheral skin MC1R antagonist was discovered when the disulfide bridge formed by Cys110-Cys117 of Y-c[CRFFNAFC]-Y was replaced by a lactam bridge through the use of Glu and Dpr (diaminopropionic acid), which is interesting since the endogenous AGRP protein does not bind, agonize or antagonize at this receptor. It is also an antagonist at the MC4R, however, it was not functional at the MC3R or MC5R.[84]

Subsequent structure activity studies were performed using this decapeptide template to regain MC3R pharmacology; peptides were synthesized in which the N- and/or C-terminus were extended or included more than one cyclization based on previous studies done by AMGEN.[85] This resulted in the identification of two monocyclic peptide sequences consisting of 14 amino acids with both MC3R and MC4R antagonistic activity. From these two peptides, Yc[CRFFNAFC] YARKL-NH$_2$ and TAYc[CRFFNAFC]YAR-NH$_2$, it was hypothesized that the extension of the C-terminus of the decapeptide template is necessary to re-establish MC3R antagonism.[86] In addition, it was proposed that Arg-120 is important for activity at MC3R due to a postulated participation in a β-hairpin secondary structure involving hAGRP106-120 as indicated by NMR.[81,87]

Stereochemical modifications of the Arg-Phe-Phe region were examined in the monocyclic hAGRP(103-133, C105A, C108A, C119A), DPAATAY-c[CRFFNAFC]YARKL.[88] Both ends of the decapeptide template were extended beyond the minimal sequence; in addition, it contained the β-hairpin motif hAGRP(106-120) and the proposed active loop. This peptide displayed high nM antagonism at the MC3R and MC4R and was a full agonist at the MC1R. A D-amino acid scan was performed in hopes of increasing antagonistic potency at the MC3R and MC4R; however, it actually resulted in the conversion of an antagonist to an agonist. The addition of the D-stereo isomers resulted in the loss of antagonistic activity at the MC3R and MC4R, except for the DPhe[112] analogue. This analogue showed a reduction in maximal stimulation at the MC3R and MC4R. In comparison to the control lacking D-amino acids, the DArg[111] peptide was shown to be a 6-fold less potent mMC1R agonist, became a MC5R agonist, was only able to stimulate MC3R to 70% maximal stimulation, however, it possessed µM mMC4R full agonist pharmacology. An 8-fold increase in potency at the mMC1R was observed for the DPhe[113] analogue and was a full µM agonist at both the mMC3R and mMC4R. The observation that the D-amino acids converted these analogues into full µM or partial agonists leading to the hypothesis that L-amino acids are needed to maintain potent antagonism of AGRP derived peptides at MC3R and MC4R.[88] Agonist activity may be attributed to putative interactions between the mMC4R Asn115—hAGRP DArg in TM3 and mMC4R Phe176-h-AGRP DPhe[113] that were observed when homology modeling studies were conducted using these analogues and the mMC4R.[88,89]

Two bicyclic hAGRP derived compounds presented by AMGEN were further examined by the Haskell-Luevano lab to determine the minimal sequence needed for maintaining MC4R antagonism.[85,90] The bicyclic compounds were constructed by extending both ends of the decapeptide beyond the active central loop, hAGRP(110-117), contained two out of the five disulfide bonds with the substitution of pseudo isotere α-aminobutyric acid (Abu, U) for the Cys residues not participating in disulfide bonds. The hAGRP (91-122) analogue displayed decreased antagonistic activity at the MC3R and MC4R, even though it did not include the disulfide bond containing the active loop, RFFNAFC. The other bicyclic analogue, hAGRP(101-122) exhibited binding affinity that was equipotent to hAGRP (87-132), however, was a 80-fold less potent mMC4R antagonist.[90] Modeling studies postulate that the decreased potency of this analogue may be due to the presence of an additional interaction of the Arg111 with mMC4R Asn115 that was not observed for hAGRP(87-132) in modeling studies.

Through the use of NMR, mutagenesis and pharmacological studies, mini-AGRP (Fig. 3) was designed by Jackson et al based on the hypothesis that the ICK domain found in the C-terminal region of AGRP can maintain the antagonistic activity of this region.[87] This mini-protein, Nα-acetyl-AGRP(87-120, C105A), encompasses four of the five disulfide bridges found with the C-terminal domain and demonstrated a similar ICK folding motif. When assayed it was found to exhibit nearly identical pharmacological profiles to the full length C-terminal, hAGRP(87-132) for the melanocortin receptors. The design of this mini-protein confirmed the hypothesis that N-terminal loop of this ICK region and the tri-peptide were sufficient for full biological activity.

Development of Chimeric Peptide Analogues

Another approach for SAR is to place key structural moieties into novel templates or link them together on alternate templates to produce chimeric analogues to examine selectivity and/or potency. Recent examples in this context are the novel chimeric melanotropin-deltorphin analogues by Han et al[91] Chimeric melanocortin-AGRP peptides were synthesized to test the hypothesis that the Arg-Phe-Phe motif hAGRP(111-113) mimics the DPhe-Arg-Trp of the melanocortin agonists in interactions with melanocortin receptors. Agonist activity was observed at the mMC1R, mMC3-5Rs when the DPhe-Arg-Trp residues in NDP-MSH and MTII were substituted with the AGRP Arg-Phe-Phe residues in a study conducted by Joseph et al.[92] The NDP-MSH analogue, Ac-Ser-Tyr-Ser-Nle-Glu-His-Arg-DPhe-Phe-Gly-Lys-Pro-Val-NH$_2$ exhibited nanomolar agonist potency at the mMC1R and was selective for the mMC1R over the mMC3R, mMC4R and mMC5R. The results of this study support the hypothesis that the Arg-Phe-Phe residues of AGRP mimics the agonist residues Phe-Arg-Trp.

Wilczynski et al substituted different combinations of the agonist tetrapeptide, His-Phe-Arg-Trp, for the Arg-Phe-Phe triplet in the antagonist hAGRP(109-118) template Tyr-c[Asp-Arg-Phe-Phe-Asn-Phe-Phe-Ans-Ala-Phe-Dpr]-Tyr-NH$_2$, that contains a lactam bridge rather than a disulfide bridge.[93] The peptide, Tyr-c[Asp-His-DPhe-Arg-Trp-Asn-Ala-Phe-Dpr]-Tyr-NH$_2$, exhibited sub nM agonist activity equipotent to α-MSH at the mMC1R, mMC3R and mMC4R, however, at the mMC4R it was 30-fold more potent than the endogenous α-MSH peptide. The deletion of His within that peptide resulted in an analogue that was 200 fold more- selective for MC4R versus MC3R. Further SAR studies were conducted in this chimeric peptide template by Wilczynski et al to find out if the chimeric peptides exhibit pharmacological profiles similar to the melanocortin agonists and antagonists. Unexpected results were observed with the replacement of His with Pro and Phe at the mMC3R. It was found that these peptides were nM antagonists with partial agonist activity. In addition, they were found to display equipotent agonist activity at the mMC4R compared to the control template. The mixed pharmacology observed for the peptide with the Phe replacement of His, Tyr-c[β-Asp-Phe-DPhe-Arg-Trp-Asn-Ala-Phe-Dpr]-Tyr-NH$_2$, may be explained by the presence of a γ-turn with the DPhe as indicated by NMR studies.[93] Modifications at the His position have been previously shown to differentiate between MC3R and MC4R selective agonist activity. The replacement of DPhe with Ala and DNal(1') resulted in 730- and 560-fold, respectively, mMC4R selective agonists versus mMC3R. Also, they displayed nM agonist activity at the mMC1R and mMC5R.[93]

A potent nanomolar agonist was identified when His-DPhe-Arg-Trp replaced the Arg-Phe-Phe triplet in mini-AGRP (hAGRP 87-120, C105A).[89] A study conducted by Jackson et al involved the design of ligands based on the substitution of the active loop region, RFFNAF, of mini-hAGRP. Modeling studies postulated that the HFRW tetrapeptide of α-MSH and RFF of AGRP overlap in binding sites within the MC4R.[94] It was hypothesized that mini-AGRP containing the HFRW sequence should function as an agonist; however, it should maintain mini-AGRP receptor selectivity, binding only to MC3R and MC4R. The substitution of amino acids did result in the conversion of pharmacology from antagonist to agonist; however, differences in receptor selectivity were noticed among the eleven analogues in which they were active at MC1R, MC3R and MC4R. This led to the hypothesis that the overlapping binding sites are not exactly aligned, it is more of a partial overlap of the agonist and antagonist postulated binding pockets within the MC4R.[94]

Conclusion

Significant effort has been made in attempt to understand the ligand-receptor interactions and its outcome to design more efficient compounds that mimic the biological properties of the endogenous melanocortin peptides. The task of designing receptor targeted ligands that are selective, potent and drug-like metabolically is very challenging and demanding. Continuous research and new discoveries will emerge in the approach and strategies to design novel compounds. The results from SAR studies have enhanced our understanding of the melanocortin system and ongoing efforts may aid in finding novel ligands with increased stability, potency and receptor subtype selectivity.

Acknowledgements

We would like to acknowledge financial support from NIH Grants RO1DK57080, RO1DK64250, RO1DK063974 and an American Diabetes Research Award.

References

1. Chhajlani V, Wikberg JES. Molecular cloning and expression of the human melanocyte stimulating hormone receptor cDNA. FEBS Lett 1992; 309(3):417-420.
2. Mountjoy KG, Robbins LS, Mortrud MT et al. The cloning of a family of genes that encode the melanocortin receptors. Science 1992; 257:1248-1251.
3. Roselli-Rehfuss L, Mountjoy KG, Robbins LS et al. Identification of a receptor for g melanotropin and other proopiomelanocortin peptides in the hypothalamus and limbic system. Proc Natl Acad Sci USA 1993; 90:8856-8860.
4. Mountjoy KG, Mortrud MT, Low MJ et al. Localization of the melanocortin-4 receptor (MC4-R) in neuroendocrine and autonomic control circuits in the brain. Mol Endo 1994; 8:1298-1308.
5. Gantz I, Konda Y, Tashiro T et al. Molecular cloning of a novel melanocortin receptor. J Biol Chem 1993; 268(11):8246-8250.

6. Gantz I, Miwa H, Konda Y et al. Molecular cloning, expression and gene localization of a fourth melanocortin receptor. J Biol Chem 1993; 268(20):15174-15179.

7. Gantz I, Shimoto Y, Konda Y et al. Molecular cloning, expression and characterization of a fifth melanocortin receptor. Biochem Biophys Res Commun 1994; 200(3):1214-1220.

8. Eipper BA, Mains RE. Structure and biosynthesis of Pro-ACTH/Endorphin and related peptides. Endocrin Rev 1980; 1:1-26.

9. Hruby VJ, Wilkes BC, Cody WL et al. Melanotropins: Structural, conformational and biological considerations in the development of superpotent and superprolonged analogs. Peptide Protein Rev 1984; 3:1-64.

10. Haskell-Luevano C, Sawyer TK, Hendrata S et al. Truncation studies of a-melanotropin peptides identifies tripeptide analogues exhibiting prolonged agonist bioactivity. Peptides 1996; 17:995-1002.

11. Lu D, Willard D, Patel IR et al. Agouti protein is an antagonist of the melanocyte-stimulating-hormone receptor. Nature 1994; 371(6500):799-802.

12. Ollmann MM, Wilson BD, Yang Y-K et al. Antagonism of central melanocortin receptors in vitro and in vivo by agouti-related protein. Science 1997; 278:135-138.

13. Chen AS, Marsh DJ, Trumbauer ME et al. Inactivation of the mouse melanocortin-3 receptor results in increased fat mass and reduced lean body mass. Nat Genet 2000; 26(1):97-102.

14. Butler AA, Kesterson RA, Khong K et al. A unique metabolic syndrome causes obesity in the melanocortin-3 receptor-deficient mouse. Endocrinology 2000; 141(9):3518-3521.

15. Huszar D, Lynch CA, Fairchild-Huntress V et al. Targeted disruption of the melanocortin-4 receptor results in obesity in mice. Cell 1997; 88:131-141.

16. Chen W, Kelly MA, Opitz-Araya X et al. Exocrine gland dysfunction in MC5-R deficient mice: Evidence for coordinated regulation of exocrine gland functions by melanocortin peptides. Cell 1997; 91:789-798.

17. Harrold JA, Widdowson PS, Williams G. b-MSH: A functional ligand that regulated energy homeostasis via hypothalamic MC4-R? Peptides 2003; 24(3):397-405.

18. Eberle AN. The melanotropins: Chemistry, physiology and mechanisms of action. Basel: Karger; 1988.

19. Holder JR, Haskell-Luevano C. Melanocortin Ligands: 30 Years of structure-activity relationship (SAR) studies. Med Res Rev 2004; 24(3):325-356.

20. Irani BG, Holder JR, Todorovic A et al. Progress in the development of melanocortin receptor selective ligands. Curr Pharm Des 2004; 10(28):3443-3479.

21. Sawyer TK, Sanfillippo PJ, Hruby VJ et al. 4-Norleucine, 7-D-Phenylalanine-a-melanocyte-stimulating hormone: A highly potent a-melanotropin with ultra long biological activity. Proc Natl Acad Sci USA 1980; 77:5754-5758.

22. Hruby VJ, Wilkes BC, Hadley ME et al. a-Melanotropin: The minimal active sequence in the frog skin bioassay. J Med Chem 1987; 30:2126-2130.

23. Castrucci AML, Hadley ME, Sawyer TK et al. a-Melanotropin: The minimal active sequence in the lizard skin bioassay. Gen Comp Endocrinol 1989; 73:157-163.

24. Haslach EM, Schaub JW, Haskell-Luevano C. b-Turn secondary structure and melanocortin ligands. Bioorg Med Chem 2009; 17:952-958.

25. Haskell-Luevano C, Rosenquist Å, Souers A et al. Compounds that activate the mouse melanocortin-1 receptor identified by screening a small molecule library based upon the b-turn. J Med Chem 1999; 42:4380-4387.

26. Haskell-Luevano C, Holder JR, Monck EK et al. Characterization of melanocortin ndp-msh agonist peptide fragments at the mouse central and peripheral melanocortin receptors. J Med Chem 2001; 44:2247-2252.

27. Sahm UG, Olivier GWJ, Branch SK et al. Synthesis and biological evaluation of a-MSH analogs substituted with alanine. Peptides 1994; 15(7):1297-1302.

28. Holder JR, Bauzo RM, Xiang Z et al. Structure-activity relationships of the melanocortin tetrapeptide Ac-His-DPhe-Arg-Trp-NH$_2$ at the mouse melanocortin receptors: I modifications at the his position. J Med Chem 2002; 45:2801-2810.

29. Holder JR, Xiang Z, Bauzo RM et al. Structure-activity relationships of the melanocortin tetrapeptide Ac-His-DPhe-Arg-Trp-NH$_2$ at the mouse melanocortin receptors: Part 3 modifications at the Arg position. Peptides 2003; 24:73-82.

30. Holder JR, Xiang Z, Bauzo RM et al. Structure-activity relationships of the melanocortin tetrapeptide Ac-His-DPhe-Arg-Trp-NH$_2$ at the mouse melanocortin receptors: Part 4 modifications at the Trp position. J Med Chem 2002; 45:5736-5744.

31. Holder JR, Bauzo RM, Xiang Z et al. Structure-activity relationships of the melanocortin tetrapeptide Ac-His-DPhe-Arg-Trp-NH$_2$ at the mouse melanocortin receptors: Part 2 modifications at the Phe position. J Med Chem 2002; 45:3073-3081.

32. Proneth B, Pogozheva ID, Portillo FP et al. Melanocortin tetrapeptide Ac-His-DPhe-Arg-Trp-NH$_2$ modified at the para position of the benzyl side chain (DPhe): Importance for mouse melanocortin-3 receptor agonist versus antagonist activity. J Med Chem 2008; 51(18):5585-5593.

33. Joseph CG, Sorensen NB, Wood MS et al. Modified melanocortin tetrapeptide Ac-His-DPhe-Arg-Trp-NH$_2$ at the arginine side chain with ureas and thioureas. J Pept Res 2005; 66(5):297-307.

34. Danho W, Swistok J, Wai-Hing Cheung A et al. Structure-activity relationship of linear peptide Bu-His(6)-DPhe(7)-Arg(8)-Trp(9)-Gly(10)-NH(2) at the human melanocortin-1 and -4 receptors: DPhe(7) and Trp(9) substitution. Bioorg Med Chem Lett 2003; 13(4):649-652.

35. Cheung AW, Danho W, Swistok J et al. Structure-activity relationship of linear peptide Bu-His-DPhe-Arg-Trp-Gly-NH(2) at the human melanocortin-1 and -4 receptors: histidine substitution. Bioorg Med Chem Lett 2003; 13(1):133-137.

36. Cheung A, Danho W, Swistok J et al. Structure-activity relationship of linear peptide Bu-His-DPhe-Arg-Trp-Gly-NH(2) at the human melanocortin-1 and -4 receptors: arginine substitution. Bioorg Med Chem Lett 2002; 12(17):2407-2410.

37. Al-Obeidi F, Castrucci AM, Hadley ME et al. Potent and prolonged acting cyclic lactam analogues of a-melanotropin: Design based on molecular dynamics. J Med Chem 1989; 32:2555-2561.

38. Hruby VJ, Lu D, Sharma SD et al. Cyclic lactam a-melanotropin analogues of Ac-Nle^4-c[Asp^5, DPhe^7, Lys^{10}]-a-MSH(4-10)-NH$_2$ with bulky aromatic amino acids at position 7 show high antagonist potency and selectivity at specific melanocortin receptors. J Med Chem 1995; 38:3454-3461.

39. Al-Obeidi F, Hruby VJ, Yaghoubi N et al. Synthesis and biological activities of fatty acid conjugates of a cyclic lactam a-melanotropin. J Med Chem 1992; 35:118-123.

40. Todorovic A, Holder JR, Bauzo RM et al. N-terminal fatty acylated His-DPhe-Arg-Trp-NH$_2$ tetrapeptides: Influence of fatty acid chain length on potency and selectivity at the mouse melanocortin receptors and human melanocytes. J Med Chem 2005; 48(9):3328-3336.

41. Chaturvedi DN, Knittel JJ, Hruby VJ et al. Synthesis and biological actions of highly potent and prolonged acting biotin-labeled melanotropins. J Med Chem 1984; 27:1406-1410.

42. Chaturvedi DN, Hruby VJ, Castrucci AM et al. Synthesis and biological evaluation of the superagonist [Na-Chlorotriazinylaminofluorescein-Ser^1, Nle^4, D-Phe^7]-a-MSH. J of Pharmaceutical Sciences 1985; 74:237-240.

43. Bowen M, Monguchi Y, Sankaranarayanan R et al. Design, synthesis and validation of a branched flexible linker for bioactive peptides. J Org Chem 2007; 72:1675-1680.

44. Holder JR, Marques FF, Xiang Z et al. Characterization of aliphatic, cyclic and aromatic N-terminally "Capped" His-DPhe-Arg-Trp-NH$_2$ melanocortin tetrapeptides at the melanocortin receptors. Eur J Pharmacol 2003; 462:41-52.

45. Koikov LN, Ebetino FH, Solinsky MG et al. Sub-nanomolar hMC1R agonists by end-capping of the melanocortin tetrapeptide His-D-Phe-Arg-Trp-NH(2). Bioorg Med Chem Lett 2003; 13(16):2647-2650.

46. Koikov LN, Ebetino FH, Hayes JC et al. End-capping of the modified melanocortin tetrapeptide (p-Cl)Phe-D-Phe-Arg-Trp-NH$_2$ as a route to hMC4R agonists. Bioorg Med Chem Lett 2004; 14(19):4839-4842.

47. Koikov LN, Ebetino FH, Solinsky MG et al. Analogs of sub-nanomolar hMC1R agonist LK-184 [Ph(CH2)3CO-His-D-Phe-Arg-Trp-NH$_2$]. An additional binding site within the human melanocortin receptor 1? Bioorg Med Chem Lett 2004; 14(15):3997-4000.

48. Haskell-Luevano C, Sawyer TK, Trumpp-Kallmeyer S et al. Three-dimensional molecular models of the hMC1R melanocortin receptor: Complexes with melanotropin peptide agonists. Drug Design and Discovery 1996; 14:197-211.

49. Haskell-Luevano C, Cone RD, Monck EK et al. Structure activity studies of the melanocortin-4 receptor by in vitro mutagenesis: identification of agouti-related protein (AGRP), melanocortin agonist and synthetic peptide antagonist interaction determinants. Biochemistry 2001; 40(20):6164-6179.

50. Sargent DF, Schwyzer R. Membrane lipid phase as catalyst for peptide-receptor interactions. Proc Natl Acad Sci USA 1986; 83:5774-5778.

51. Yan LZ, Hsiung HM, Heiman M. Structure-activity relationships of β-MSH derived melanocortin-4 receptor peptide agonists. Current Topics in Med Chem 2007; 7:1052-1067.

52. Balse-Srinivasan P, Grieco P, Cai M et al. Structure-activity relationships of novel cyclic α-MSH/ β-MSH hybrid analogues that lead to potent and selective ligands for the human MC3R and human MC5R. J Med Chem 2003; 46(17):3728-3733.

53. Grieco P, Balse-Srinivasan P, Han G et al. Synthesis and biological evaluation on hMC3, hMC4 and hMC5 receptors of g-MSH analogs substituted with L-Alanine. J Pept Res 2002; 59(5):203-210.

54. Grieco P, Balse PM, Weinberg D et al. D-Amino acid scan of g-Melanocyte-stimulating hormone: Importance of Trp(8) on human MC3 receptor selectivity. J Med Chem 2000; 43(26):4998-5002.

55. Balse-Srinivasan P, Grieco P, Cai M et al. Structure-activity relationships of g-MSH analogues at the human melanocortin MC3, MC4 and MC5 receptors. Discovery of highly selective hMC3R, hMC4R and hMC5R analogues. J Med Chem 2003; 46(23):4965-4973.

56. Oosterom J, Burbach JP, Gispen WH et al. Asp10 in Lys-Gamma2-MSH fetermines delective activation of the melanocortin MC3 receptor. Eur J Pharmacol 1998; 354(1):R9-11.

57. Schwyzer R. ACTH: A short introductory review. Ann N Y Acad Sci 1977; 297:3-26.

58. Blake J, Wang KT, Li CH. Adrenocorticotropin. Solid-phase synthesis of 1-19 -adrenocorticotropic hormone, Alanyl- 1-19 -adrenocorticotropic hormone and Prolyl- 1-19 -adrenocorticotropic hormone and their adrenocorticotropic activity. Biochemistry 1972; 11:438-442.

59. Li CH, Hemmasi B. Adrenocorticotropin. 40. The Synthesis of a protected nonapeptide and of a biologically active nonadecapeptide related to adrenocorticotropic hormone. (5-glutamine) adrenocorticotropin-(1-19). J Med Chem 1972; 15:217-219.

60. Ramachandran J, Chung D, Li CH. Adrenocorticotropins. Xxxiv. Aspects of structure-activity relationships of the ACTH molecule. Synthesis of a heptadecapeptide amide, an octadecapeptide amide and a nonadecapeptide amide possessing high biological activities. J Am Chem Soc 1965; 87:2696-2708.

61. Haskell-Luevano C, Todorovic A, Gridley K et al. The melanocortin pathway: Effects of voluntary exercise on melanocortin-4 receptor knockout mice and ACTH(1-24) ligand structure activity relationships at the melanocortin-2 receptor. Endocrine Res 2004; 30:591-597.

62. Seelig S, Sayers G, Schwyzer R et al. Isolated adrenal cells: ACTH(11-24), a competitive antagonist of ACTH(1-39) and ACTH(1-10). FEBS Lett 1971; 19(3):232-234.

63. Engel MH, Sawyer TK, Hadley ME et al. Quantitative determination of amino acid racemization in Heat-Alkali-Treated melanotropins: Implications for peptide hormone strucute-function studies. Anal Biochem 1981; 116:303-311.

64. Bednarek M, MacNeil T, Tang R et al. Analogs of a-melanocyte stimulating hormone with high agonist potency and selectivity at human melanocortin receptor 1b: The role of Trp9 in molecular recognition. Biopolymers 2007; 89:401-408.

65. Bednarek M, MacNeil T, Tang R et al. Potent and selective agonists of α-melanotropin (αMSH) action at human melanocortin receptor 5; linear analogs of α-melanotropin. Peptides 2007; 28:1020-1028.

66. Hruby VJ, Mosberg HI. Conformational and dynamic considerations in peptide structure-function studies. Peptides 1982; 3(3):329-336.

67. Hruby V. Designing peptide receptor agonists and antagonists. Nat Rev Drug Discov 2002; 1:847-858.

68. Sawyer TK, Hruby VJ, Darman PS et al. [half-Cys⁴,half-Cys¹⁰]-a-Melanocyte-stimulating hormone: A cyclic a-melanotropin exhibiting superagonist biological activity. Proc Natl Acad Sci USA 1982; 79:1751-1755.

69. Schioth HB, Muceniece R, Mutulis F et al. Selectivity of cyclic [DNal7] and [DPhe7] substituted MSH analogues for the melanocortin receptor subtypes. Peptides 1997; 18(7):1009-1013.

70. Schioth HB, Mutulis F, Muceniece R et al. Discovery of novel melanocortin4 receptor selective MSH analogues. Br J Pharmacol 1998; 124(1):75-82.

71. Skuladottir GV, Jonsson L, Skarphedinsson JO et al. Long term orexigenic effect of a novel melanocortin 4 receptor selective antagonist. Br J Pharmacol 1999; 126(1):27-34.

72. Al-Obeidi F, Hruby VJ, Castrucci AM et al. Design of potent linear a-Melanotropin 4-10 analogues modified in positions 5 and 10. J Med Chem 1989; 32(1):174-179.

73. Fan W, Boston BA, Kesterson RA et al. Role of melanocortinergic neurons in feeding and the agouti obesity syndrome. Nature 1997; 385:165-168.

74. Hess S, Linde Y, Ovadia O et al. Backbone cyclic peptidomimetic melanocortin-4 receptor agonist as a novel orally administrated drug lead for treating obesity. J Med Chem 2008; 51(4):1026-1034.

75. Linde Y, Ovadia O, Safrai E et al. Structure-activity relationship and metabolic stability studies of backbone cyclization and N-methylation of melanocortin peptides. Biopolymers 2008; 90:671-690.

76. Todorovic A, Holder JR, Scott JW et al. Synthesis and activity of the melanocortin Xaa-DPhe-Arg-Trp-NH₂ tetrapeptides with amide bond modifications. J Pept Res 2004; 63(3):270-278.

77. McNulty JC, Jackson PJ, Thompson DA et al. Structures of the agouti signaling protein. J Mol Biol 2005; 346(4):1059-1070.

78. Shutter JR, Graham M, Kinsey AC et al. Hypothalamic expression of ART, a novel gene related to agouti, is up-regulated in obese and diabetic mutant mice. Genes and Development 1997; 11(5):593-602.

79. Haskell-Luevano C, Monck EK. Agouti-related protein (AGRP) functions as an inverse agonist at a constitutively active brain melanocortin-4 receptor. Regulatory Peptides 2001; 99:1-7.

80. Nijenhuis WA, Oosterom J, Adan RA. AGRP(83-132) Acts as an inverse agonist on the human-melanocortin-4 receptor. Mol Endocrinol 2001; 15(1):164-171.

81. McNulty JC, Thompson DA, Bolin KA et al. High-resolution NMR structure of the chemically-synthesized melanocortin receptor binding domain AGRP(87-132) of the agouti-related protein. Biochemistry 2001; 40:15520-15527.

82. Tota MR, Smith TS, Mao C et al. Molecular interaction of agouti protein and agouti-related protein with human melanocortin receptors. Biochemistry 1999; 38(3):897-904.

83. Haskell-Luevano C, Monck EK, Wan YP et al. The agouti-related protein decapeptide (Yc[CRFFNAFC]Y) possesses agonist activity at the murine melanocortin-1 receptor. Peptides 2000; 21(5):683-689.

84. Thirumoorthy R, Holder JR, Bauzo RM et al. Novel agouti-related protein (AGRP) based melanocortin-1 receptor antagonist. J Med Chem 2001; 44:4114-4124.

85. Jarosinski MA, Dodson SW, Harding BJ et al. Design and synthesis of simplified AGRP(65-112) analogues: Protein-mimetics with affinity at the melanocortin receptors. 2nd International and 17th American Peptide Symposium. San Diego, CA; 2001:Poster #322.

86. Joseph CG, Bauzo RM, Xiang Z et al. Elongation studies of the human agouti-related protein (AGRP) core decapeptide (Yc[CRFFNAFC]Y) results in antagonism at the mouse melanocortin-3 receptor. Peptides 2003; 27:263-270.

87. Jackson PJ, McNulty JC, Yang YK et al. Design, pharmacology and NMR structure of a minimized cystine knot with agouti-related protein activity. Biochemistry 2002; 41(24):7565-7572.

88. Joseph CG, Wang XS, Scott JW et al. Stereochemical studies of the monocyclic agouti-related protein (103-122) Arg-Phe-Phe residues: Conversion of a melanocortin-4 receptor antagonist into an agonist and results in the discovery of a potent and selective melanocortin-1 agonist. J Med Chem 2004; 47(27):6702-6710.

89. Wilczynski A, Wang XS, Joseph CG et al. Identification of putative agouti-related protein(87-132)-Melanocortin-4 receptor interactions by homology molecular modeling and validation using chimeric peptide ligands. J Med Chem 2004; 47(9):2194-2207.

90. Wilczynski AM, Wang XS, Bauzo RM et al. Structural characterization of a potent (Cys101-Cys119, Cys110-Cys117) bicyclic agouti-related protein (AGRP) melanocortin receptor antagonist. J Med Chem 2004; 47:5662-5673.

91. Han G, Quillan J, Carlson K et al. Design of novel vhimeric melanotropin-deltorphin analogues. Discovery of the first potent human melanocortin 1 receptor antagonist. J Med Chem 2003; 46:810-819.

92. Joseph CG, Wilczynski AM, Holder JR et al. Chimeric NDP-MSH and MTII melanocortin peptides with agouti-related protein (AGRP) Arg-Phe-Phe amino acids possess agonist melanocortin receptor activity. Peptides 2003; 24:1899-1908.

93. Wilczynski A, Wilson KR, Scott JW et al. Structure-activity relationships of the unique and potent agouti-related protein (AGRP)-melanocortin chimeric Tyr-c[β-Asp-His-DPhe-Arg-Trp-Asn-Ala-Phe-Dpr]-Tyr-NH₂ peptide template. J Med Chem 2005; 48(8):3060-3075.

94. Jackson PJ, Yu B, Hunrichs B et al. Chimeras of the agouti-related protein: Insights into agonist and antagonist selectivity of melanocortin receptors. Peptides 2005; 26(10):1978-1987.

95. Bures, EJ, Hui, JO; Young, Y et al. Determination of disulfide structure in agouti-related protein (AGRP) by stepwise reduction and alkylation. Biochemistry 1998; 37:12172-12177.

CHAPTER 2

Melanocortin Signalling Mechanisms

Paula C. Eves and John W. Haycock*

Abstract

The melanocortin family are a series of very potent neuropeptides that derive from a parent propopiomelanocortin molecule (POMC). They are expressed predominantly in the brain, specifically the pituitary gland and also in the central nervous system. Interestingly, recent research also suggests the existence of regulatory functions outside of the brain, in a wide range of peripheral tissues. Several important melanocortin peptides with differing functions are created by the tissue-specific proteolytic cleavage of POMC, generating peptides including ACTH and α-MSH. For many years the major recognised function of α-MSH was an ability to stimulate melanocyte cells of the skin to pigment. However, a number of parallel functions unrelated to melanogenesis have been described in the literature for several years. A more complete understanding of this work arose after the discovery and cloning of the melanocortin receptors in 1992, which lead to the recognition of many wider roles of the melanocortin peptides. The knowledge of the tissue in which a given receptor subtype was expressed could now be combined with functional downstream studies. From these studies, we know that α-MSH has a very significant role in controlling inflammation and immunomodulation, with other roles including control over energy homeostasis and exocrine secretion, an ability to trigger erectile functions and the control of sexual behaviour. This chapter will briefly review the melanocortin system and melanocortin receptors, with a focus on the key signalling mechanisms of α-MSH and how these link receptors through to function.

Introduction

The melanocortin peptides adrenocorticotrophic hormone (ACTH), α-, β- and γ-melanocyte stimulating hormone (α-, β- and γ-MSH) are derived from the postranslational processing of proopiomelanocortin (POMC), summarised in Figure 1.[1] Prohormone convertase Type 1 (PC1, also known as PC3) is a serine type proteinase that initially cleaves POMC to produce pro-ACTH and β-lipotropin (β-LPH). PC1 then acts on the pro-ACTH molecule to produce an N-terminal peptide (N-POC) and a joining peptide (JP). A second serine proteinase called prohormone convertase 2 (PC2) has a number of target substrates and acts on the β-LPH molecule to form γ-lipotropin (γ-LPH) and β-endorphin (β-END). It also acts on ACTH to form ACTH 1-17, corticotrophin-like intermediate lobe peptide (CLIP) and importantly α-melanocyte-stimulating hormone (α-MSH), after modification by a CPE peptidase. Other target sites for PC2 include the cleavage of γ-LPH to form β-MSH and N-POC to form γ-MSH. The predominant body site for production of the melanocortin peptides is the pituitary gland, however extra-pituitary sites for melanocortin peptide production are also reported and include the skin.[2,3]

*Corresponding Author: John W. Haycock—Kroto Research Institute, Department of Engineering Materials, The University of Sheffield, Broad Lane, Sheffield, S3 7AU, UK.
Email: j.w.haycock@sheffield.ac.uk

Melanocortins: Multiple Actions and Therapeutic Potential, edited by Anna Catania.
©2010 Landes Bioscience and Springer Science+Business Media.

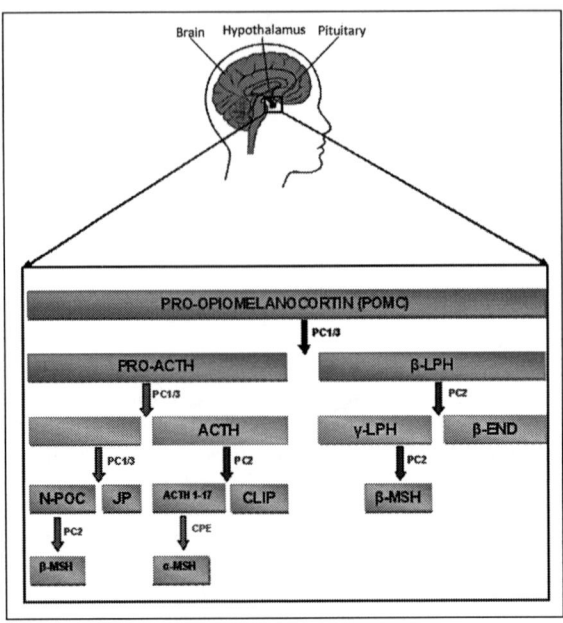

Figure 1. The processing of proopiomelanocortin arises in the pituitary gland within the brain. A series of proteolytic cleavage events generate shorter active peptides including α-MSH, ACTH and β-endorphin.

Melanocortin Receptors

The many functions of the melanocortin peptides are elicited through the tissue specific expression of five melanocortin receptors, named MC1R to MC5R. Each receptor type has a very similar structure and is comprised of a seven-pass transmembrane structure linked to a G-protein. The receptors have N-glycosylated regions at the amino termini, conserved cysteine residues at the carboxyl termini and recognition sites for interaction with protein kinase A (PKA) and protein kinase C (PKC). The conformation of each receptor enables individual ligands to bind to the extracellular domain with specificity which in turn activates an intracellular domain resulting in a secondary signalling pathway. The intracellular pathways activated thereafter lead towards resultant functions. However, specific functions are controlled not just by a given ligand, but also by interactions between a ligand and a receptor sub-type. Furthermore the tissue-specific expression of receptor sub-types provides an additional level of control.

The MC1 receptor (MC1R) is 317 amino acids in length and has a very high affinity for α-MSH. It was the first of the receptors to be cloned[4] and is expressed in a wide range of cells including the skin (keratinocytes, melanocytes and fibroblasts), melanoma cells, immune cells (neutrophils, monocytes, dendritic cells, B-lymphocytes), glial cells and endothelial cells.[5] MC1R spans the plasma membrane seven times and links the extracelluar ligand-binding domain with a G-protein on the intracellular side. The major recognised function of the MC1 receptor resulting from its interaction with α-MSH is the synthesis of pigmentation (or melanogenesis) and the regulation of skin physiology.[6] It has been widely documented that when α-MSH binds to melanocytes, an intracellular elevation of cyclic AMP arises from the activation of adenylyl cyclase which in turn activates the enzyme tyrosinase, resulting in the synthesis of eumelanin.[6] Of particular interest is that MC1R is expressed on many nonpigmentary cells and a role for this receptor during inflammation and immunoregulation is now supported by a large number of studies.

The MC2 receptor binds most melanotropic peptides, but has highest affinity for ACTH. It is 297 amino acids in length, spans the membrane seven times and links to a G-protein complex on the intracellular side. MC2R is predominantly expressed in the adrenal cortex and is concentrated in the zona glomerulosa and zona fasiculata.[7] In addition to the adrenal cortex, MC2R is expressed in the skin, on human keratinocytes, melanoma cells and in murine adipocytes.[8-11] Activation of MC2R results in the secretion of adrenal steroids which have a predominant role in stress function. ACTH binding activates adenylyl cyclase and the elevation of cyclic AMP, which in turn activates PKA. Interestingly, ACTH is reported to upregulate the expression of its own MC2 receptors.[12]

The MC3 receptor is 361 amino acids in length and is expressed in the CNS, stomach, duodenum, kidneys, placenta, heart, human monocytes and murine macrophages.[13-16] Unusually it binds the γ-MSH peptide and has a comparable affinity between this and ACTH. Activation of the receptor results in the elevation of cyclic AMP, but in addition an inositol Ca^{2+}-phospholipid signalling system is present under certain conditions (discussed in further detail below).[17] MC3R is involved in anti-inflammatory responses,[16,18,19] the control of feeding behaviour and has a role in autonomic functions and energy homeostasis.[20,21] Interestingly, mice which are deficient in MC3R demonstrate an increase in the amount of basal adipose tissue compared to wild type and also display a higher weight gain to food intake ratio.[20]

The MC4 receptor is 332 amino acids in length and has the highest affinity for α-MSH and ACTH, with a lesser affinity for β-MSH and γ-MSH. It is predominantly expressed in the CNS and whilst it is expressed widely throughout the CNS tissue (including the spinal cord, brainstem, hypothalamus, thalamus and cortex) it has not been found in other peripheral body tissues to date.[4,12] Activation of MC4R results in the elevation of cyclic AMP through adenylyl cyclase, which primarily causes changes in the neuroendocrine and autonomic system, in particular control over food intake and alterations in energy homeostasis. Mice which a have loss-of-function of the MC4 receptor do not respond to α-MSH with a predictable decrease in weight compared to wild type[22] and in this respect are similar to MC3R-deficient mice in that they more readily convert food in to adipose tissue.[23] It has also been demonstrated that MC4R is involved in penile erection and sexual function, thought to arise via expression of this receptor in the spinal cord.[24]

The MC5 receptor is 325 amino acids in length and is widespread in many peripheral tissues including exocrine glands, the spleen, skin, lung, gut, sexual organs, bone marrow and adipose tissue.[14] It has the highest binding affinity for α-MSH, slightly less affinity for ACTH and does not bind γ-MSH at all. The predominant functions arising from MC5R are a regulation of the exocrine glands and control over the secretion of sebum. Thus, mice with a disruption in this receptor display an inability to repel water effectively and have problems with regulating body temperature.[25] Interestingly, it has been shown that MC5R is expressed on B-lymphocytes and that α-MSH acting through this receptor can switch on the Jak/STAT phosphorylation pathway.[26] This second messenger pathway typically communicates pro-inflammatory cytokine and growth factor signals.[26]

Melanocortins and Pigmentation

The ability of melanocortins to stimulate human skin pigmentation was demonstrated by Lerner and McGuire[27] and Levine and colleagues,[28] who showed that injection of α-MSH, β-MSH or ACTH can produce measurable skin darkening in humans. Local immunoreactivity for POMC and MSH peptides is reported in human skin,[29-32] with the largest concentrations of α-MSH being found in the epidermis.[29,30] α-MSH in particular plays an important role in modulating the ratio of phaeomelanin (yellow/red pigment) to eumelanin (brown/black pigment) in humans. Ultraviolet radiation stimulates human skin keratinocytes to produce and secrete α-MSH and ACTH which then act predominantly on MC1Rs to stimulate melanocytes to produce eumelanin. This production of eumelanin helps protect melanocytes from UV-induced apoptosis and DNA damage. However, studies on the pigmentary effects of α-MSH on human skin melanocytes in vitro do not give a clear consensus on the function of this hormone. Some investigators report that cultured human melanocytes do not pigment in response to α-MSH,[33-35] while others report significant melanogenic responses to this peptide.[6,36]

A significant finding in the field of skin pigmentation biology was the discovery that the MC1R is highly polymorphic.[37] Both loss-of-function and gain-of-function MC1R mutations have been demonstrated in a large number of species. In humans, MC1R gene variations correlating with loss of receptor function are associated with red haired individuals who have an inability to tan when exposed to sunlight.[37-40] Epidemiological data has also suggested for many years that melanoma incidence in the Northern hemisphere correlates with individuals who display such traits. It has been generally accepted that eumelanogenic skin pigmentation arising in response to UV-light protects skin cells from DNA mutations and neoplasia. It is therefore highly relevant that some polymorphic variations of the MC1R have been associated with human cutaneous melanoma,[40-44] although not all studies confirm a positive association.[45] Structure-activity studies of the MC1R using human melanoma as a model demonstrate that polymorphic loss-of-function variations of the extracellular domain interrupt ligand binding, whereas variations confined to the intracellular domain permit ligand binding, but interrupt second message activation.[46]

Melanocortin Anti-Inflammatory and Immunomodulatory Roles

An unambiguous role for MSH peptides in the regulation of inflammatory responses has been reviewed expertly and in detail previously.[47,48] In these studies the anti-inflammatory effects of α-MSH in particular have been demonstrated to occur in the brain and central neurogenic pathways, but also in migratory immune cells and many peripheral tissues. Inflammatory responses elicited in the body are largely mediated by the release of proinflammatory cytokines such as interleukin-1 (IL-1), IL-6 and tumour necrosis factor-α (TNF-α), as well as immunostimulatory cytokines such as interferon-γ (IFN-γ). A large number of studies have now demonstrated that α-MSH and other melanocortins, by binding to melanocortin receptors both in the CNS and peripheral tissues can exert potent anti-cytokine and anti-inflammatory effects. α-MSH has also been demonstrated to antagonise many of the biological effects of surface bacterial endotoxins, such as lipopolyssaccharide (LPS). These anti-inflammatory effects include reduction of body temperature, suppression of fever and immune and neuroendocrine functions. In addition to counteracting the effect of proinflammatory cytokines, α-MSH also upregulates the production of immunosuppressive cytokines such as IL-10.[49] It is therefore suggested that the downregulation of proinflammatory cytokines and upregulation of immunosuppressive factors supports a pivotal role for α-MSH in regulating anti-inflammatory responses within the body.

The anti-inflammatory biology of α-MSH is mediated in the periphery by altering the expression of key adhesion molecules, such as intercellular adhesion molecule-1 (ICAM-1). ICAM-1 has a central role controlling immunologic and inflammatory reactions by physically linking interactions between T-lymphocytes and target cells.[50] Levels of ICAM-1 are normally very low in human cells,[50-52] but are upregulated dramatically when cells and tissues are exposed to a wide range of proinflammatory cytokines (e.g., IFN-γ, IL-1, IL-6 and TNF-α).[50-53] Studies have shown that α-MSH can significantly inhibit the upregulation of ICAM-1 in a wide range of cells (e.g., melanocytes and melanoma cells).[54,55] When investigating the intracellular mechanism of how this arises, chemicals such as isobutylmethylxanthine (IBMX) and forskolin are found to mimic the action of α-MSH. IBMX is a phosphodiester inhibitor which prevents the breakdown of cyclic AMP. Forskolin is a labdane diterpene produced by the Indian coleus plant and activates adenylyl cyclase, which in turn raises cyclic AMP levels. This suggests that α-MSH inhibits inflammatory signalling by the cyclic AMP pathway. Interestingly, the extent of α-MSH inhibition of ICAM-1 correlates with the relative number of MSH receptors.[55]

Intracellular Signalling of Melanocortin Peptides

The predominant signalling pathway of the five melanocortin receptors is through the activation of adenylyl cyclase and elevation of cyclic AMP. The multitudes of potential functions which arise thereafter are primarily dictated by the individual melanocortin ligand (e.g., α-MSH verses γ-MSH), the receptor subtype and the tissue in which that receptor is expressed. Of particular interest is that additional second messenger pathways have been reported e.g., intracellular calcium elevation has been detected from MC1R and MC3R in response to α-MSH and Jak/STAT activation from MC5R.[11,17,56] Thus evidence is appearing that suggests the presence of alternative or additional pathways. It would appear that activation of these pathways is under physiological control and that individual pathways can communicate with each other, known as receptor 'cross-talk'. Thus, if the cyclic AMP pathway is inhibited pharmacologically by the use of agents such as N6-phenylisopropyl adenosine (R-PIA) α-MSH can be demonstrated to stimulate an acute intracellular calcium signal instead.[11,17,56] R-PIA is a specific agonist of the A1 adenosine receptor which links to a class of $G_{i/o}$ proteins that inhibit adenylyl cyclase.

These findings would therefore suggest that the MC1 receptor is linked to both adenylyl cyclase and the Ca^{2+}/diacylglycerol/inositol trisphosphate pathways (summarised in Fig. 2). The response to R-PIA/α-MSH has been reported in detail for a number human melanoma cell types[11] and human keratinocyte cells[56] and it is suggested that in fact all five receptor subtypes are linked to a Ca^{2+} signalling system.[57] The data on human melanoma cells and keratinocytes would suggest that α-MSH acts through a 'dominant' cyclic AMP pathway, but under conditions where this pathway is inhibited, a resultant Ca^{2+} signal arises instead. It has also been found that ACTH plus R-PIA and ACTH derivatives (e.g., ACTH 1-17) plus R-PIA can elevate intracellular calcium in normal human keratinocytes,[56] supporting a similar link between MC2R and a calcium pathway in these cells. The specificity of the MC1 receptor on calcium signalling has been demonstrated by transfection of the MC-1R into CHO-K1 cells, where wild type CHO-K1 cells do not express MC1R or respond to combinations of α-MSH/R-PIA. However transfected CHO-K1/MC1R cells elevate calcium when stimulated with α-MSH/R-PIA.[56] The functional significance of an interaction between these pathways is not fully understood. However in keratinocyte cells it has been shown that if intracellular calcium levels were elevated using ionomycin the NF-κB transcription factor could be inhibited in the presence of TNF-α.[56] This is an important finding, as it is now widely accepted that α-MSH acts as an anti-inflammatory and immunomodulatory molecule by inhibition of NF-κB, a transcription factor that exists in virtually all cell types.[58] Whilst, most studies report that this arises via the cyclic AMP pathway, it would appear that acute elevation of intracellular calcium can also inhibit this pathway.

NF-κB plays a critical role in the immune system by regulating the expression of several proinflammatory cytokines and genes.[58] It has a major role in controlling gene expression in response to TNF-α, a very common proinflammatory cytokine. In practice the activation of NF-κB arises in response to a very wide range of pro-inflammatory stimuli. This triggers the proteolysis of a cytoplasmic inhibitory component (IκB) and unmasks a nuclear localization signal, enabling the translocation of a p50-p65 heterodimeric complex into the nucleus. It is here that a highly specific interaction arises between NF-κB and certain gene promoter regions facilitating RNA polymerase II activation and mRNA synthesis.[58]

Manna and Aggarwal first described that α-MSH could inhibit activated NF-κB in immune cells in a dose and time-dependent manner.[59] These findings have been confirmed and extended to show that α-MSH can inhibit TNF-α-induced activation of NF-κB in human cutaneous and ocular melanocytes and melanoma cells,[60,61] human dermal fibroblasts[5,62,63] and keratinocytes,[8,56] olfactory ensheathing cells of the central nervous systems,[64] Schwann cells of the peripheral nervous system[65] and endothelial cells.[66] The mechanism is widely agreed to arise via the elevation of cyclic AMP, as the use of IBMX or forskolin for elevating cyclic AMP was found to inhibit NFκB. However, a more precise mechanism linking α-MSH with NF-κB was not understood until 2000 when it was shown that human melanoma cells and keratinocytes responded to TNF-α stimulation (or sub-toxic hydrogen peroxide stimulation) with rapid activation of the enzyme glutathione peroxidise (GPx).[61] This rapid activation was inhibited in the presence of α-MSH.[61] GPx is a key antioxidant enzyme that enables cells to specifically remove peroxide species, more generally referred to as 'oxidative stress'. Early studies have suggested that the generation of peroxide species (and related oxygen free radicals) are cytotoxic. However, it is more generally agreed that only an excessive or unregulated production of these species is

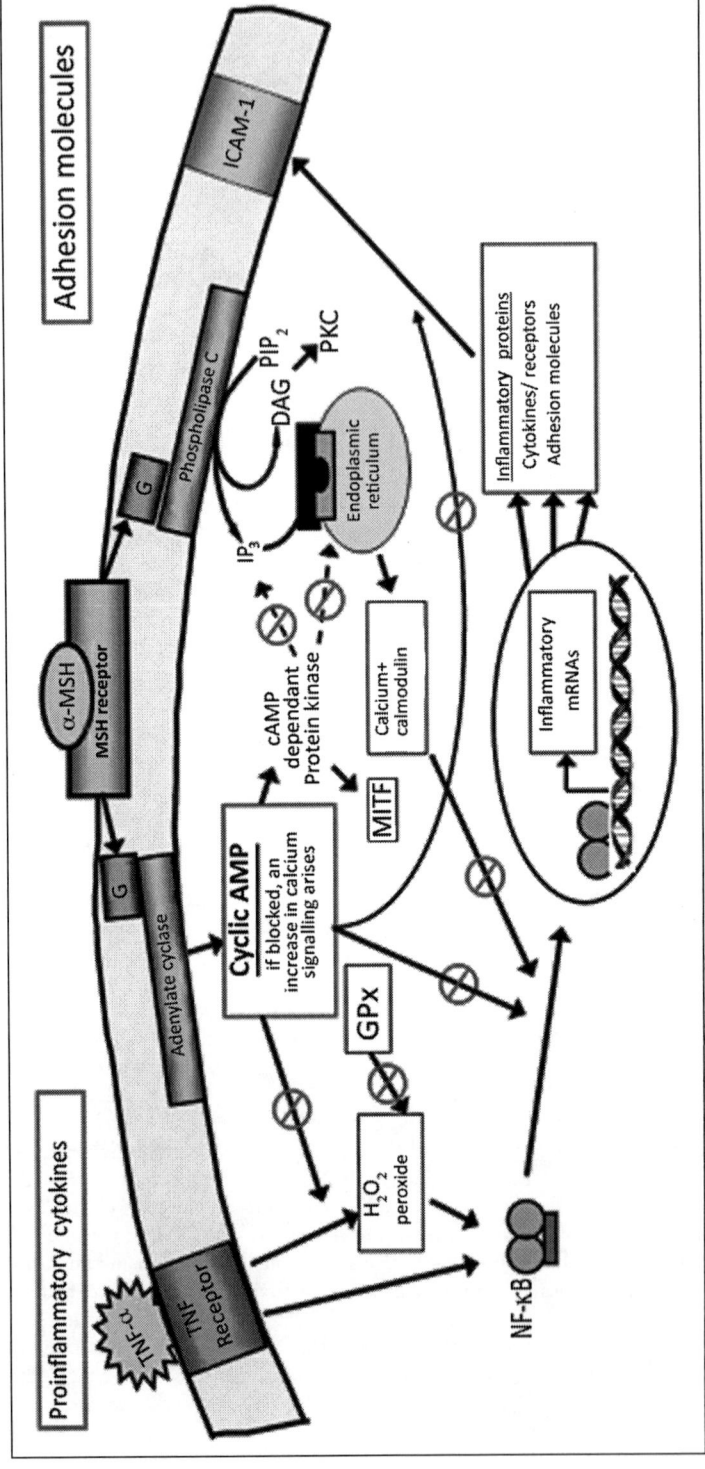

Figure 2. The relationship between α-MSH, the MC receptors and signalling pathways arising via G-protein signalling. Inflammatory activation at the cell membrane is shown by TNF-α and the interactions of the resultant pathways summarised diagrammatically.

damaging and that regulated levels control transcription factor activation and cell signalling.[67] Thus, NF-κB can be activated by both TNF-α or hydrogen peroxide (as peroxide species can activate NF-κB directly). It is long been reported that TNF-α can signal by transiently elevating intracellular peroxide species[67] and so if α-MSH can inhibit the generation of these species, inhibition of NF-κB is expected to result.[61]

Studies have also shown that α-MSH can down regulate NF-κB activation in human immunodeficiency virus (HIV) infected monocytes.[68] This suppression of NF-κB by α-MSH, which is not believed to have any pharmacologic toxicity in humans, makes it an interesting candidate for the potential treatment of pathogenic conditions initiated through NF-κB activation, such as inflammatory diseases and HIV replication in AIDs. The potent ability of α-MSH to inhibit NF-κB activation may also make it potentially useful for ischemic injuries, particularly relevant for tissue of the brain and heart (reviewed in ref. 48).

The discovery that melanocortins can control NF-κB infers that any gene under the control of NF-κB is under potential regulation. NF-κB controls the expression of about 150 genes, which are grouped according to function and include cytokines, cytokine receptors and adhesion molecules.[58] A number of functional studies have shown the link between melanocortins, NF-κB and the relative expression of several down-stream proteins. Of particular note is work on the relative expression of adhesion molecules such as ICAM-1 and E-Selectin, as an interaction between these adhesion molecules and immune cells is required for a primary inflammatory or immune response. For example, TNF-α can upregulate the expression of ICAM-1 in human melanoma cells and α-MSH can inhibit this increase.[54] Similarly, LPS mediated upregulation of E-selectin in endothelial cells is inhibited by α-MSH.[66] However, these detailed studies represent only a small proportion of potential candidate proteins that are under the complete control of melanocortins via NF-κB. In addition to NF-κB, intracellular signalling mechanisms have also been shown to involve activation of the cyclic AMP response element-binding protein (CREB).[69,70] As CREB plays an important role in cell survival during metabolic and oxidative stress, it is thought that activation of this intracellular signalling pathway provides cells with anti-inflammatory and anti-apoptotic capabilities.

The key anti-inflammatory signalling pathways mediated by the melanocortins are thought to arise predominantly via the MC1 and MC3 receptors in peripheral tissues and by the MC4 receptor in the CNS.[68] In this respect other signalling pathways involving α-MSH or MSH agonists have included phosphorylation of mitogen-activated protein kinase/extracellular signal-regulated kinase (MAPK/ERK). This includes work showing attenuation of p38 MAPK phosphorylation and a decrease in activation of the stress-activated kinase, JNK3. It is also reported that activation of cyclic AMP via MC4R, followed by attenuation of p38 MAPK or MAPK/JNK results in the decreased production of TNF-α and inhibition of NF-κB.[68] Although it is not yet clear what definitive roles MAPKs play following MC4R activation by α-MSH, they have been suggested by Lasagna and colleagues to participate in the anti-inflammatory biology of α-MSH.

Melanocortin Receptor Antagonists and Agonists

In addition to melanocortin peptide derivatives of POMC which serve as agonists to the five melanocortin receptors, there are also two naturally occurring antagonists. These include the agouti signalling protein (ASP) and the agouti-related protein (AGRP).[71,72] Both antagonists play important roles in preventing agonist-induced G-protein activation and upregulation of cyclic AMP by competitively binding to the receptors. This antagonism has been clearly demonstrated in mice. For example, activation of MC1Rs by α-MSH results in the synthesis of the black/brown eumelanin pigment, whereas antagonism of melanocyte MC1R by agouti in mice switches pigment production to the yellow/orange pheomelanin pigment resulting in a yellow/orange coat colour.[73] Whilst a definitive role for this endogenous antagonist in human pigmentation has not been fully elucidated, recent work has shown that in humans, a 3'UTR ASP polymorhphism has been found at a higher frequency in darker-skinned populations compared to Caucasians and has been associated with dark hair and eye colour (reviewed in ref. 74).

Conclusion

The present chapter summarises the key signalling mechanisms that arise between melanocortin peptides and their receptors, focussing predominantly on α-MSH. It covers functional studies with respect to melanocortins, pigmentation and inflammation in a breadth of cell types including those of the skin, nervous tissue and the vasculature. Importantly, α-MSH assists many cells to resist the actions of proinflammatory cytokines, in particular TNF-α, which serves to trigger inflammation in a wide range of tissues via the activation of NF-κB. The role of how the melanocortins, the melanocortin receptors and signalling pathways interact are discussed in relation to attenuating inflammation, in light of the predominant second messenger pathways and how these link to the control of major proteins such as ICAM-1 and E-Selectin in regulating the immune response. Finally, the roles of antagonists are considered as modulators of receptor function.

Acknowledgements

The authors wish to acknowledge support from the EPSRC and BBSRC (UK).

References

1. Eberle AN. The melanotropins: chemistry, physiology and mechanisms of action. 1988; 1-439. Karger: Basel.
2. Chakraborty AK, Funsaka Y, Slominski A et al. Production and release of proopiomelanocortin (POMC) derived peptides by human melanocytes and keratinocytes in culture: regulation by ultraviolet B. Biochim Biophys Acta 1996; 313:130-8.
3. Slominski A, Wortsman J, Luger T et al. Corticotropin releasing hormone and proopiomelanocortin involvement in the cutaneous response to stress. Physiol Rev 2000; 80:979-1020.
4. Mountjoy KG, Robbins LS, Mortrud MT et al. The cloning of a family of genes that encode the melanocortin receptors. Science 1992; 257:1248-51.
5. Bohm M, Metze D, Schulte U et al. Detection of melanocortin-1 receptor antigenicity on human skin cells in culture and in situ. Exp Dermatol 1999; 8:453-61.
6. Hunt G, Todd, Cresswell JE et al. α-melanocyte stimulating hormone and its analogue Nle⁴DPhe⁷ α-MSH affect morphology, tyrosinase activity and melanogenesis in cultured human melanocytes. J Cell Sci 1994; 107:205-11.
7. Liakos P, Chambaz EM, Feige JJ et al. Expression of ACTH receptors (MC2-R and MC5-R) in the glomerulosa and the fasciculata-reticularis zones of bovine adrenal cortex. Endocr Res 1998; 24:427-32.
8. Moustafa M, Szabo M, Ghanem GE et al. Inhibition of tumour necrosis factor-alpha stimulated NFkappaB/p65 in human keratinocytes by alpha-melanocyte stimulating hormone and adrenocorticotrophic hormone peptides. J Invest Dermatol 2002; 119:1244-53.
9. Slominski A, Ermak G, Mihm M. ACTH receptor, CYP11A1, CYP17 and CYP21A2 genes are expressed in skin. J Clin Endocrinol Metab 1996; 81:2746-9.
10. Boston BA, Cone RD. Characterization of melanocortin receptor subtype expression in murine adipose tissues and in the 3T3-L1 cell line. Endocrinology 1996; 137:2043-50.
11. Eves P, Haycock JW, Layton C et al. Anti-inflammatory and anti-invasive effects of α-melanocyte-stimulating hormone in human melanoma cells. Br J Cancer 2003; 89:2004-15.
12. Mountjoy KG. The human melanocyte stimulating hormone receptor has evolved to become "super-sensitive" to melanocortin peptides. Mol Cell Endocrinol 1994; 102(1-2):R7-11.
13. Gantz I, Konda Y, Tashiro T et al. Molecular cloning of a novel melanocortin receptor. J Biol Chem 1993; 268:8246-50.
14. Chhajlani V. Distribution of cDNA for melanocortin receptor subtypes in human tissues. Biochem Mol Biol Int 1996; 38(1):73-80.
15. Taherzadeh S, Sharma S, Chhajlani V et al. Alpha-MSH and its receptors in regulation of tumor necrosis factor-alpha production by human monocyte/macrophages. Am J Physiol 1999; 276:289-94.
16. Getting SJ, Gibbs L, Clark AJ et al. POMC gene-derived peptides activate melanocortin type 3 receptor on murine macrophages, suppress cytokine release and inhibit neutrophil migration in acute experimental inflammation. J Immunol 1999; 162:7446-53.
17. Konda Y, Gantz I, DelValle J et al. Interaction of dual intracellular signaling pathways activated by the melanocortin-3 receptor. J Biol Chem 1994; 269:13162-6.
18. Getting SJ, Perretti M. MC3-R as a novel target for antiinflammatory therapy. Drug News Perspect 2000; 13:19-27.
19. Getting SJ. Melanocortin peptides and their receptors: new targets for anti-inflammatory therapy. Trends Pharmacol Sci 2002; 23:447-9.

20. Chen AS, Marsh DJ, Trumbauer ME et al. Inactivation of the mouse melanocortin-3 receptor results in increased fat mass and reduced lean body mass. Nat Genet 2000; 26:97-102.
21. Getting SJ. Targeting melanocortin receptors as potential novel therapeutics. Pharmacol Ther 2006; 111:1-15.
22. Marsh DJ, Hollopeter G, Huszar D et al. Response of melanocortin-4 receptor-deficient mice to anorectic and orexigenic peptides. Nat Genet 1999; 21:119-22.
23. Ste Marie L, Miura GI, Marsh DJ et al. A metabolic defect promotes obesity in mice lacking melanocortin-4 receptors. Proc Natl Acad Sci 2000; 97:12339-44.
24. Wessells H, Gralnek D, Dorr R et al. Effect of an α-melanocyte-stimulating hormone analogue on penile erection and sexual desire in men with organic erectile dysfunction. Urology 2000; 56:641-46.
25. Chen W, Kelly MA, Optiz-ArayaX et al. Exocrine gland dysfunction in MC5-R-deficient mice: evidence for coordinated regulation of exocrine gland function by melanocortin peptides. Cell 1997; 91:789-98.
26. Buggy JJ. Binding of α-melanocyte-stimulating hormone to its G-protein coupled receptor on B-lymphocytes activates the Jak/STAT pathway. Biochem J 1998; 331:211-16.
27. Lerner AB, McGuire JS. Effect of α- and β-melanocyte stimulating hormones on skin colour of man. Nature 1961; 21:176-9.
28. Levine N, Sheftel SN, Eytan T et al. Induction of skin tanning by subcutaneous administration of a potent synthetic melanotropin. JAMA 1991; 266:2730-6.
29. Thody AJ, Hunt G, Donatien PD et al. Human melanocytes express functional melanocyte-stimulating hormone receptors. Ann N Y Acad Sci 1993; 680:381-90.
30. Bhardwaj RS, Luger TA. Proopiomelanocortin production by epidermal cells: evidence for an immune neuroendocrine network in the epidermis. Arch Dermatol Res 1994; 287:85-90.
31. Can G, Abdel-Malek Z, Porter-Gill PA et al. Identification and sequencing of a putative variant of proopiomelanocortin in human epidermis and epidermal cells in culture. J Invest Dermatol 1998; 111:485-91.
32. Wakamatsu K, Graham A, Cook D et al. Characterisation of ACTH peptides in human skin and their activation of the melanocortin-1 receptor. Pigment Cell Res 1997; 10:288-97.
33. Halaban R, Pomerantz SH, Marshall S et al. Regulation of tyrosinase in human melanocytes grown in culture. J Cell Biol 1983; 97(2):480-8.
34. Hedley SJ, Gawkrodger DJ, Weetman AP et al. α-MSH and melanogenesis in normal human adult melanocytes. Pigment Cell Res 1998; 11:45-56.
35. De Luca M, Siegrist W, Bondanza S et al. α-melanocyte stimulating hormone (αMSH) stimulates normal human melanocyte growth by binding to high-affinity receptors. J Cell Science 1993; 105:1079-84.
36. Abdel-Malek Z, Swope VB, Suzuki I et al. Mitogenic and melanogenic stimulation of normal human melanocytes by melanotropic peptides. Proc Natl Acad Sci USA 1995; 92:1789-93.
37. Valverde P, Healy E, Jackson I et al. Variants of the melanocyte-stimulating hormone receptor gene are associated with red hair and fair skin in humans. Nat Genet 1995; 11:328-30.
38. Schiöth HB, Phillips SR, Rudzish R et al. Loss of function mutations of the human melanocortin 1 receptor are common and are associated with red hair. Biochem Biophys Res Commun 1999; 260:488-91.
39. Rees JL, Birch-Machin M, Flanagan N et al. Genetic studies of the human melanocortin-1 receptor. Ann NY Acad Sci 1999; 885:34-42.
40. Schaffer JV, Bolognia JL. The melanocortin-1 receptor: red hair and beyond. Arch Dermatol 2001; 137:1477-85.
41. Palmer JS, Duffy DL, Box NF et al. Melanocortin-1 receptor polymorphisms and risk of melanoma: is the association explained solely by pigmentation phenotype? Am J Hum Genet 2000; 66:176-86.
42. Rees JL. The melanocortin I receptor (MC1R): more than just red hair. Pigment Cell Res 2000; 3:135-40.
43. Jimenez-Cervantes C, Olivares C, Gonzalez P et al. The Pro162 variant is a loss-of-function mutation of the human melanocortin 1 receptor gene. J Invest Dermatol 2001; 117:156-8.
44. Sturm RA, Duffy DL, Box NF et al. The role of melanocortin-1 receptor polymorphism in skin cancer risk phenotypes. Pigment Cell Res 2003; 16:266-72.
45. Ichii-Jones F, Lear JT, Heagerty AH et al. Susceptibility to melanoma: influence of skin type and polymorphism in the melanocyte stimulating hormone receptor gene. J Invest Dermatol 1998; 111:218-21.
46. Oliva ABP, Fernenez LP, DeTorre C et al. Identification and functional analysis of novel variants of the human melanocortin 1 receptor found in melanoma patients. Human Mut 2009; 30:811-22.
47. Lipton JM, Catania A. Anti-inflammatory actions of the neuroimmunomodulator α-MSH. Immunol Today 1997; 18:140-5.
48. Catania A, Gatti S, Columbo G et al. Targetting melanocortin receptors as a novel strategy to control inflammation. Pharm Rev 2004; 56:1-24.
49. Bhardwaj RS, Shwarz A, Becher E et al. Pro-opiomelanocortin-derived peptides induce IL-10 production in human monocytes. J Immunol 1996; 156:2517-21.

50. Kirnbauer R, Charvat B, Schauer E et al. Modulation of intercellular adhesion molecule-1 expression on human melanocytes and melanoma cells: evidence for a regulatory role of IL-6, IL-7, TNFβ and UVB light. J Invest Dermatol 1992; 98:320-6.
51. Vejlsgaard GL, Ralfkiaer E, Avnstorp C et al. Kinetics and characterisation of intercellular adhesion molecule-1 (ICAM-1) expression on keratinocytes in various inflammatory skin lesions and malignant cutaneous lymphomas. J Am Acad Dermatol 1989; 20:782-90.
52. Singer KH, Tuck DT, Sampson HA et al. Epidermal keratinocytes express the adhesion molecule intercellular adhesion molecule-1 in inflammatory dermatoses. J Invest Dermatol 1989; 92:746-50.
53. Krutmann J, Kock A, Schauer E et al. Tumour necrosis factor beta and ultraviolet radiation are potent regulators of human keratinocyte ICAM-1 expression. J Invest Dermatol 1990; 95:127-31.
54. Hedley SJ, Gawkrodger DJ, Weetman AP et al. α-melanocyte stimulating hormone inhibits tumour necrosis factor-α stimulated intercellular adhesion molecule-1 expression in normal cutaneous human melanocytes and in melanoma cell lines. Br J Dermatol 1998; 138:536-43.
55. Morandini R, Boeynaems JM, Hedley SJ et al. Modulation of ICAM-1 expression by α-MSH in human melanoma cells and melanocytes. J Cell Physiol 1998; 175:276-82.
56. Elliott RJ, Szabo M, Wagner MJ et al. Alpha-melanocyte-stimulating hormone, MSH 11-13 KPV and adrenocorticotrophic hormone signalling in human keratinocyte cells. J Invest Dermatol 2004; 122:1010-19.
57. Hoogduijn MJ, McGurk S, Smit NPM et al. Ligand-dependent activation of the melanocortin 5 receptor: cAMP production and ryanodine receptor-dependent elevations of (Ca^{2+}). Biochem Biophys Res Commun 2002; 290:844-50.
58. Baeuerle PA, Henkel T. Function and activation of NF-κB in the immune system. Ann Rev Immunol 1994; 12:141-79.
59. Manna SK, Aggarwal BB. Alpha-melanocyte-stimulating hormone inhibits the nuclear transcription factor NF-kappa B activation induced by various inflammatory agents. J Immunol 1998; 161:2873-80.
60. Haycock JW, Wagner M, Morandini R et al. α-melanocyte stimulating hormone inhibits NF-κB activation in human melanocytes and melanoma cells. J Invest Dermatol 1999; 113:560-6.
61. Haycock JW, Rowe ST, Cartledge S et al. α-melanocyte stimulating hormone reduces impact of proinflammatory cytokine and peroxide-generated oxidative stress on keratinocyte and melanoma cell lines. J Biol Chem 2000; 275:15629-36.
62. Hill RP, MacNeil S, Haycock JW. Melanocyte stimulating hormone peptides inhibit TNF-α signalling in human dermal fibroblast cells. Peptides 2006; 27:421-30.
63. Hill RP, Wheeler P, MacNeil S et al. Alpha-melanocyte stimulating hormone cytoprotective biology in human dermal fibroblast cells. Peptides 2005; 26:1150-8.
64. Teare KA, Pearson RG, Shakesheff KM et al. α-MSH inhibits inflammatory signalling in olfactory ensheathing cells. NeuroReport 2003; 14:2171-6.
65. Teare KA, Pearson RG, Shakesheff KM et al. α-MSH inhibits inflammatory signalling in Schwann cells. NeuroReport 2004; 15:493-8.
66. Scholzen TE, Sunderkotter C, Kalden DH et al. Alpha-melanocyte stimulating hormone prevents lipopolysaccharide-induced vasculitis by down-regulating endothelial cell adhesion molecule expression. Endocrinol 2003; 144:360-70.
67. Schulzeosthoff K, Bakker AC, Vanhaesebroeck B et al. Cytotoxic activity of tumor-necrosis-factor is mediated by early damage of mitochondrial functions—evidence for the involvement of mitochondrial radical generation. J Biol Chem 1992; 267:5317-23.
68. Lasaga M, Debeljuk L, Durand D et al. Role of alpha-melanocyte stimulating hormone and melanocortin 4 receptor in brain inflammation. Peptides 2008; 29:1825-35.
69. Busca R, Ballotti R. CyclicAMP a key messenger in the regulation of skin pigmentation. Pigment Cell Res 2000; 13:60-9.
70. Sarkar S, Legradi G, Lechan RM. Intracerebroventricular administration of α-melanocyte stimulating hormone increases phosphorylation of CREB in TRH and CRH-producing neurons of the hypothalamic paraventricular nucleus. Brain Res 2002; 945:50-9.
71. Ollman MM, Wilson BD, Yang YK et al. Interaction of Agouti protein with the melanocortin 1 receptor in vitro and in vivo. Genes Dev 1998; 12:316-30.
72. Wikberg JE, Muceniece R, Mandrika I et al. New aspects on the melanocortins and their receptors. Pharmacol Res 2000; 42:398-420.
73. Lu D, Willard D, Patel IR et al. Agouti protein is an antagonist of the melanocyte-stimulating-hormone receptor. Nature 1994; 371:799-802.
74. Carroll L, Voisey J, van Daal A. Gene polymorphisms and their effects in the melanocortin system. Peptides 2005; 26:1871-85.

CHAPTER 3

Distribution and Function of Melanocortin Receptors within the Brain

Kathleen G. Mountjoy*

Abstract

Biological responses to pro-opiomelanocortin (POMC)-derived peptides administered in the brain were documented in the 1950s but their molecular mechanisms of action only began to be resolved with the mapping of melanocortin receptor subtypes to specific brain regions in the 1990s. Out of the five melanocortin receptor subtypes, MC3R and MC4R are widely recognised as 'neural' melanocortin receptors. In situ hybridization anatomical mapping of these receptor subtypes to distinct hypothalamic nuclei first indicated their roles in energy homeostasis, roles that were later confirmed with the obese phenotypes exhibited by *Mc3R* and *Mc4R* knockout mice. It is perhaps less well known however, that all five melanocortin receptor subtypes have been detected in developing and/or adult brains of various species. This chapter provides a comprehensive summary of the detection and mapping of each melanocortin receptor subtype in mammalian, chicken and fish brains and relates the sites of expression to functions that are either known or proposed for each receptor subtype.

Introduction

Melanocortin peptides derived from pro-opiomelanocortin (POMC) have been known to have many diverse functions in the brain since the 1950s.[1,2] Melanocortin peptide-induced stretching and yawning response and grooming in the rat, were among the first described behaviors. Grooming behavior is thought to regulate body temperature and to reduce mild stress-induced arousal.[3] Melanocortins injected into rat brain were also shown to exhibit potent antipyretic activity,[4] affect brain development,[5] learning, memory, sexual behavior, attention and motivation and functional recovery from central nervous system (CNS) lesions.[3,6] Functional recovery from impaired motor activity caused by 6-hydroxydopamine lesions in the nucleus accumbens was accelerated by adrenocorticotropin$_{4-10}$ (ACTH$_{4-10}$) and α-melanocyte stimulating hormone (α-MSH).[5] Melanocortins were first shown to regulate appetite when α-MSH and ACTH$_{1-24}$ were injected into rat brain either intracerebroventricular (icv) or directly into the hypothalamus and resulted in a significant decrease in food intake.[7]

The cloning of the melanocortin receptors in the 1990s[8,9] stimulated intense interest in melanocortin peptide signaling in the brain and a great deal of this interest has since focused on roles for melanocortin peptides in energy homeostasis.[10] This led large pharmaceutical companies to search for small molecule agonists and antagonists of specific brain melanocortin receptors.[11,12]

*Kathleen G. Mountjoy—Departments of Physiology and Molecular Medicine and Pathology, School of Medical Sciences, Faculty of Medical and Health Sciences, University of Auckland, Private Bag 92019, Auckland 1023, New Zealand. Email: kmountjoy@auckland.ac.nz

Melanocortins: Multiple Actions and Therapeutic Potential, edited by Anna Catania.
©2010 Landes Bioscience and Springer Science+Business Media.

Although none of these have yet translated into therapeutics for energy homeostasis, the development of these drugs has helped to identify functions for specific brain melanocortin receptors. This knowledge identified other potential therapeutic interventions targeting melanocortin receptors, such as treatment for brain inflammation[13] and erectile function.[14]

Of the five melanocortin receptor subtypes, the melanocortin 3 (MC3R) and melanocortin 4 (MC4R) receptors are widely recognised as the 'neural' melanocortin receptors. These brain receptors have been extensively characterised for expression and function since obese phenotypes developed in either *Mc3R* or *Mc4R* knockout mice.[10] However, while the central MC3R and MC4R proteins play critical roles in regulating energy homeostasis, they are not the only melanocortin receptors expressed in the brain. All five melanocortin receptor subtypes have been detected in the brain of various species although the MC3R and MC4R are the most abundant central melanocortin receptors. Mapping the mRNA expression of Mc3R and Mc4R in rat or mouse brain led to predictions for melanocortin peptide roles in energy homeostasis and other physiological functions. The aim of this chapter is to provide a comprehensive summary of the mapping of each melanocortin receptor subtype in mammalian, chicken and fish brains. These sites of receptor expression are then related to functions that are either known, or proposed, for each receptor subtype.

MC1R Is Expressed in the Periaqueductal Gray and the MC1R Regulates Pain and Analgesia

The MC1R is well known for its expression in melanocytes where it plays a critical role in pigmentation. Recessive defective mutations in the MC1R result in red hair and fair skin.[15] However, the MC1R is expressed in other tissues and has functions beyond pigmentation. Mc1R mRNA has been detected by reverse transcriptase polymerase chain reaction (RT-PCR) in BALB/c mouse brain.[16] In rat and human brain, MC1R mRNA and protein is expressed in neurons in the periaqueductal gray (PAG) region as shown using in situ hybridization and immunohistochemistry, respectively.[17] This expression suggested a functional role for the MC1R in analgesia since the PAG region is a midline locus of crucial relevance to endogenous analgesic circuitry.[18] The Mc1R has also been shown to be present in teleost fish (platyfish, medaka and zebrafish) and the Japanese pufferfish (*Fugu*) brain using RT-PCR.[19,20] In *Fugu*, weak Mc1R expression was seen in the telencephalon, optic tectum and hypothalamus following southern blotting of the RT-PCR products. The functional roles of the Mc1R in teleost brain are unknown.

Evidence supporting a role for MC1R mediated analgesia in mouse and human was provided when a quantitative trait locus for stress-induced analgesia mapped to the mouse chromosome 8 where the Mc1R is encoded.[21] This association was observed in females but not in males, thus reflecting reported sex differences in pain and analgesic sensitivity.[22] Confirmation that the Mc1R mediates κ-opioid analgesia in female mice was provided when female but not male Mc1R$^{e/e}$ mutant mice displayed altered κ-opioid analgesia[21] and red haired and fair skinned women with two defective MC1R alleles displayed greater analgesia from κ-opioid, pentazocine, than red haired men with variant MC1R alleles, or men and women with all other hair colors.[21] Pentazocine produced increases in ischemic pain thresholds and tolerance, decreases in rating of ischemic pain intensity and decreases in thermal pain intensity ratings and these responses were robust in red haired women with variant MC1R alleles. Proof that the MC1R affects pain and μ-opioid analgesia in mice and humans was provided when Mogil et al[23] demonstrated that Mc1R$^{e/e}$ mutant mice and human red heads with two defective MC1R alleles displayed reduced sensitivity to noxious stimuli and increased analgesic responsiveness to the μ-opioid selective metabolite, M6G. These effects were similar in both male and female mice and there was no effect of gender in humans, in contrast to the sex dependent responses observed for κ-opioid analgesia.[21]

MC1R expression in the PAG is likely responsible for mediating MC1R regulation of pain and analgesia but its mechanism of action is unclear. Mogil et al[21] were unable to produce reliable effects on nociceptive sensitivity in either gender when they injected α-MSH icv into mice. These authors raised the possibility that the κ-opioid receptor ligands such as dynorphin may be involved. Metabolites of dynorphin derived from cleavage of the amino terminal Tyr residue (des-Tyr derivatives) bind and antagonise the MC1R in vitro, with potencies that parallel those reported for pharmacological non-opioid effects of dynorphins in vivo.[24]

The MC1R may also have an immunomodulatory role in the brain. MC1R mRNA has been detected in a human glioma cell line (A-172, anaplastic astrocytoma cells) and α-MSH has potent anti-cytokine effects on these cells.[25] However, it is unknown whether the MC1R is expressed in glioma cells and astrocytes in vivo. If it is, then it could modulate inflammatory responses in the CNS.

MC2R Is Expressed in Teleost Fish Brain and Fetal Mouse Brain, but Not in Adult Mammalian Brain

The MC2R is recognised as the ACTH receptor in the adrenal cortex where it regulates glucocorticoid, aldosterone and androgen production. MC2R mRNA has also been detected in fetal mouse brain[26] and in teleost fish brain.[19] Immunohistochemical studies showed that Mc2R protein is expressed in the developing mouse embryo in a wide number of tissues, including the brain and spinal cord. Mc2R protein is present in the mouse telencephalon, mesencephalon, metencephalon, myelencephalon and spinal cord from E11.5 to E13.5.[26] The expression of Mc2R in adult *Fugu* brain is very low but was detected using RT-PCR in total RNA prepared from telencephalon and hypothalamus, as seen with ethidium bromide staining.[19] Southern blotting of the RT-PCR products also showed Mc2R mRNA expression in cerebellum and brain stem. Like *Fugu* brain, the hypothalamus of Rainbow trout also expresses low levels of Mc2R mRNA as detected by quantitative real-time PCR on cDNA prepared from total RNA.[27]

The presence of Mc2R in the brain at late stages of mouse organogenesis suggests that the Mc2R plays a role in brain development. The Mc2R has not been found in adult brain of any mammal despite extensive searches for this receptor in brain.[28,29] It has been proposed that the Mc2R in teleost brain may exist as a central negative feedback loop for ACTH, a role later taken over by the MC3R in mammals.[19] Interestingly, only four melanocortin receptor subtypes are present in *Fugu*, medaka and stickleback genomes; the MC3R gene is missing.[19] Not only is the MC3R missing in these fish, but the natural mammalian MC3R ligand, γ-MSH, is also missing. Zebrafish however, do have a Mc3R gene and therefore Mc3R expression is variable in fish.[20]

MC3R Is Specifically Expressed in Hypothalamus and the Limbic System Where Its Functions Are Not Clearly Understood

Adult Brain

The Mc3R is the most abundantly expressed melanocortin receptor subtype in the rat brain. It was first cloned in 1993 from rat by Roselli-Rehfuss et al[30] and from human by Gantz et al.[31] In both instances, MC3R mRNA expression was detected by Northern blotting using 4-5 μg of rat hypothalamic tissue poly (A)⁺ RNA. Nevertheless, MC3R gene expression is relatively low in the brain as poly (A)⁺ RNA was required for its detection. Expression of Mc3R mRNA is restricted in the adult rat brain, with highest densities being found in the hypothalamus and limbic systems. In situ hybridization mapping of Mc3R mRNA in rat brain determined the anatomical localization for this melanocortin receptor subtype in approximately 30 different nuclei[30,31] (Fig. 1). The greatest density of Mc3R containing neurons in the hypothalamus were found in the arcuate nucleus (ARH), the dorsomedial portion of the ventromedial nucleus (VMHdl), anteroventral preoptic area, posterior hypothalamic area and the medial preoptic area (MPO). Outside of the hypothalamus, relatively dense signal was observed in the intermediate part of the lateral nucleus of the septum, in the medial habenula nucleus of the thalamus (MHb), in the ventral tegmental area (VTA) and in the central linear nucleus of raphe.[30] Weak signals were present in the hippocampus, the piriform cortex and a few brainstem nuclei.

Autoradiographs of [¹²⁵I]-NDP-MSH binding (binds both MC3R and MC4R similarly) and displacement with nonradioactive γ1-MSH (40 fold selective for MC3R) was used as a method

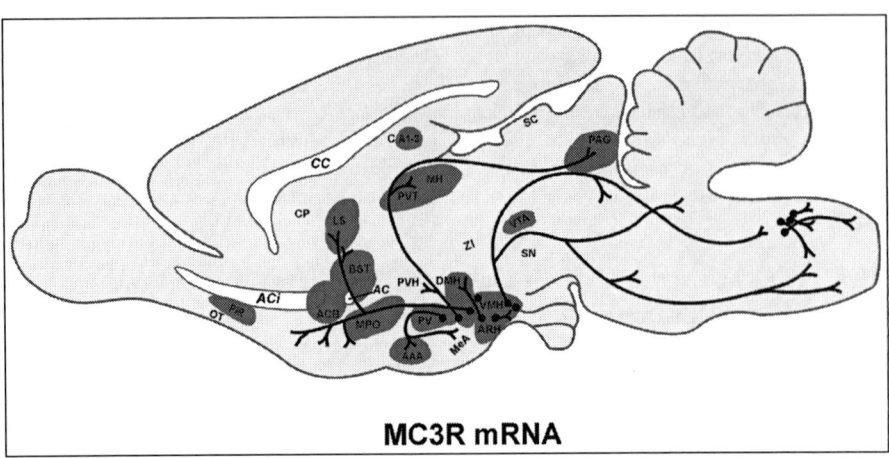

MC3R mRNA

Figure 1. Schematic of rat adult brain sagittal section showing regions expressing Mc3R mRNA. POMC neurons shown as black dots and POMC projections shown as black lines. Shading represents regions in situ hybridization mapped for Mc3R mRNA expression.[30] (Modified from ref. 142 with permission.) Abbreviations: AAA: anterior amygdala; AC: anterior commissure; ACB: nucleus accumbens; ACi: Anterior commissure, intrabulbar; ARH: arcuate nucleus hypothalamus; BST: bed nuclei of the stria terminalis; CA1-3: hippocampus; CC: corpus callosum; CP: caudate putamen; DMH: dorsomedial nucleus, hypothalamus; DMX: dorsal motor nucleus of the vagus; LS: lateral septal area; LSd: lateral septal area, dorsal aspects; MeA: medial amygdala; MH: medial habenula; MPO: medial preoptic area; OT: olfactory tubercle; PAG: periaqueductal gray; PIR: piriform cortex; PV: periventricular zone; PVH: paraventricular nucleus, hypothalamus; PVT: paraventricular nucleus, thalamus; RN: red nucleus; SC: superior colliculus; SN: substantia nigra; VMH: ventromedial nucleus, hypothalamus; VTA: ventral tegmental area; ZI: zona incerta. A color version of this image is available at www.landesbioscience.com/curie.

to discriminate between Mc3R and Mc4R in rat brain.[32] The autoradiographs showed dominant expression of Mc3R in the nucleus accumbens shell, MPO and VMH.

In the ARH, Mc3R mRNA is expressed in both POMC and agouti-related peptide (AgRP) neurons.[33,34] Double labelling in situ hybridization was used to show that a large portion of POMC neurons in the rostral ARH are positive for Mc3R mRNA[33,34] as are a large proportion of AgRP expressing neurons.[34] Mc3R was detected in 31% POMC and 44% AgRP expressing neurons. Many AgRP expressing neurons also express neuropeptide Y (NPY) and therefore it is not surprising that double labelling in situ hybridization also showed that 38% of NPY neurons in rat ARH express Mc3R mRNA.[35] Mc3R mRNA expression was mapped in Spiny dogfish (Squalus acanthias) brain using southern blotting of RT-PCR products. Mc3R mRNA mapped to hypothalamus and telencephalon in Spiny dogfish brain[19] and interestingly dogfish contains γ-MSH, like mammals.[19] In contrast to *Fugu*, zebrafish do have a Mc3R gene but its expression in zebrafish brain has not been mapped.[36] Interestingly in chicken, the Mc3R is not expressed in brain, but it is expressed in adrenal gland.[37]

Fetal and Postnatal Brain

No Mc3R mRNA was detected in the developing rat embryo.[38] Expression of this receptor first appeared in the rat brain at postnatal (PN) day 0 when weak signal was seen in the hypothalamus.[39] The diencephalon and mesencephalon expressed Mc3R mRNA by PN day 7 and by PN day 21 the expression was similar to adult Mc3R mRNA expression with intense signals seen in the VMH, ARH, MHb and VTA regions.[38,39]

Functions for MC3R in Brain

Mapping Mc3R mRNA expression in adult rat brain indicated several physiological functions for the MC3R, many of which have either not yet been confirmed, or are poorly understood. First, strong Mc3R protein but not mRNA expression in the nucleus accumbens (ACB) suggested that the MC3R is working presynaptically in nerve terminals of long projecting neurons. Expression of Mc3R mRNA in ARH POMC neurons also suggested that MC3R functions presynaptically as an auto-receptor to control the release of POMC-derived peptides. Electrophysiological studies on neurons expressing green fluorescent protein under the control of the POMC promoter indeed showed that melanocortin peptides have an autoinhibitory effect on POMC neurons.[40] Second, co-expression of Mc3R with POMC, AgRP and NPY in the ARH was evidence that the MC3R plays a role in complex interactions controlling energy homeostasis, since all three molecules play critical roles regulating body weight. Indeed, the phenotype of the *Mc3R* knockout mouse is modest obesity, resulting in large part from increased feed efficiency and a reduction in locomotor activity.[41,42] The expression of MC3R in AgRP neurons might serve as a negative feedback control through MC3R autoregulation of POMC-derived peptides since AgRP is an antagonist of MC3R signaling in the brain.

The *Mc3R* knockout mouse model as well as the development of MC3R specific ligands has enabled MC3R specific functions to be identified. *Mc3R* knockout mice exhibit abnormal daily patterns of feeding behavior and this led to the discovery that the Mc3R is critical for entrainment of anticipatory behavior to feeding time.[43] Maintaining circadian rhythms in energy consumption and expenditure is dependent on synchronisation of oscillating clock genes in the forebrain[44-46] and Mc3R deficiency results in impaired synchronisation of clock genes.[43] While the master pacemaker clock for light entrainable oscillation is located in the suprachiasmatic nucleus (SCN), the location of the food entrainable oscillator is uncertain. The VMHdl shares strong connections with regions involved in appetite regulation, such as paraventricular and dorsomedial hypothalamic nuclei[47] and the dense Mc3R expression in this brain region[30] may be responsible for maintaining entrainment to feeding time. Similar dense Mc3R mRNA expression is observed in the MHb, a site of melatonin synthesis in addition to the pineal gland.[48] The MHb is a key bridge between limbic forebrain and midbrain monoaminergic centers and has been associated with functional roles involved in the regulation of sleep, circadian rhythm, stress response, pain, feeding and reproductive behaviour.[49] It is possible that Mc3R expression in the MHb is involved in circadian rhythms and possibly entrainment of anticipatory behavior to feeding.

A potential role for CNS Mc3R in the seasonal regulation of Siberian hamster body weight was identified when Mc3R mRNA was found to be photoperiodically regulated in the dorsomedial posterior arcuate nucleus (dmpARC).[50] Mc3R mRNA is expressed only under short photoperiod. A change in the duration of melatonin secretion from the pineal gland is the main driver relaying a response to photoperiod to the dmpARC.[51] The changing photoperiod triggers seasonal adaptations including altered food intake and body mass, annual reproductive activity cycle and changes in pelage color and insulation.[52] Short days drive a reduction in food intake and a corresponding loss in body weight and are associated with increased posttranslational endoproteolytic POMC processing to increase the relative abundance of α-MSH.[53] It is possible that photoperiod-induced increased MC3R expression in the dmpARC regulates this posttranslational processing of POMC during short days since the MC3R acts as an autoreceptor.

The VTA and ACB are important brain structures involved in the dopaminergic mesolimbic reward system involved in drug dependence and motivational processes.[54,55] Regulation of the rat dopaminergic mesolimbic system may be a function for MC3R expressed in the VTA and ACB.[56] Gamma 1-MSH shows 4-fold selectivity for the MC3R over the MC4R and when γ1MSH was injected into rat brain VTA, it caused an increase in the release of extracellular dopamine and its metabolite in the ACB together with pronounced grooming and vertical activity. Interestingly, γ2MSH also selectively binds the MC3R but it had the opposite effect and decreased extracellular dopamine. The mechanism of action for these opposing effects of γ1MSH and γ2MSH is unknown.

MC4R Is Expressed in Distinct Nuclei in Every Region of the Brain Reflecting It's Many Diverse Functions in the Brain

The MC4R has attracted much attention in recent years due to its involvement in the regulation of appetite and energy homeostasis.[57] The MC4R is one of the most well characterised monogenic factors causing human obesity. Single point mutations in the MC4R coding region account for about 5% morbid human obesity while two polymorphisms in the human MC4R coding region are associated with protection from human obesity.[58,59] The phenotype of the *Mc4R* knockout mouse first identified the *MC4R* gene with physiological roles in regulation of appetite, body weight, linear growth, lean body mass, glucose homeostasis, insulin secretion and sensitivity, bone mineral content and sympathetic nervous system responses.[57] Because of the critical role that the MC4R plays in energy homeostasis, more attention has been given to investigating specific CNS functions for the MC4R than has been given to the other MCR subtypes and this has included the development of MC4R-specific agonists and antagonists.[11,12] The MC4R is the second most highly expressed melanocortin receptor subtype in the mammalian brain. In contrast to the Mc3R mRNA, Mc4R mRNA has not been detected in any rat brain region by Northern blotting. It is however, much more widely expressed in the brain compared with the Mc3R.[60] Although we know a lot more about specific functions for the CNS MC4R than we do for the CNS MC3R, there is still a great deal that we do not know about specific physiological roles for MC4R in the brain. Understanding roles for this receptor until now has focused largely around energy homeostasis and brain inflammation as there is huge potential for pharmaceutical interventions in these areas.

Adult Brain

The MC4R was first cloned in 1993[60,61] and although its expression was originally reported to be only in the brain, it has since been detected at low levels in the periphery where its functions are probably numerous, but not yet determined.[62-64] The MC4R in mammals is not therefore brain specific, but most of our knowledge about the MC4R today relates to MC4R expression and function in the brain. In situ hybridization studies mapped the brain anatomical localization of the Mc4R in rat[60,61,65] and mouse[66,67] to over 100 different nuclei (Fig. 2) and remarkably, in the mouse ~1 kb Mc4R promoter drives this pattern of expression.[66] The hypothalamus and brainstem contain the highest Mc4R mRNA expression. Hypothalamic sites expressing Mc4R mRNA include the periventricular zone of the hypothalamus with strongest expression in the suprachiasmatic preoptic nucleus, anteroventral periventricular nucleus (AVPV), supraoptic nucleus (SO), paraventricular nucleus of the hypothalamus (PVH), MPO, anteroventral preoptic nucleus, anterior hypothalamic nucleus, ventromedial nucleus of the hypothalamus (VMH), dorsomedial nucleus of the hypothalamus (DMH), tuberomammillary nucleus and lateral hypothalamic area. Brain stem sites expressing the highest Mc4R mRNA expression include the superior colliculus, in particular the optic layer and nucleus of the optic tract, dorsal motor nucleus of the vagus nerve (DMX), substantia nigra (SN), red nucleus (RN), raphe, and reticular formation in particular parvicellular reticular nucleus. After the hypothalamus and brain stem the strongest Mc4R mRNA signals are seen in several nuclei of the amygdala including the anterodorsal part of the medial nucleus of amygdala, the medial zone of cortical nucleus of the amygdala and the capsular part of the cental nucleus of the amygdala.

Regions in the isocortex expressing Mc4R mRNA include the primary auditory area, agranular insular and anterior cingulate areas of isocortex. Mc4R mRNA is also expressed in regions of cortex involved in olfactory responses, such as the anterior olfactory nucleus, the taenia tecta, olfactory tubercle and the piriform area. In the hippocampus relatively high levels of expression are seen in the lateral part of the entorhinal area and ventral part of the subiculum with lower levels present in the parasubiculum and fields CA1, CA2 and CA3 of Ammon's horn. The lateral septal nucleus is among those regions with relatively high densities of MC4R mRNA, especially the lateral septal nucleus and the medial septal nucleus. Moderate levels of Mc4R mRNA expression are present throughout the bed nuclei of the stria terminalis (BST) and

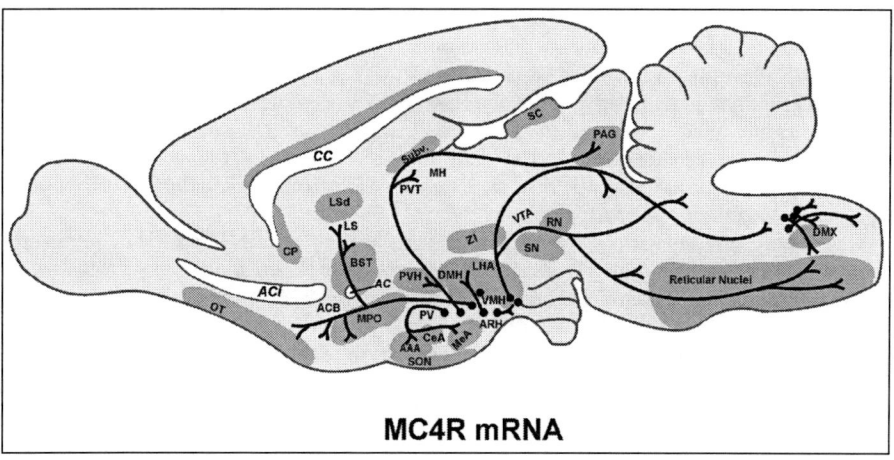

MC4R mRNA

Figure 2. Schematic of rat adult brain sagittal showing regions expressing Mc4R mRNA. POMC neurons shown as black dots and POMC projections shown as black lines. Gray shading represents regions in situ hybridization mapped for Mc4R mRNA expression.[60] (Modified from ref. 142 with permission.) Abbreviations used as in Figure 1 legend.

higher levels of expression are seen in the septohippocampal nucleus, subfornical organ (SFO) and fundus of the striatum. Weak Mc4R expression is present in the thalamus and mostly seen in the suprageniculate nucleus, zona incerta and the peripeduncular nucleus. In the striatum, Mc4R mRNA signal is present in the entire rostrocaudal extent of the caudate-putamen and in the ACB.

The Mc4R has also been detected in fish and in chicken brains. In chicken, RT-PCR detected Mc4R in the brain but anatomical mapping was not performed.[68] In the gold fish however, Mc4R mRNA has been mapped using in situ hybridization.[69] High Mc4R expression was found in the telencephalon, preoptic area, ventral thalamus, tuberal hypothalamus and hypothalamic inferior lobe. RT-PCR also detected low levels of Mc4R expression in goldfish cerebellum. Detailed brain mapping using RT-PCR showed Mc4R mRNA expression in Sea bass, *Dicentrarchus labrax,* and found this receptor to be expressed in telencephalon, preoptic area, hypothalamus, ventral thalamus, tectum mesencephalon and rombencephalon regions of the brain.[70] RT-PCR was also used to detect Mc4R mRNA in brains of barfin flounder, *Verasper moseri*[71] and in *Fugu* brain.[19] RT-PCR detected expression in *Fugu* brain in the telencephalon, optic tectum, hypothalamus and cerebellum, but not in the brain stem. Overall, the distribution of MC4R in teleost and mammalian brains is very similar.

Fetal and Postnatal Brain

Mapping of Mc4R mRNA during rat development showed strong expression in the brain from E14 in diencephalon neuroepithelia, telencephalon, lamina terminalis and spinal trigeminal nucleus.[38,62] By E19, the pattern of CNS Mc4R mRNA expression is similar to that seen in adult rat brain. As seen in the developing embryo, postnatally Mc4R mRNA also predominates and continues to show a distinct temporal and spatial pattern of expression.[38]

Functions for MC4R in the Brain

The unique neuronal distribution of Mc4R mRNA in fetal and adult rat brains indicated specific and complex physiological roles for the MC4R in neuroendocrine and autonomic control. Mc4R mRNA expression in hypothalamic and brain stem nuclei suggested roles in control of energy homeostasis, stress and reproduction, all of which have been confirmed, although still poorly understood. Characterisation of the phenotype of the *Mc4R* gene knockout mouse first exposed the critical role MC4R plays in appetite control and body weight regulation in mammals.[72] However, it is only recent experiments using a conditional *Mc4R* knockout mouse in which Mc4R expression was rescued specifically in the PVH and amygdala brain regions, that started to shed light on the relative contribution of MC4R signaling in individual CNS sites.[73] These studies identified Mc4R expression in the PVH and possibly the amygdala, as critical for appetite regulation. Further evidence that Mc4R in the PVH is critical for appetite regulation was provided when adeno-associated virus-mediated knockdown of Mc4R in the PVH promoted hyperphagia in adult rats fed a high fat diet.[74]

Mc4R is co-expressed with corticotrophin releasing hormone (CRH) on PVH neurons and administration of CRH to rodent brain inhibits appetite.[75] CRH also inhibits appetite in *Mc4R* knockout mice indicating that CRH may act downstream of the MC4R in the PVH to regulate appetite.[76] In addition, single-minded gene 1 (Sim1), brain derived growth factor (BDNF) and oxytocin may also be mediators of MC4R signaling in the PVH. Sim1 is a transcriptional factor expressed in the PVH and amygdala and *Sim1* knockout mice are obese and resistant to melanocortin peptide inhibition of appetite.[77] Activation of Mc4R in the PVH magnocellular neurons results in mobilisation of intracellular calcium and induction of c-Fos, followed by dendritic oxytocin release.[78] Oxytocin deficiency is responsible for much of the hyperphagia in obese Sim$^{+/-}$ mice[79] and therefore oxytocin likely mediates at least some of the MC4R driven inhibition of appetite. The synthetic melanocortin peptide, MTII, stimulates BDNF expression in the VMH of wild type mice and BDNF suppresses feeding in *Mc4R* knockout mice,[80] all of which suggests a role for BDNF also mediating MC4R regulation of appetite. In the brainstem, feeding and body weight are controlled by the DMX, a region of high MC4R mRNA density that receives afferent projections from the gastrointestinal tract.[81] Activation of brainstem Mc4R reduces meal size[81] without affecting meal frequency.[82] A critical role for the Mc4R in satiety suppression of food intake by cholecystokinin (CCK) mediated by melanocortin neurons in the brainstem was demonstrated using *Mc4R* knockout mice.[83] BDNF is also a downstream mediator of brainstem MC4R induced appetite suppression.[84] However, it remains to be determined how MC4R satiety signaling in the brainstem integrates with MC4R suppression of appetite initiated in the PVH. Mc4R mRNA was found in the nodose ganglia and electrophysiological and biochemical methods were used to provide evidence that MC4R signaling in the caudal brainstem leads to mainly presynaptic modulation of glutamatergic synaptic transmission.[85] Presynaptic MC4R may therefore modulate vagal glutamatergic inputs to nucleus of the solitary tract (NTS) neurons.[85]

Rescue of MC4R in PVH/amygdala restored appetite control and linear growth but not energy expenditure.[73] The neuroanatomical sites critical for MC4R mediated energy expenditure are not yet identified. It is known however, that MC4R regulation of energy expenditure is mediated through activation of the sympathetic nervous system involving sites in the hypothalamus and brain stem.[86,87] MC4R mRNA expression in the intermediolateral cell column (IML) of the spinal cord[62,65] first implicated the sympathetic nervous system in MC4R regulation of energy expenditure. The IML projects to postganglionic neurons innervating brown adipose tissue (BAT). BAT also receives inputs from other autonomic control regions expressing Mc4R mRNA such as the ventro-medial preoptic nucleus, PVH, LHA and rostral ventrolateral medulla. Transneuronal viral retrograde tract tracer, the pseudorabies virus (PRV), was used to map brain regions where sympathetic outflow to white adipose tissue (WAT) and BAT originate.[88] Highest percentages of PRV infected cells that co-express Mc4R mRNA are laterodorsal tegmental nucleus and the rostral raphe pallidus following PRV injection into BAT and the PVH following PRV injection into WAT. In addition to regulating cellular thermogenesis in BAT, the CNS MC4R through activation of the sympathetic nervous system controls peripheral nutrient partitioning by promoting fat storage via direct actions on liver, muscle and fat metabolism.[89,90] Some of these central MC4R mediated actions can be pharmacologically manipulated and in future may lead to treatments for Type 2 diabetes.[91]

Expression of Mc4R in parabrachial neurons (PBN) located in the dorsolateral of the pons in the brainstem suggested that this receptor might be involved in illness-related suppression of feeding. The PBN is a relay centre for signals from the NTS to the forebrain and has been implicated in mechanisms underlying anorexia and food aversion during disease. Dual labelling in situ hybridization showed MC4R mRNA on neurons in the external lateral parabrachial subnucleus that displayed lipopolysaccharide- or lithium chloride- induced expression of c-fos mRNA.[92] Activation of brain structures by systemic administration of lipopolysaccharide models acute systemic infection associated with anorexia, while activation of brain structures by systemic administration of lithium chloride is representative of conditioned taste aversion (CTA). Furthermore, these Mc4R expressing neurons all co-express calcitonin gene related peptide (CGRP) and it has been suggested that there is a MC4R regulated CGRP-positive pathway from the external lateral parabrachial subnucleus to the amygdala that relays information to forebrain responses to certain aspects of sickness behavior.[92] CGRP is anorectic and induces CTA.

Further neuroendocrine roles for Mc4R expressed in the PVH include inhibition of oxytocin release from their terminals in the neurohypophysis[78] and stimulation of CRH[75] and thyroid releasing hormone (TRH)[93] with subsequent increased anterior pituitary gland production of ACTH/α-MSH (94) and thyroid stimulating hormone,[95] respectively. Mc4R mRNA is expressed in both the magnocellular and parvocellular divisions of the PVH and it may therefore play a role in the release of arginine vasopressin (AVP) followed by anterior pituitary production of ACTH. In hypothalamic explants, α-MSH significantly increased AVP release[96,97] and AVP is a potent stimulator of ACTH release.[98] CNS Mc4R is also associated with mediating leptin stimulation of luteinizing hormone and prolactin secretion in rats, but the sites of brain MC4R expression responsible for these responses are unknown.[99,100] In the ACB, MC4R mediates α-MSH induced release of dopamine.[101] Elevations in dopamine were observed in the caudate putamen and ACB after α-MSH was administered into rat VTA, a dopamine synthesising brain region where Mc4R mRNA is weakly expressed. Pretreatment with a MC4R selective antagonist blocked the α-MSH induced dopamine response.[101] This Mc4R mediated increase in dopamine may be involved in Mc4R regulation of appetite and behaviors such as excessive grooming[102] and stretching and yawning.[101,103]

Mc4R expressed in the parvocellular division of the PVN participates in the stress response through stimulation of CRH followed by release in rats of pituitary derived ACTH and increased circulating corticosteroids.[97] Central melanocortins also activate, stress-induced behavior such as excessive grooming independent of adrenal derived corticosteroid and these behavioral effects are mediated through the Mc4R.[94] ACTH$_{1-24}$ administered into the PAG,[104] the periventricular nucleus[105] and the substantia nigra[106] induced excessive grooming behavior. MC4R is expressed in all of these brain regions where it may be modulating the dopamine response. MC4R expressed in the amygdala plays an important role in morphine tolerance, a response that is mediated through dopamine signalling.[107,108] Morphine down regulated MC4R expression in the ACB and the PAG, brain regions that mediate opiate addiction.[109] Furthermore, the MC4R modulates the behavioral effects of cocaine. Chronic, but not acute, cocaine treatment increased Mc4R mRNA expression in the striatum and hippocampus and antagonism of MC4R in the amygdala reversed morphine tolerance.[108]

Central MC4R not only plays an important role in the stress response but it also plays a role in the regulation of emotional behaviour.[97] Stimulation of Mc4R causes anxiogenic-like activity in rats.[110] Administration of α-MSH into the MPO and ventromedial nucleus, areas where Mc4R is expressed, significantly increased aggressive behaviour.[111] Intraventricular ACTH reduced social interaction in male rats and the septum was identified as a brain region mediating the anxiogenic-like effects of ACTH.[112] The relatively high expression of Mc4R mRNA in the lateral septum likely plays an important role in this anxiety-like behavior. Mc4R mRNA expression is also relatively high in the amygdala, a brain region that plays a role in orchestrating various aspects of emotional output and fear-related behaviours.[113] MC4R mRNA is increased in the amygdala and in the hypothalamus by electrical foot shock stress.[114] The central nucleus of the amygdala where Mc4R mRNA is expressed also contains a relatively high concentration of CRH, which may mediate the MC4R effects of stress.[115] MC4R-mediated stimulation of PVH CRH and the subsequent activation of the hypothalamic-pituitary-axis are also believed to play a role in melanocortin anxiogenic-like effects.[116] Mc4R mRNA in the dorsal raphe nucleus and locus coeruleus may modulate serotoninergic and noradrenergic signaling with stimulation of the MC4R associated with anxiety-like behavior and MC4R antagonism associated with antidepressant-like effects.[97,117]

A physiological role for MC4R in reproductive function was demonstrated by difficulties with breeding homozygous MC4R null mice.[118] Melanocortin peptides play a significant role in regulation of penile erection through activation of the MC4R centrally and peripherally. Central administration of the MC4R selective agonist, THIQ, into the 3rd ventricle of rats increased reflective penile erections.[119] The brain regions responsible for these MC4R mediated effects on erection are unknown but may reside in the MPO and PVH, regions known to be involved with copulatory behaviors.

A functional role for the MC4R in neuroprotection was first identified when Mc4R mRNA was found to be up-regulated in the striatum in the nondamaged hemisphere within 24 hour after severe unilateral hypoxic ischemic brain injury.[120] This Mc4R up-regulation may be involved in transfer of function to the uninjured hemisphere following unilateral brain injury. Intracerebral events contributing to ischemia- and stroke-induced brain damage promote an inflammatory response. The neuroprotective effect of melanocortin peptides could be mediated through the modulation of mechanisms such as inflammatory reaction and apoptosis associated with neuroinflammatory diseases.[13,121-123] Mc4R expressed in the brainstem DMX and ventral division of the nucleus ambiguous may mediate the melanocortin protective effects in rats against hemorrhagic shock.[124]

The CNS MC4R modulates heart rate and blood pressure in humans and mice and this involves enhanced sympathetic nerve activity.[125-127] $Mc4R^{-/-}$ mice maintain normal blood pressure despite marked obesity and MC4R deficiency in humans results in lower heart rate and blood pressure and lower urinary norepinephrine excretion than in control subjects. Acute central administration of α-MSH in mice increased mean arterial pressure and heart rate, except in $Mc4R^{-/-}$ mice.[126] The MC4R expressing brain regions responsible for melanocortin peptide regulation of cardiovascular function have not been identified but are likely to involve MC4R expressed in the PVH and/or in the NTS. Both PVH and NTS brain regions can lead to activation of sympathetic nerve activity.

MC5R Expression and Function in the Brain Is Unclear

The MC5R is the most widely expressed melanocortin receptor in the periphery where it likely has many functions that are not yet identified.[128,129] Analysis of the Mc5R knockout mouse phenotype exposed the role for MC5R in exocrine function, regulating sebaceous gland secretion.[130] Expression of the MC5R was initially recognised in human,[131] mouse[129] and rat[128] brain using RT-PCR and/or RNase protection assay. Rat brain Mc5R mRNA expression was reported to be in the olfactory tubercle, substantia nigra, striatum, medulla, cerebellum, hypothalamus, hippocampus, midbrain and cerebral cortex. However, attempts to map Mc5R mRNA in rat or mouse adult brain using in situ hybridization have failed to detect this receptor.[120,128] In the mouse embryo during the organogenetic period, Mc5R protein was detected using immunohistochemistry in the telencephalon (cerebral cortex) from E16.5 to R18.5.[26]

Mc5R mRNA has been detected in brains of birds and fish. RT-PCR detected Mc5R expression in brain of adult White Leghorn chickens.[68] Southern blotting of RT-PCR products detected Mc5R mRNA expression in Spiny dogfish (*Squalus acanthias*) brain where it mapped to hypothalamus, telencephalon and weakly in the brain stem.[19] In *Cyprinus carpio*, Mc5R mRNA is expressed in brain as shown by RT-PCR.[132] In situ hybridization studies revealed Mc5R mRNA expression in many regions of goldfish brain, including ventral telencephalon, nucleus lateralis tuberis and nucleus preopticus.[133] MC5R mRNA has also been detected in Rainbow trout brain using RT-PCR.[134]

The function of MC5R in adult brain of any species is not understood, but expression of Mc5R in mouse embryo suggests that it may play a role in the development of brain cerebral cortex. The sites of Mc5R expression in goldfish brain suggest MC5R has neuroendocrine and behavioral roles in goldfish some of which overlap with roles for the MC4R.[133] It is possible that the mammalian MC4R has taken over these roles that were once the functions of MC5R.

Melanocortin Receptor Accessory Proteins (MRAPs)

It is likely that the biological activity of each melanocortin receptor subtype expressed in the brain is modified by receptor interacting-proteins in ways that we do not yet understand. One or more G protein coupled receptor (GPCR)-interacting proteins modify the biological activity of most, if not all, GPCRs expressed in the brain.[135] GPCRs have long been known to mediate many of their effects through interacting with heterotrimeric G proteins. However, a large number of proteins in addition to G proteins have recently been recognised to interact with various GPCRs. These interacting proteins include GPCRs themselves as homo- or hetero-dimers, multi-domain scaffolding proteins and accessory/chaperone molecules. They provide diverse molecular mechanisms for ligand recognition, signaling specificity and receptor trafficking.[135] Recently, a family of novel accessory proteins for the melanocortin receptors have been discovered and in humans they comprise two splice variants, MRAPα and MRAPβ and a second gene, MRAP2.[136-138] MRAPα is essential for the MC2R to functionally express in the adrenal cortex and in heterologous cells, but it is not essential for the other melanocortin receptor subtypes to functionally express. Nevertheless, MRAPα and MRAP2 have been found to interact with all five receptor subtypes in vitro and in contrast to the MC2R, these MRAPs reduce the responsiveness of MC1R, MC3R, MC4R and MC5R to melanocortin peptide coupling to adenylyl cyclase.[136,139] These MRAPs are expressed in the brain as well as in the periphery, but it is unknown whether they modify brain melanocortin receptor signaling. MRAPs may be functioning similar to receptor activity modifying proteins (RAMPs) that are required for calcitonin-like receptor expression in the plasma membrane and functioning as either the calcitonin gene-related peptide or adrenomedullin receptor.[140] However, there are no structural similarities between RAMPs and MRAPs. There is structural, but not sequence, similarity with accessory proteins described for the olfactory receptors, receptor-transporting protein (RTP) 1 and 2 and receptor-expression enhancing protein (REEP).[140] However, the structure of MRAPs is unique among GPCR accessory proteins since MRAPs form antiparallel homo- and hetero-dimmers.[136,141] It is unknown at present, precisely where MRAPs are expressed in the brain. However, if they co-express with melanocortin receptors in the brain they are likely to be important modulators of central melanocortin functions and may themselves become targets for therapeutic interventions.

Conclusion

MC3R and MC4R have long been recognised as the 'neural' melanocortin receptor subtypes. However, all five melanocortin receptor subtypes have been detected in developing and in adult brains of various species. Their distinct receptor subtype-dependent pattern and region-specific expression refects different functions for each melanocortin receptor subtype in the brain (Table 1). These functions include brain development; regulation of neuropeptide and pituitary-derived hormones, the stress response, appetite and feeding behavior, reproduction, pain, analgesia, anxiety, cardiovascular function and neuroprotection (Table 2).

Molecular biological techniques and genetically engineered mice have played critical roles in exposing functions for melanocortin receptors expressed in the brain. The many diverse functions for melanocortin peptides in the brain makes these receptors attractive drug targets for diseases, dysfunctional behaviors, analgesia and brain inflammation. There is a great deal yet to be revealed about specific functions and mechanisms of action for melanocortin receptors expressed

Table 1. Expression of melanocortin receptors in adult mammalian, chicken and fish brains

Receptor	Species	Brain Location	Detection Method	Reference
MC1R	Mouse	PAG	RT-PCR	16
	Human	PAG	RT-PCR, immuno-histochemistry	17
	Fish (playfish, medaka, Zebrafish, *Fugu*)	Telencephalon, optic tectum, hypothalamus (shown for *Fugu* only)	RT-PCR	19, 20
MC2R	Fish (*Fugu*, Rainbow trout)	Telencephalon, hypothalamus, cerebellum, brain stem	RT-PCR	19, 27
MC3R	Rat	~30 distinct nuclei including: ARH, VMHdl, anteroventral preoptic area, posterior hypothalamic area, MPO, ACB, intermediate part of the lateral nucleus of the septum, MHb, VTA, central linear nucleus of raphe, hippocampus, piriform cortex	Northern blotting, RT-PCR, in situ hyridisation	30, 31
	Fish (Spiny dogfish, Zebrafish)	Hypothalamus, telencephalon	RT-PCR and Southern blotting	19, 36
MC4R	Rat	>100 distinct nuclei including:	In situ hybridisation	60, 61, 65
	Mouse	periventricular zone of the hypothalamus, suprachiasmatic preoptic nucleus, AVPV, SO, PVH, MPO, anteroventral preoptic nucleus, anterior hypothalamic nucleus, VMH, DMH, tuberomammillary nucleus, lateral hypothalamic area, superior colliculus, nucleus of the optic tract, DMX, SN, RN, raphe, and reticular formation in particular parvicellular reticular nucleus, anterodorsal part of the medial nucleus of amygdala, the medial zone of cortical nucleus of the amygdala, the capsular part of the cental nucleus of the amygdala, the primary auditory area, agranular insular, anterior cingulate areas of isocortex, anterior olfactory nucleus, the taenia tecta, olfactory tubercle, piriform area, entorhinal area, ventral part of the subiculum,		66, 67

continued on next page

Table 1. *Continued*

Receptor	Species	Brain Location	Detection Method	Reference
	Chicken	parasubiculum and fields CA1, CA2, and CA3 of Ammon's horn, lateral septal nucleus, medial septal nucleus, BST, septohippocampal nucleus, SFO, fundus of the striatum, suprageniculate nucleus, zona incerta, peripeduncular nucleus, entire rostrocaudal extent of the caudate-putamen, ACB	RT-PCR	68
	Fish Goldfish	Telencephalon, preoptic area, ventral thalamus, tuberal hypothalamus, hypothalamic inferior lobe, cerebellum	RT-PCR, in situ hybridisation	69
	Sea bass	Telencephalon, preoptic area, hypothalamus, ventral thalamus, tectum mesencephalon, rombencephalon	RT-PCR	70
	Barfin flounder		RT-PCR	71
	Fugu	Telencephalon, optic tectum, hypothalamus and cerebellum	RT-PCR	19
MC5R	Rat	olfactory tubercle, substantia nigra, striatum, medulla, cerebellum, hypothalamus, hippocampus, midbrain, cerebral cortex	RT-PCR	128
	Mouse		RT-PCR	129
	Human		RT-PCR	131
	Chicken		RT-PCR	68
	Fish			
	Spiny dogfish	Hypothalamus, telencephalon, brain stem	RT-PCR	19
	Carp		RT-PCR	132
	Goldfish	Ventral telencephalon, nucleus lateralis tuberis, nucleus preopticus	In situ hybridisation	133
	Rainbow trout		RT-PCR	134

**Table 2. Functional roles for melanocortin receptors expressed in mammalian brain
(* function is predicted)**

Receptor	Functions	Reference
MC1R	• Pain and analgesia (mediates κ-opioid analgesia in females and μ-opioid analgesia in males and females)	21, 23
	• Neuroprotection*	25
MC2R	• Brain development*	
MC3R	• Brain development*	
	• Auto-receptor controlling release of POMC-derived peptides	40
	• Nutrient partitioning	41, 42
	• Locomotor activity	41, 42
	• Food entrainable feeding behaviour	43
	• Seasonal regulation of body weight*	50
	• Reward system involved in drug dependence and motivation*	56
MC4R	• Brain development*	
	• Neuroendocrine regulation (stress response, growth and reproduction)	75, 78, 93-97, 99-101, 119
	• Autonomic nervous system control (thermogenesis, insulin sensitivity, nutrient partitioning)	86, 87, 89, 90
	• Appetite regulation including food aversion and satiety	73, 74, 83, 92
	• Morphine tolerance and opiate addiction	107-109
	• Anxiety-like behaviour	97, 110, 111, 113, 116, 117
	• Neuroprotection	13, 120-124
	• Blood pressure and heart rate	125-127
MC5R	• Brain development*	

in specific brain nuclei that will underpin future targeted interventions. Understanding specific functions for the melanocortin receptors expressed in avian and teleost brains will contribute to this knowledge. Furthermore, MRAPs are relatively new players in the melanocortin system and their significance for melanocortin receptor signaling in the brain is unknown.

Importantly, future therapeutics targeting any of the brain melanocortin receptors should consider potential harmful side effects of these drugs on fetal development since at least four melanocortin receptor subtypes are expressed in the developing mammalian brain.

References
1. de Wied D. Behavioral pharmacology of neuropeptides related to melanocortins and the neurohypophyseal hormones. Eur J Pharmacol 1999; 375(1-3):1-11.
2. De Wied D, Jolles J. Neuropeptides derived from pro-opiocortin: behavioral, physiological and neurochemical effects. Physiological Reviews 1982; 62(3):976-1059.
3. Adan RAH. Effects of melanocortins in the nervous system. In: Cone RD, ed. The Melanocortin Receptors. Totowa: Humana Press, 2000:109-41.

4. Catania A, Lipton JM. α-Melanocyte stimulating hormone in the modulation of host reactions. Endocr Rev 1993; 14(5):564-76.
5. Strand FL, Rose KJ, Zuccarelli LA et al. Neuropeptide hormones as neurotrophic factors. Physiol Rev 1991; 71:1017-46.
6. Tatro JB. Melanotropin receptors in the brain are differentially distributed and recognize both corticotropin and α-melanocyte stimulating hormone. Brain Res 1990; 536:124-32.
7. Poggioli R, Vergoni AV, Bertolini A. ACTH-(1-24) and alpha-MSH antagonize feeding behavior stimulated by kappa opiate agonists. Peptides 1986; 7(5):843-8.
8. Mountjoy KG. Cloning of the melanocortin receptors. In: Cone RD, ed. The Melanocortin Receptors. Totowa: Humana Press Inc., 2000:209-35.
9. Cone RD, Mountjoy KG, Robbins LS et al. Cloning and functional characterization of a family of receptors for the melanotropic peptides. Ann N Y Acad Sci 1993; 680:342-63.
10. Cone RD. The Central Melanocortin System and Energy Homeostasis. Trends Endocrinol Metab 1999; 10(6):211-6.
11. Van der Ploeg LH, Kanatani A, MacNeil D et al. Design and synthesis of (ant)-agonists that alter appetite and adiposity. Prog Brain Res 2006; 153(17):107-18.
12. Schioth HB, Kask A, Mutulis F et al. Novel selective melanocortin 4 receptor antagonist induces food intake after peripheral administration. Biochem Biophys Res Commun 2003; 301(2):399-405.
13. Catania A. Neuroprotective actions of melanocortins: a therapeutic opportunity. Trends Neurosci 2008; 31(7):353-60.
14. Van der Ploeg LH, Martin WJ, Howard AD et al. A role for the melanocortin 4 receptor in sexual function. Proc Natl Acad Sci USA 2002; 99(17):11381-6.
15. Rees JL. Genetics of hair and skin color. Annu Rev Genet 2003; 37:67-90.
16. Rajora N, Boccoli G, Burns D et al. α-MSH modulates local and circulating TNFα in experimental brain inflammation. J Neurosci 1997; 17(6):2181-6.
17. Xia Y, Wikberg JE, Chhajlani V. Expression of melanocortin 1 receptor in periaqueductal gray matter. Neuroreport 1995; 6(16):2193-6.
18. Sandkuhler J. The organization and function of endogenous antinociceptive systems. Prog Neurobiol 1996; 50(1):49-81.
19. Klovins J, Haitina T, Fridmanis D et al. The melanocortin system in Fugu: determination of POMC/AGRP/MCR gene repertoire and synteny, as well as pharmacology and anatomical distribution of the MCRs. Mol Biol Evol 2004; 21(3):563-79.
20. Selz Y, Braasch I, Hoffmann C et al. Evolution of melanocortin receptors in teleost fish: the melanocortin type 1 receptor. Gene 2007; 401(1-2):114-22.
21. Mogil JS, Wilson SG, Chesler EJ et al. The melanocortin-1 receptor gene mediates female-specific mechanisms of analgesia in mice and humans. Proc Natl Acad Sci USA 2003; 100(8):4867-72.
22. Berkley KJ, Zalcman SS, Simon VR. Sex and gender differences in pain and inflammation: a rapidly maturing field. Am J Physiol Regul Integr Comp Physiol 2006; 291(2):R241-4.
23. Mogil JS, Ritchie J, Smith SB et al. Melanocortin-1 receptor gene variants affect pain and mu-opioid analgesia in mice and humans. J Med Genet 2005; 42(7):583-7.
24. Quillan JM, Sadee W. Dynorphin peptides: antagonists of melanocortin receptors. Pharm Res 1997; 14(6):713-9.
25. Wong KY, Rajora N, Boccoli G et al. A potential mechanism of local anti-inflammatory action of alpha-melanocyte-stimulating hormone within the brain: modulation of tumor necrosis factor-alpha production by human astrocytic cells. Neuroimmunomodulation 1997; 4(1):37-41.
26. Nimura M, Udagawa J, Hatta T et al. Spatial and temporal patterns of expression of melanocortin type 2 and 5 receptors in the fetal mouse tissues and organs. Anat Embryol 2006; 211(2):109-17.
27. Aluru N, Vijayan MM. Molecular characterization, tissue-specific expression and regulation of melanocortin 2 receptor in rainbow trout. Endocrinology 2008; 149(9):4577-88.
28. Xia Y, Wikberg JES. Localization of ACTH receptor mRNA by in situ hybridization in mouse drenal gland. Cell Tissue Res 1996; 286:63-8.
29. Chhajlani V. Distribution of cDNA for melanocortin receptor subtypes in human tissues. Biochem Mol Biol Int 1996; 38:73-80.
30. Roselli-Rehfuss L, Mountjoy KG, Robbins LS et al. Identification of a receptor for gamma melanotropin and other proopiomelanocortin peptides in the hypothalamus and limbic system. Proc Natl Acad Sci USA 1993; 90(19):8856-60.
31. Gantz I, Konda K, Tashiro T et al. Molecular cloning of a novel melanocortin receptor. J Biol Chem 1993; 265(11):8246-50.
32. Lindblom J, Schioth HB, Larsson A et al. Autoradiographic discrimination of melanocortin receptors indicates that the MC3 subtype dominates in the medial rat brain. Brain Res 1998; 810:161-71.

33. Jegou S, Boutelet I, Vaudry H. Melanocortin-3 receptor mRNA expression in pro-opiomelanocortin neurones of the rat arcuate nucleus. J Neuroendocrinol 2000; 12(6):501-5.
34. Bagnol D, Lu XY, Kaelin CB et al. Anatomy of an endogenous antagonist: relationship between Agouti-related protein and proopiomelanocortin in brain. J Neurosci 1999; 19(18):RC26.
35. Mounien L, Bizet P, Boutelet I et al. Expression of melanocortin MC3 and MC4 receptor mRNAs by neuropeptide Y neurons in the rat arcuate nucleus. Neuroendocrinology 2005; 82(3-4):164-70.
36. Logan DW, Bryson-Richardson RJ, Pagan KE et al. The structure and evolution of the melanocortin and MCH receptors in fish and mammals. Genomics 2003; 81(2):184-91.
37. Takeuchi S, Takahashi S. A possible involvement of melanocortin 3 receptor in the regulation of adrenal gland function in the chicken. Biochim Biophys Acta 1999; 1448(3):512-8.
38. Kistler-Heer V, Lauber ME, Lichtensteiger W. Different developmental patterns of melanocortin MC3 and MC4 receptor mRNA: predominance of Mc4 in fetal rat nervous system. J Neuroendocrinol 1998; 10(2):133-46.
39. Xia Y, Wikberg JES. Postnatal expression of melanocortin-3 receptor in rat diencephalon and mesencephalon. Neuropharmacology 1997; 36:217-24.
40. Cowley MA, Smart JL, Rubinstein M et al. Leptin activates anorexigenic POMC neurons through a neural network in the arcuate nucleus. Nature 2001; 411(6836):480-4.
41. Chen AS, Marsh DJ, Trumbauer ME et al. Inactivation of the mouse melanocortin-3 receptor results in increased fat mass and reduced lean body mass. Nat Genet 2000; 26(1):97-102.
42. Butler AA, Kesterson RA, Khong K et al. A unique metabolic syndrome causes obesity in the melanocortin-3 receptor-deficient mouse. Endocrinology 2000; 141(9):3518-21.
43. Sutton GM, Perez-Tilve D, Nogueiras R et al. The melanocortin-3 receptor is required for entrainment to meal intake. J Neurosci 2008; 28(48):12946-55.
44. Hirota T, Fukada Y. Resetting mechanism of central and peripheral circadian clocks in mammals. Zoolog Sci 2004; 21(4):359-68.
45. Mistlberger RE. Circadian rhythms: perturbing a food-entrained clock. Curr Biol 2006; 16(22):R968-9.
46. Verwey M, Khoja Z, Stewart J et al. Differential regulation of the expression of Period2 protein in the limbic forebrain and dorsomedial hypothalamus by daily limited access to highly palatable food in food-deprived and free-fed rats. Neuroscience 2007; 147(2):277-85.
47. Canteras NS, Simerly RB, Swanson LW. Organization of projections from the ventromedial nucleus of the hypothalamus: a Phaseolus vulgaris-leucoagglutinin study in the rat. J Comp Neurol 1994; 348(1):41-79.
48. Yu EZ, Hallenbeck JM, Cai D et al. Elevated arylalkylamine-N-acetyltransferase (AA-NAT) gene expression in medial habenular and suprachiasmatic nuclei of hibernating ground squirrels. Brain Res 2002; Molecular Brain Research(1-2):9-17.
49. Qin C, Luo M. Neurochemical phenotypes of the afferent and efferent projections of the mouse medial habenula. Neuroscience 2009; 161(3):827-37.
50. Nilaweera KN, Archer ZA, Campbell G et al. Photoperiod regulates genes encoding melanocortin 3 and serotonin receptors and secretogranins in the dorsomedial posterior arcuate of the Siberian hamster. J Neuroendocrinol 2009; 21(2):123-31.
51. Bartness TJ, Demas GE, Song CK. Seasonal changes in adiposity: the roles of the photoperiod, melatonin and other hormones and sympathetic nervous system. Exp Biol Med 2002; 227(6):363-76.
52. Helwig M, Archer ZA, Heldmaier G et al. Photoperiodic regulation of satiety mediating neuropeptides in the brainstem of the seasonal Siberian hamster (Phodopus sungorus). J Comp Physiol [A] 2009; 195(7):631-42.
53. Helwig M, Khorooshi RM, Tups A et al. PC1/3 and PC2 gene expression and posttranslational endoproteolytic pro-opiomelanocortin processing is regulated by photoperiod in the seasonal Siberian hamster (Phodopus sungorus). J Neuroendocrinol 2006; 18(6):413-25.
54. Spanagel R, Herz A, Shippenberg TS. Opposing tonically active endogenous opioid systems modulate the mesolimbic dopaminergic pathway. Proc Natl Acad Sci USA 1992; 89(6):2046-50.
55. Bromberg-Martin ES, Hikosaka O. Midbrain dopamine neurons signal preference for advance information about upcoming rewards. Neuron 2009; 63(1):119-26.
56. Jansone B, Bergstrom L, Svirskis S et al. Opposite effects of gamma(1)- and gamma(2)-melanocyte stimulating hormone on regulation of the dopaminergic mesolimbic system in rats. Neurosci Lett 2004; 361(1-3):68-71.
57. Cone RD. Studies on the physiological functions of the melanocortin system. Endocr Rev 2006; 27(7):736-49.
58. Geller F, Reichwald K, Dempfle A et al. Melanocortin-4 receptor gene variant I103 is negatively associated with obesity. Am J Hum Genet 2004; 74(3):572-81.
59. Stutzmann F, Vatin V, Cauchi S et al. Nonsynonymous polymorphisms in melanocortin-4 receptor protect against obesity: the two facets of a Janus obesity gene. Hum Mol Genet 2007; 16(15):1837-44.

60. Mountjoy KG, Mortrud MT, Low MJ et al. Localization of the melanocortin-4 receptor (MC4-R) in neuroendocrine and autonomic control circuits in the brain. Mol Endocrinol 1994; 8(10):1298-308.
61. Gantz I, Miwa H, Konda Y et al. Molecular cloning, expression and gene localization of a fourth melanocortin receptor. J Biol Chem 1993; 268:15174-9.
62. Mountjoy KG, Wild JM. Melanocortin-4 receptor mRNA expression in the developing autonomic and central nervous systems. Brain Res Dev Brain Res 1998; 107(2):309-14.
63. Mountjoy KG, Jenny Wu CS, Dumont LM et al. Melanocortin-4 receptor messenger ribonucleic acid expression in rat cardiorespiratory, musculoskeletal and integumentary systems. Endocrinology 2003; 144(12):5488-96.
64. Dumont LM, Wu C-SJ, Tatnell MA et al. Evidence for direct actions of melanocortin peptides on bone metabolism. Peptides 2004; 26(10):1929-35.
65. Kishi T, Aschkenasi C, Lee C et al. Expression of melanocortin 4 receptor mRNA in the cental nervous system of the rat. J Comp Neurol 2003; 457:213-35.
66. Daniel PB, Fernando C, Wu CS et al. 1 kb of 5' flanking sequence from mouse MC4R gene is sufficient for tissue specific expression in a transgenic mouse. Mol Cell Endocrinol 2005; 239(1-2):63-71.
67. Liu H, Kishi T, Roseberry AG et al. Transgenic mice expressing green fluorescent protein under the control of the melanocortin-4 receptor promoter. J Neurosci 2003; 23(18):7143-54.
68. Takeuchi S, Takahashi S. Melanocortin receptor genes in the chicken—tissue distributions. Gen Comp Endocrinol 1998; 112(2):220-31.
69. Cerda-Reverter JM, Ringholm A, Schioth HB et al. Molecular Cloning, Pharmacological Characterization and Brain Mapping of the Melanocortin 4 Receptor in the Goldfish: Involvement in the Control of Food Intake. Endocrinology 2003; 144(6):2336-49.
70. Sanchez E, Rubio VC, Thompson D et al. Phosphodiesterase inhibitor-dependent inverse agonism of agouti-related protein on melanocortin 4 receptor in sea bass (Dicentrarchus labrax). Am J Physiol Regul Integr Comp Physiol 2009; 296(5):R1293-306.
71. Kobayashi Y, Tsuchiya K, Yamanome T et al. Food deprivation increases the expression of melanocortin-4 receptor in the liver of barfin flounder, Verasper moseri. Gen Comp Endocrinol 2008; 155:280-7.
72. Huszar D, Lynch CA, Fairchild-Huntress V et al. Targeted disruption of the melanocortin-4 receptor results in obesity in mice. Cell 1997; 88(1):131-41.
73. Balthasar N, Dalgaard LT, Lee CE et al. Divergence of melanocortin pathways in the control of food intake and energy expenditure. Cell 2005; 123(3):493-505.
74. Garza JC, Kim CS, Liu J et al. Adeno-associated virus-mediated knockdown of melanocortin-4 receptor in the paraventricular nucleus of the hypothalamus promotes high-fat diet-induced hyperphagia and obesity. J Endocrinol 2008; 197(3):471-82.
75. Lu XY, Barsh GS, Akil H et al. Interaction between alpha-melanocyte-stimulating hormone and corticotropin-releasing hormone in the regulation of feeding and hypothalamo-pituitary-adrenal responses. J Neurosci 2003; 23(21):7863-72.
76. Marsh DJ, Hollopeter G, Huszar D et al. Response of melanocortin-4 receptor-deficient mice to anorectic and orexigenic peptides. Nat Genet 1999; 21(1):119-22.
77. Kublaoui BM, Holder JL Jr, Gemelli T et al. Sim1 haploinsufficiency impairs melanocortin-mediated anorexia and activation of paraventricular nucleus neurons 10.1210/me.2005-0483. Mol Endocrinol 2006;me.2005-0483.
78. Sabatier N, Caquineau C, Dayanithi G et al. Alpha-melanocyte-stimulating hormone stimulates oxytocin release from the dendrites of hypothalamic neurons while inhibiting oxytocin release from their terminals in the neurohypophysis. J Neurosci 2003; 23(32):10351-8.
79. Kublaoui BM, Gemelli T, Tolson KP et al. Oxytocin deficiency mediates hyperphagic obesity of Sim1 haploinsufficient mice. Mol Endocrinol 2008; 22(7):1723-34.
80. Xu B, Goulding EH, Zang K et al. Brain-derived neurotrophic factor regulates energy balance downstream of melanocortin-4 receptor.[see comment]. Nat Neurosci 2003; 6(7):736-42.
81. Grill HJ, Ginsberg AB, Seeley RJ et al. Brainstem application of melanocortin receptor ligands produces long-lasting effects on feeding and body weight. J Neurosci 1998; 18(23):10128-35.
82. Zheng H, Patterson LM, Phifer CB et al. Brain stem melanocortinergic modulation of meal size and identification of hypothalamic POMC projections.[see comment]. Am J Physiol Regul Integr Comp Physiol 2005; 289(1):R247-58.
83. Fan W, Ellacott KL, Halatchev IG et al. Cholecystokinin-mediated suppression of feeding involves the brainstem melanocortin system. Nat Neurosci 2004; 7(4):335-6.
84. Bariohay B, Roux J, Tardivel C et al. Brain-derived neurotrophic factor/tropomyosin-related kinase receptor type B signaling is a downstream effector of the brainstem melanocortin system in food intake control. Endocrinology 2009; 150(6):2646-53.
85. Wan S, Browning KN, Coleman FH et al. Presynaptic melanocortin-4 receptors on vagal afferent fibers modulate the excitability of rat nucleus tractus solitarius neurons. J Neurosci 2008; 28(19):4957-66.

86. Williams DL, Bowers RR, Bartness TJ et al. Brainstem melanocortin 3/4 receptor stimulation increases uncoupling protein gene expression in brown fat. Endocrinology 2003; 144(11):4692-7.
87. Elmquist JK. Hypothalamic pathways underlying the endocrine, autonomic and behavioral effects of leptin. International Journal of Obesity and Related Metabolic Disorders: Int J Obes Relat Metab Disord 2001; 25(Suppl 5):S78-82.
88. Song CK, Vaughan CH, Keen-Rhinehart E et al. Melanocortin-4 receptor mRNA expressed in sympathetic outflow neurons to brown adipose tissue: neuroanatomical and functional evidence. Am J Physiol Regul Integr Comp Physiol 2008; 295(2):R417-28.
89. Nogueiras R, Wiedmer P, Perez-Tilve D et al. The central melanocortin system directly controls peripheral lipid metabolism. J Clin Invest 2007; 117(11):3475-88.
90. Obici S, Feng Z, Tan J et al. Central melanocortin receptors regulate insulin action. J Clin Invest 2001; 108(7):1079-85.
91. Zhou L, Sutton GM, Rochford JJ et al. Serotonin 2C receptor agonists improve type 2 diabetes via melanocortin-4 receptor signaling pathways.[see comment]. Cell Metab 2007; 6(5):398-405.
92. Paues J, Mackerlova L, Blomqvist A. Expression of melanocortin-4 receptor by rat parabrachial neurons responsive to immune and aversive stimuli. Neuroscience 2006; 141(1):287-97.
93. Harris M, Aschkenasi C, Elias CF et al. Transcriptional regulation of the thyrotropin-releasing hormone gene by leptin and melanocortin signaling. J Clin Invest 2001; 107(1):111-20.
94. Von Frijtag JC, Croiset G, Gispen WH et al. The role of central melanocortin receptors in the activation of the hypothalamus-pituitary-adrenal-axis and the induction of excessive grooming. Br J Pharmacol 1998; 123(8):1503-8.
95. Martin NM, Small CJ, Sajedi A et al. Abnormalities of the hypothalamo-pituitary-thyroid axis in the pro-opiomelanocortin deficient mouse. Regul Pept 2004; 122(3):169-72.
96. Dhillo WS, Small CJ, Seal LJ et al. The hypothalamic melanocortin system stimulates the hypothalamo-pituitary-adrenal axis in vitro and in vivo in male rats. Neuroendocrinology 2002; 75(4):209-16.
97. Chaki S, Okuyama S. Involvement of melanocortin-4 receptor in anxiety and depression. Peptides 2005; 26(10):1952-64.
98. Papadimitriou A, Priftis KN. Regulation of the hypothalamic-pituitary-adrenal axis. Neuroimmunomodulation 2009; 16(5):265-71.
99. Watanobe H, Schioth HB, Izumi J. Pivotal roles of alpha-melanocyte-stimulating hormone and the melanocortin 4 receptor in leptin stimulation of prolactin secretion in rats. J Neurochem 2003; 85(2):338-47.
100. Watanobe H, Schioth HB, Wikberg JE et al. The melanocortin 4 receptor mediates leptin stimulation of luteinizing hormone and prolactin surges in steroid-primed ovariectomized rats. Biochem Biophys Res Commun 1999; 257(3):860-4.
101. Lindblom J, Opmane B, Mutulis F et al. The MC4 receptor mediates alpha-MSH induced release of nucleus accumbens dopamine. Neuroreport 2001; 12(10):2155-8.
102. Spruijt BM, Cools AR, Ellenbroek BA et al. Dopaminergic modulation of ACTH-induced grooming. Eur J Pharmacol 1986; 120(3):249-56.
103. Wikberg JE, Muceniece R, Mandrika I et al. New aspects on the melanocortins and their receptors. Pharmacol Res 2000; 42(5):393-420.
104. Spruijt BM, Cools AR, Gispen WH. The periaqueductal gray: a prerequisite for ACTH-induced excessive grooming. Behav Brain Res 1986; 20(1):19-25.
105. Van Erp AM, Kruk MR, Willekens-Bramer DC et al. Grooming induced by intrahypothalamic injection of ACTH in the rat: Comparison with grooming induced by intrahypothalamic electrical stimulation and i.c.v. injections of ACTH. Brain Res 1991; 538:203-10.
106. Wiegant VM, Cools AR, Gispen WH. ACTH-induced excessive grooming involves brain dopamine. Eur J Pharmacol 1977; 41:343-5.
107. Starowicz K, Sieja A, Bilecki W et al. The effect of morphine on MC4 and CRF receptor mRNAs in the rat amygdala and attenuation of tolerance after their blockade. Brain Res 2003; 990(1-2):113-9.
108. Alvaro JD, Taylor JR, Duman RS. Molecular and behavioral interactions between central melanocortins and cocaine. J Pharmacol Exp Ther 2003; 304(1):391-9.
109. Alvaro JD, Tatro JB, Quillan JM et al. Morphine down-regulates melanocortin-4 receptor expression in brain. Molecular Pharmacology 1996.
110. Chaki S, Hirota S, Funakoshi T et al. Anxiolytic-like and antidepressant-like activities of MCL0129 (1-[(S)-2-(4-fluorophenyl)-2-(4-isopropylpiperadin-1-yl)ethyl]-4-[4-(2-methoxynaphthalen-1-yl)butyl] piperazine), a novel and potent nonpeptide antagonist of the melanocortin-4 receptor. J Pharmacol Exp Ther 2003; 304(2):818-26.
111. Gonzalez MI. Behavioral effects of alpha-MSH and MCH after central administration in the female rat. Peptides 1996; 17:171-7.

112. File SE, Clarke A. Intraventricular ACTH reduces social interaction in male rats. Pharmacol Biochem Behav 1980; 12(5):711-5.
113. Seymour B, Dolan R. Emotion, decision making and the amygdala. Neuron 2008; 58(5):662-71.
114. Yamano Y, Yoshioka M, Toda Y et al. Regulation of CRF, POMC and MC4R gene expression after electrical foot shock stress in the rat amygdala and hypothalamus. J Vet Med Sci 2004; 66(11):1323-7.
115. Richter RM, Pich EM, Koob GF et al. Sensitization of cocaine-stimulated increase in extracellular levels of corticotropin-releasing factor from the rat amygdala after repeated administration as determined by intracranial microdialysis. Neurosci Lett 1995; 187:169-72.
116. Vecsernyes M, Biro E, Gardi J et al. Involvement of endogenous corticotropin-releasing factor in mediation of neuroendocrine and behavioral effects to alpha-melanocyte-stimulating hormone. Endocr Res 2000; 26(3):347-56.
117. Kawashima N, Chaki S, Okuyama S. Electrophysiological effects of melanocortin receptor ligands on neuronal activities of monoaminergic neurons in rats. Neurosci Lett 2003; 353(2):119-22.
118. Irani BG, Xiang Z, Moore MC et al. Voluntary exercise delays monogenetic obesity and overcomes reproductive dysfunction of the melanocortin-4 receptor knockout mouse. Biochem Biophys Res Commun 2005; 326(3):638-44.
119. King SH, Mayorov AV, Balse-Srinivasan P et al. Melanocortin receptors, melanotropic peptides and penile erection. Curr Top Med Chem 2007; 7(11):1098-106.
120. Mountjoy KG, Guan J, Elia CJ et al. Melanocortin-4 receptor messenger RNA expression is up-regulated in the nondamaged striatum following unilateral hypoxic-ischaemic brain injury. Neuroscience 1999; 89(1):183-90.
121. Giuliani D, Mioni C, Altavilla D et al. Both early and delayed treatment with melanocortin 4 Receptor-Stimulating Melanocortins Produces Neuroprotection in Cerebral Ischemia. Endocrinology 2006; 147(3):1126-35.
122. Lasaga M, Debeljuk L, Durand D et al. Role of alpha-melanocyte stimulating hormone and melanocortin 4 receptor in brain inflammation. Peptides 2008; 29(10):1825-35.
123. Tatro JB. Melanocortins defend their territory: multifaceted neuroprotection in cerebral ischemia.[comment]. Endocrinology 2006; 147(3):1122-5.
124. Guarini S, Cainazzo MM, Giuliani D et al. Adrenocorticotropin reverses hemorrhagic shock in anesthetized rats through the rapid activation of a vagal anti-inflammatory pathway. Cardiovasc Res 2004; 63(2):357-65.
125. Nordheim U, Nicholson JR, Dokladny K et al. Cardiovascular responses to melanocortin 4-receptor stimulation in conscious unrestrained normotensive rats. Peptides 2006; 27:438-43.
126. Ni X, Butler A, Cone R et al. Central receptors mediating the cardiovascular actions of melanocyte stimulating hormones. J Hypertens 2006; 24(11):2239-46.
127. Greenfield JR, Miller JW, Keogh JM et al. Modulation of blood pressure by central melanocortinergic pathways. N Engl J Med 2009; 360(1):44-52.
128. Griffon N, Mignon V, Facchinetti P et al. Molecular cloning and characterisation of the rat fifth melanocortin receptor. Biochem Biophys Res Commun 1994; 200:1007-14.
129. Labbe O, Desarnaud F, Eggerickx D et al. Molecular cloning of a mouse melanocortin 5 receptor gene widely expressed in peripheral tissues. Biochemistry 1994; 33:4543-9.
130. Chen W, Kelly MA, Opitz-Araya X et al. Exocrine gland dysfunction in MC5-R-deficient mice: evidence for coordinated regulation of exocrine gland function by melanocortin peptides. Cell 1997; 91(6):789-98.
131. Chhajlani V, Muceniece R, Wikberg JE. Molecular cloning of a novel human melanocortin receptor [published erratum appears in Biochem Biophys Res Commun 1996 17; 218(2):638]. Biochem Biophys Res Commun 1993; 195(2):866-73.
132. Metz JR, Geven EJ, van den Burg EH et al. ACTH, alpha-MSH and control of cortisol release: cloning, sequencing and functional expression of the melanocortin-2 and melanocortin-5 receptor in Cyprinus carpio. Am J Physiol Regul Integr Comp Physiol 2005; 289(3):R814-26.
133. Cerda-Reverter JM, Ling MK, Schioth HB et al. Molecular cloning, characterization and brain mapping of the melanocortin 5 receptor in the goldfish. J Neurochem 2003; 87(6):1354-67.
134. Haitina T, Klovins J, Andersson J et al. Cloning, tissue distribution, pharmacology and three-dimensional modelling of melanocortin receptors 4 and 5 in rainbow trout suggest close evolutionary relationship of these subtypes. Biochem J 2004; 380(Pt 2):475-86.
135. Brady AE, Limbird LE. G protein-coupled receptor interacting proteins: emerging roles in localization and signal transduction. Cellular Signalling 2002; 14(4):297-309.
136. Chan LF, Webb TR, Chung TT et al. MRAP and MRAP2 are bidirectional regulators of the melanocortin receptor family. Proc Natl Acad Sci USA 2009; 106(15):6146-51.

137. Roy S, Rached M, Gallo-Payet N. Differential regulation of the human adrenocorticotropin receptor [melanocortin-2 receptor (MC2R)] by human MC2R accessory protein isoforms alpha and beta in isogenic human embryonic kidney 293 cells. Mol Endocrinol 2007; 21(7):1656-69.
138. Metherell LA, Chapple JP, Cooray S et al. Mutations in MRAP, encoding a new interacting partner of the ACTH receptor, cause familial glucocorticoid deficiency type 2. Nat Genet 2005; 37(2):166-70.
139. Sebag JA, Hinkle PM. Opposite effects of melanocortin-2 (MC2) receptor accesory protein MRAP on C2 and MC5 receptor dimerization and trafficking. J Biol Chem 2009; 284:22641-8.
140. Clark AJ, Metherell LA, Cheetham ME et al. Inherited ACTH insensitivity illuminates the mechanisms of ACTH action. Trends Endocrinol Metab 2005; 16(10):451-7.
141. Sebag JA, Hinkle PM. Regions of melanocortin 2 (MC2) receptor accessory protein necessary for dual topology and MC2 receptor trafficking and signaling. J Biol Chem 2009; 284(1):610-8.
142. Low MJ, Simerly RB, Cone RD. Receptors for the melanocortin peptides in the central nervous system. Curr Opin Endo Diabetes 1994; 1:79-88.

CHAPTER 4

Drugs, Exercise, and the Melanocortin-4 Receptor—
Different Means, Same Ends: Treating Obesity

Jay W. Schaub, Erin B. Bruce, and Carrie Haskell-Luevano*

Abstract

As the percentage of obese humans expands, new options for weight loss are being explored. Body weight homeostasis is the result of a balance between energy intake (food) and expenditure (activity). A shift in homeostasis into a negative balance results in weight loss. Two potential options available for the management of body weight, as related to the melanocortin system, are exercise (increase energy expenditure) and drugs targeting the melanocortin-4 receptors for satiety.

Introduction

The metabolic syndrome is a topic of great interest to the healthcare community. Obesity is defined as having the excessive accumulation of adipose tissue leading to detrimental health conditions[1] and is measured using the body mass index scale (BMI). The BMI is calculated using a ratio between an individual's weight and the square of their height. BMI is considered to be a general indicator of the amount of adipose tissue in the body. Adults are considered overweight if they possess a BMI of 25 greater and are considered to be obese if their BMI equals or exceeds 30.[2] While BMI is an indicator of body fat, it is not a direct measurement of adipose tissue. Since BMI is an arbitrary scale, it is not an accurate indicator of obesity for all individuals notable such as professional athletes and pregnant women who might have a high BMI, but low body fat composition. Obese individuals with abdominally localized fat deposits are at a higher risk for diseases associated with obesity such as diabetes, cardiovascular diseases and some cancers.[2,3]

With the increasing incidence of obesity, significant research is being conducted to study the cause and effects as well as the impact on healthcare. Viewed from a total body standpoint, an increase in adipose tissue weight represents a net increase in the body's energy stores (Fig. 1). However, there are many causes for this shift in energy homeostasis and often multiple factors act together to cause the increase of adipose tissue that leads to obesity. The cause most popularly linked to the rapid increase in obesity worldwide is the increase of energy dense diets and a decrease in physical activity resulting in a positive energy balance with the understanding that prolonged positive balances in energy homeostasis leads to weight gain and potentially obesity.[2] With the many physiological mechanisms that regulate energy homeostasis and metabolism, it is possible that some individuals may have an inherent susceptibility to obesity.[2] Obesity often runs in families, suggesting that certain characteristics, such as where the fat is located and the ability

*Corresponding Author: Carrie Haskell-Luevano—Department of Pharmacodynamics, University of Florida, PO Box 100487, Gainesville, Florida, 32610-0487 USA.
Email: carrie@cop.ufl.edu

Melanocortins: Multiple Actions and Therapeutic Potential, edited by Anna Catania.
©2010 Landes Bioscience and Springer Science+Business Media.

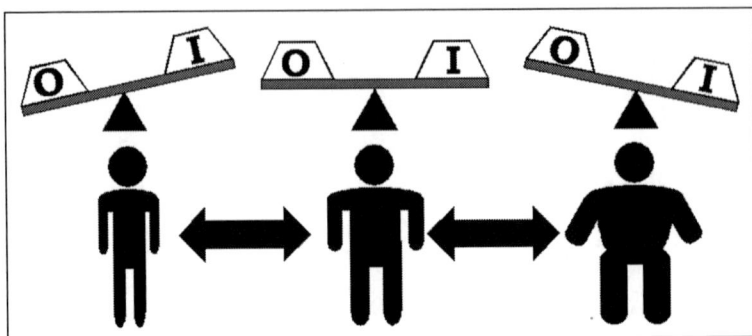

Figure 1. Observed body weight is the result of the homeostatic balance between energy input (I) and energy expenditure or output (O). Increased output or decreased input shifts the balance resulting in a decreased body weight. Weight gain is the result of a shift in the other direction with either reduced output, increased input, or both.

to lose weight easily, are heritable traits.[2] Scientists have also found certain strains of mice that are sensitive to weight gain when on a high fat diet while others are resistant to weight gain and increased adiposity.[4] One type of genetic mutation that has been identified in morbidly obese humans are melanocortin-4 receptor (MC4R) polymorphisms.[5-7] Children with MC4R polymorphisms possesse excessive amounts of adipose tissue and experience increased overall growth compared to the average child.[5,8,9]

Since obesity is the result of sustained positive energy balance, in order to stabilize or reduce body weight one must achieve a neutral or negative energy balance respectively. This change in energy balance can be achieved by reducing energy intake, increasing energy output, or a combination of the two. Energy intake reduction is often achieved by diet restriction, while energy expenditure increase can be accomplished by an increase in physical activity (i.e., exercise). One method of suppressing hunger and thereby food intake, is through the chemical manipulation of the regulatory feedback systems of the brain. There are several feedback mechanisms that have been shown to affect feeding behavior, however we will focus specifically on the role of the melanocortin-4 receptor and its potential as a drug target for the suppression of hunger. In addition to pharmaceutical intervention, there are behavioral changes that can lead to weight loss. An example of such a change would be implementation of an exercise routine to increase the energy expenditure of the body. Because of the wide spread incidence of obesity, it is paramount in the development of treatments options to develop methods that could easily be made available to large subsets of the population with relative ease meaning that combination of food restriction and increased physical activity would be most successful.

Melanocortins

The melanocortin system is made up of five G-protein coupled receptors (GPCRs) consisting of seven transmembrane helical domains with three intracellular loops and three extracellular loops, an intracellular C-terminus, and an extracellular N-terminus.[10-16] The melanocortin receptors signal primarily through the adenylate cyclase and cyclic adenosine monophosphate (cAMP) pathway via the $G\alpha_s$ protein sub-unit.[17-19] However, it has been demonstrated that melanocortin receptors are also capable of signaling through the phospholipase C and calcium ion (Ca^{2+}) pathway.[20-23] The melanocortin system possesses a series of endogenous agonists derived from the proopiomelanocortin (POMC) gene transcript.[24] POMC is posttranslationally cleaved and modified into the melanocortin agonists adrenocorticotropin hormone (ACTH), α-, β- and γ-melanocyte stimulating hormones (MSH).[25] In addition to endogenous peptide hormones, the melanocortin pathway is unique in that it has the only two known endogenous antagonists for GPCRs: agouti signaling peptide and agouti related peptide (AGRP).[26-28] Central administration of either endogenous or synthetic melanocortin agonists inhibits food intake in rodent models, while antagonists elicit a strong feeding response.[29-31] The melanocortin receptors (MC1-5R) serve as regulatory units for a multitude of signaling pathways throughout the body. The MC1R is responsible for the control of skin and hair pigmentation.[10] The melanocortin-2 receptor is involved in steroidogenesis and the stress response pathway.[10,32] The MC2R is unique among the melanocortin receptors in that, of the endogenous agonists, it only responds to ACTH.[10] The MC3R is expressed in the gastrointestinal tract, the pancreas, the heart, and importantly the central nervous system and brain.[11,13,14] MC3R knockout mice are reported to possess normal body weight, but increased fat mass.[33,34] The MC4R is centrally expressed and has been demonstrated to play a role in the regulation of feeding behavior and energy homeostasis[14,16,35,36] as well as sexual function.[37] Characterization of the MC4R knockout mouse resulted in an obese, hyperphagic, hyperinsulinemic, hyperleptinemic, as well as increased body length phenotype.[38] The physiological role of the MC5R has not been fully elucidated at this point in time, though the MC5R is expressed in many tissues through out the body and is proposed to be involved in exocrine gland function.[39]

The Agouti peptide, normally expressed in skin, has been established to be a competitive antagonist of not only the MC1R, but also the MC3R and MC4R.[40,41] The agouti lethal yellow mouse (A^y/a) was identified to ectopically express agouti resulting in a light coat coloring and obesity.[42] Because of the obese phenotype of the agouti mouse, the physiologic role of the melanocortin receptors expressed in the feeding center of the brain was investigated. The MC4R is expressed throughout the brain, including high levels of expression in the hypothalamus, a region of the brain well established to be important for energy homeostasis.[14,16] The generation of the melanocortin-4 receptor knockout (KO) mouse in 1997 yielded a hyperphagic mouse with an obese phenotype, confirming the importance of the MC4R in energy homeostasis and body weight maintenance.[38] It is hypothesized that the obese phenotype of the agouti yellow mice is due to antagonism of a centrally expressed melanocortin receptor by overexpression of agouti protein.[12,14,26,40]

The MC4R KO mice have also been characterized as possessing hyperphagia, hyperglycemia, hyperinsulinemia, with elevated circulating leptin levels, but with normal basal corticosterone levels compared to the wildtype mice.[38,43-46] As a result of these findings, the MC4R KO mouse has become an important animal model for obesity and central regulation of energy homeostasis.

In addition to the MC4R, the melanocortin-3 receptor is also located in the central nervous system with highest levels of expression being in the hypothalamus.[13] Creation of a MC3R KO mouse generated mice with normal body weights (compared to WT littermates), but with increased fat mass.[33,34] These results indicate that while the MC3R appears to be involved in the regulation of energy homeostasis, the MC4R plays a more critical role in the regulation of body weight and food intake and that the MC3R might play a more subtle role in energy homeostasis.[47]

There are many receptors, ligands and pathways that are involved in aspects of energy balance, however we will focus primarily on the melanocortin system and the pathways intertwined with it. The two classes of pathways that we will discuss are the orexigenic and anorexigenic, or those that promote the intake of food and those that inhibit food intake, respectively. The primary neuropeptides of the orexigenic signaling pathway we will discuss are AGRP and neuropeptide Y (NPY). mRNA for the melanocortin antagonist, AGRP, is expressed primarily in neurons located in the arcuate nucleus (ARC) of the hypothalamus with projections to the anterioperiventricular preoptic area, the periventricular nucleus, the parvocellular portion of paraventricular nucleus (PVN), the dorsomedial nucleus, the rostral end of the posterior nucleus, the anterior hypothalamus, the lateral hypothalamus, the bed nucleus of the stria terminalis, and the ventral region of the lateral septal nucleus.[48] Neurons expressing NPY are located in the arcuate nucleus of the hypothalamus with projections to the paraventricular hypothalamus with NPY immunoreactivity being reported in the subnuclei of the paraventricular hypothalamic nucleus.[49-52] It has been shown that the majority of neurons that express AGRP coexpress NPY.[53]

The anorexigenic pathway is made up of peptides, that when secreted, reduce food intake. POMC mRNA is expressed in neurons with cell bodies in the arcuate nucleus of the hypothalamus with projections reported to extend into the preoptic nucleus, the anterior hypothalamic nucleus, the

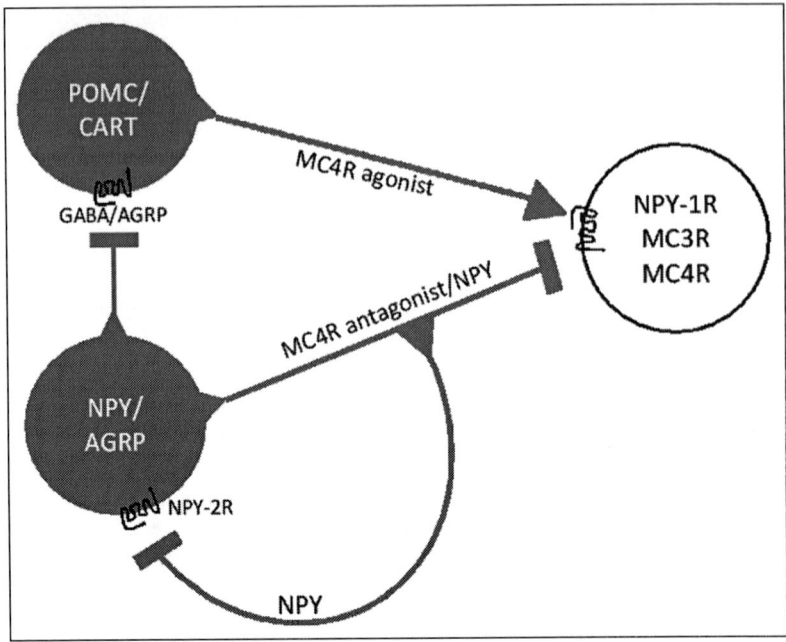

Figure 2. POMC/CART neurons stimulate MC4R expressing neurons to decrease food intake while AGRP/NPY inhibits activity of downstream neurons promoting eating. AGRP/NPY neurons also forms regulatory feedback mechanism with POMC/CART neurons.

dorsomedial nucleus, the periventricular nucleus, the amygdala, the midbrain, the cortex, the brain stem, the septum nucleus interstitialis stria terminalis, the mammillary body, the central gray matter, the cuneiform nucleus, and the nucleus of the solitary tract.[54,55] The majority of the neurons that express POMC also express Cocaine- and amphetamine-regulated transcript (CART).[56] CART mRNA expression has been reported in the Edinger-Westphal nucleus, the induseum griseum, the pariventricular nucleus, the arcuate nucleus, the supraoptic nucleus, the nucleus accumbens, the medial olfactory tubercle, the olfactory tubercle, the periformical region, the primary somatosensory area (layer 4) of the neocortex, the bed nuclei of the stria terminalis, the dorsal blade of the dentate gyrus of the rostral hippocampus, the medial region of the septal nucleus, the dorsal part of medial nucleus, the posterior cortical nucleus, and the posterior basolateral nucleus.[57,58]

In order for any of these neuropeptides to have an effect on food intake they must act on downstream neurons possessing the corresponding receptors. Neurons expressing MC4R RNA are located in many of the regions of the hypothalamus including the median preoptic nucleus, the suprachiasmatic preoptic nucleus, the periventricular nucleus, the paraventricular nucleus, the anterior hypothalamic nucleus, the ventromedial hypothalamic nucleus and the dorsomedial nucleus.[16,59] NPY-1R expression has been reported in neurons with cell bodies located in the paraventricular nucleus, the suprachiasmatic nucleus, the dorsal parvocellular region and the dorsal, ventral and anterior regions of the periventricular nucleus.[52] The NPY-2R is found on the neurons expressing NPY and AGRP.[60]

It is the interplay between these endocrine hormones and their receptors that regulates food intake (Fig. 2). Neurons expressing the MC4R are stimulated by neurons secreting POMC from the arcuate nucleus, resulting in a decrease in food intake. However, when the NPY/AGRP neurons in the ARC are stimulated, AGRP and NPY act on the MC4R/NPY-1R possessing neurons in the PVN to increase food intake. Additionally, neurons expressing AGRP inhibit neurons expressing POMC resulting in an increase in food intake both because of an increase in antagonist concentration, but

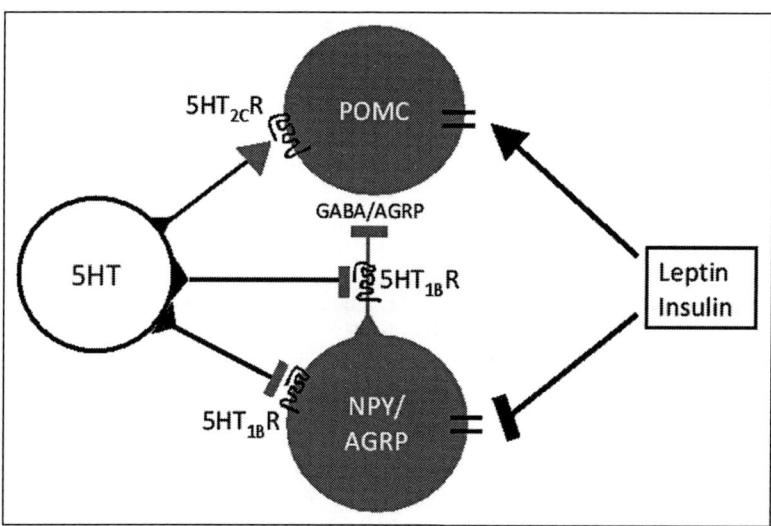

Figure 3. Serotonin, insulin, and leptin all modulate feeding behavior through melanocortin neurons. All three molecules increase POMC neuron activity while inhibiting AGRP/NPY neuron activity.

also a decrease in agonist concentration. Also, it has been shown that there is an autoregulatory feed back loop of the AGRP/NPY neurons that act on the POMC/CART expressing neurons.[60] While this system is considered to be a central mechanism involved in regulation of food intake and satiety, there are many effectors that have been shown to influence this system.

One such regulator of the central melanocortin pathway is leptin.[61] Leptin is a polypeptide hormone that is secreted from adipose tissue that acts on hypothalamic neurons to promote the release of POMC while inhibiting NPY and AGRP secretion, thereby causing a decrease in food intake.[62,63] Neurons expressing POMC have been demonstrated to coexpress the leptin receptor and are believed to mediate leptin's anorexigenic effects (Fig. 3).[63]

Insulin is secreted from the pancreas, promotes glucose uptake, and is believed to act in a similar manner to leptin in the arcuate nucleus of the hypothalamus, activating POMC and inhibiting NPY/AGRP expressing neurons (Fig. 3).[64] It has been demonstrated that leptin can inhibit insulin secretion and also increase insulin sensitivity in some tissues.[65] In 2000, using the MC4R knockout mouse, Fan et al proposed that leptin's ability to regulate insulin was via the melanocortin pathway. Fan's study proposes an that it may not be obesity that is causing diabetes in the MC4R KO mouse, it may be in part due to the disruption melanocortin system itself.[66] Furthermore, Obici showed in 2001 that the MC4R mediates the actions of insulin in the body, as well as fat distribution.[67] When the MC4R is stimulated by the agonist α-MSH the amount of abdominal fat decreased and hepatic insulin action was increased.[67] In 2002, Benoit showed that insulin receptors are colocalized with POMC in neurons of the arcuate nucleus, further demonstrating insulin's actions regulating and being regulated by the central melanocortin system.[68]

Another regulator of the melanocortin system is serotonin (5-hydroxytryptamine, or 5HT) (Fig. 3). Heisler et al demonstrated that serotonin regulates the melanocortin system via the $5HT_{1B}R$ and the $5HT_{2C}R$.[69,70] They proposed that serotonin inhibits AGRP neurons via the $5HT_{1B}R$ and decreases an inhibitory effect of AGRP on POMC neurons also through the 1B receptor. They also show that serotonin acts directly on the POMC neurons via the $5HT_{2C}R$.[70] These actions take together, cause an increase in POMC and its derivatives followed by a decrease in food intake. Lam et al showed via in situ hybridization and immunohistochemistry that the

$5HT_{2c}R$ is colocalized with POMC in neurons in the arcuate nucleus, further explaining how serotonin directly regulates the central melanocortin system.[71] It is through the manipulation of these signaling pathways that melanocortin-4 agonists could be used as effective methods of decreasing food intake. However, decreases in energy intake are only half of the energy balance picture. A decrease in body weight is achieved by shifting the homeostatic balance of the body's energy regulatory system to a negative balance. This can be accomplished by either decreasing energy intake as discussed previously, or by increasing energy expenditure.

Exercise

Exercise, defined as sustained physical activity, is being increasingly investigated to understand the mechanisms by which it causes physiological changes in the body. Physical activity in animals (in the wild) is generally a result of specific stimuli, such as the need to find food or water, migration to a breeding ground, or to escape a predator. In the laboratory setting, the physical activity associated with these needs is often eliminated and any occurring physical activity is performed voluntarily, not out of necessity. Because exercise is rarely isolated to one part of the body, it is not unexpected that multiple homeostatic systems are directly influenced by physical activity. Exercise has been demonstrated in a variety of models to positively effect thermoregulation, circulatory efficiency, metabolism, physical endurance, appetite, sleep patterns, stress pathways, mental health, and chronic diseases including obesity and Type II diabetes.[44-46,72-86] As a result, exercise is the only universally prescribed treatment for alleviation of symptoms of many chronic diseases including obesity, cardiovascular disease, and Type II diabetes.[78]

Studying the effects of voluntary exercise presents the challenge of monitoring the many parameters of interest simultaneously. For experiments involving energy homeostasis, two variables of particular interest are energy intake and expenditure. Energy intake can be monitored simply by measuring food eaten while energy expenditure presents a larger challenge with the most common methods being through the use of metabolic cages or activity monitoring systems.

Three different systems that have been used to quantitatively measure voluntary physical activity are the use of infra red beam break systems, an angled rotating running track, or alternatively, a running wheel connected to magnetic switches that are monitored by computer and software systems.[43-46,87] The computerized monitoring systems used in these studies utilize software capable of displaying and analyzing the activity data from the individual animal cages. The possibility of experimental animals either choosing to exercise or not are potential drawbacks in studies relying on paradigms of voluntary exercise.

Patterson and Levin examined the long term homeostatic effects of voluntary exercise in diet-induced obese and diet-resistant rats.[79] It was suggested that duration of the metabolic effects caused by exercise after physical activity is ceased, are dependent in part, on the age of the animal. They hypothesized that exercise lowers the defended level of adiposity and that exercise at an early age influences the formation and development of energy balance signaling pathways in the hypothalamus. The monitoring of a signaling molecule or molecules generated peripherally during exercise is suggested as a mechanism by which rats monitor their level of energy balance and determine caloric need, instead of by direct regulation of physical activity. This theory supported is supported by the finding that rats adjust their food intake rather than level of activity when allowed to exercise freely.

Flores et al studied the effects of acute exercise on the hypothalamic sensitivity to centrally administered insulin and leptin and the downstream signaling pathways.[74] Male rats were forced to swim for two three-hour sessions, after which they were centrally injected with varying doses of leptin or insulin. It was found that both leptin and insulin were more effective in reducing food intake in exercised rats versus they rested controls. It was also reported that leptin and insulin were more effective in activating the phosphorylation of downstream signaling molecules in the exercised animals, providing insight into the molecular mechanisms by which exercise is modulating food intake. The role of interleukin-6 (IL-6) in insulin and leptin signaling was investigated by central

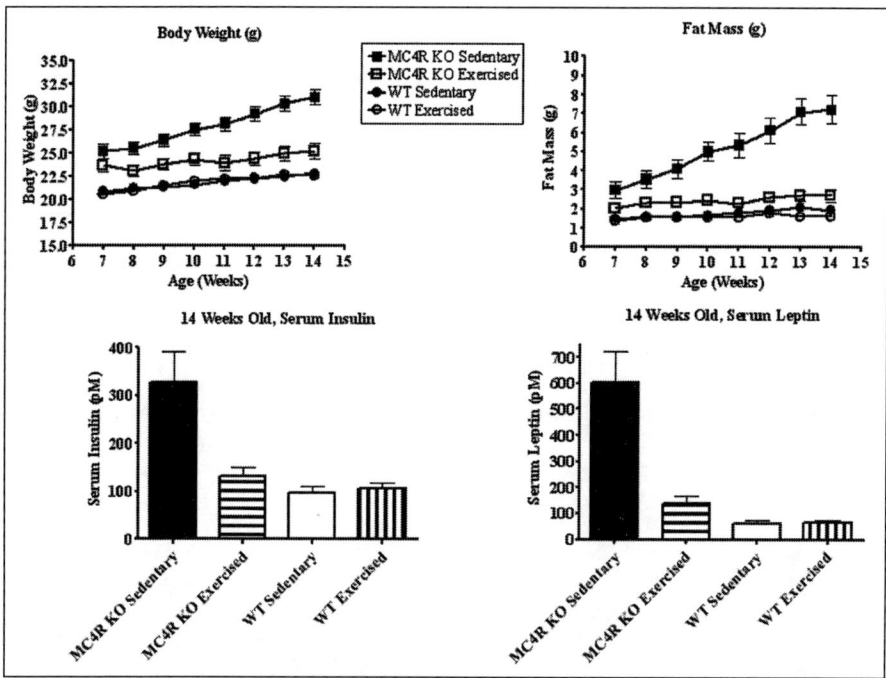

Figure 4. Illustration of the effects of voluntary exercise on body weight, fat mass and adiposity factors (insulin and leptin) of the MC4RKO mouse and wildtype littermate controls.[44]

administration of anti-IL-6. It was found that blocking the action of IL-6 prevented the increase in leptin and insulin sensitivity and the downstream signaling changes gained from exercise.

In addition to other rodent models, work has been done with the MC4R knockout mouse and the changes that occur to its phenotype as a result of exercise. The Haskell-Luevano group first reported the effects of voluntary exercise observed in the MC4R KO mouse model in 2004, which was followed by a more comprehensive study published in 2009.[44-46] It was found that when MC4RKO mice, at a young age, were allowed to exercise in cages equipped with running wheels, that the animals did not develop the obese phenotype associated with the MC4RKO mouse.[38] Parameters measured over the course of those experiments include total body weight and length, food intake, running wheel activity, reproductive success, circulating serum hormone concentrations, as well as fat and lean mass composition and distribution.[44,46] Additionally, circulating plasma levels of whole blood glucose and serum cholesterol, insulin, and leptin were monitored. Those studies found that when allowed access to voluntary exercise equipment, many of the parameters monitored as indicators of obesity were maintained at levels comparable to those of the wildtype littermate control mice. Specifically, voluntary exercise was shown to prevent the large increase in body weight and fat mass with the associated hyperinsulinemia and hyperleptinemia, typically observed for the MC4RKO mice (Fig. 4). Additionally, exercise was able to avert the decline in reproductive success seen in the obese MC4R KO mice. Changes in the hypothalamic expression levels of selected genes due to genotype, exercise, or an interaction between genotype and exercise were observed.[44] These data suggest that a change other than increased energy expenditure alone might be responsible for the lack of an obese phenotype in the MC4R KO exercised animals.

The positive effects of exercise on energy balance is not limited only to rodent models. Exercise has been shown to curb appetite and decrease unrestricted food intake in humans. This makes exercise appealing as a method of weight loss both as a method of increasing energy expenditure and also by decreasing energy intake. One of the mechanisms involved in appetite regulation is the signaling of endocrine peptide hormones from the gut on the energy sensing portion of the hypothalamus. Martins et al, using a group of human subjects, monitored the serum levels of several gut hormones in two groups (one exercised, one sedentary) to establish the effect of acute aerobic exercise on appetite and meal size and to try an establish a link between exercise, appetite and gut hormone concentration.[76] Blood was drawn at 30 minute intervals and plasma concentration for cholecystokinin (CCK), peptide YY (PYY), glucagon-like peptide-1 (GLP-1), pancreatic polypeptide (PP), non-esterified fatty acids (NEFA), and triacylglycerol (TAG) were monitored from the time of the initial meal, through the exercise or rest portion and until the start of the meal with unrestricted food access. It was reported that NEFA and TAG were significantly increased in the exercising subjects and blood glucose was decreased. This is consistent with previous theories that FFA are mobilized during exercise to reduce the amount of glucose or glycogen consumed to maintain activity and the fact that free glucose in the blood stream would be prone to uptake and oxidation during exercise. There was a significant and sustained elevation in circulating PP in the exercised individuals and an increase in PYY and GLP-1 which diminished over time. There was no reported difference in ghrelin concentration, however there was a significant decrease in insulin during the exercise and recovery periods (also consistent with theories of glucose conservation). Self-reported hunger was reduced in the exercised group compared to the sedentary group but the meal size for the exercised group was significantly larger. The authors explained this as a difference in relative energy intake (REI), calculated by subtracting estimated energy expenditure during the experimental time frame from the caloric intake of the meal. The REI of the exercised group was significantly lower than that of the sedentary group. This effect was tentatively classified as exercise-induced anorexia and the authors suggest it may be due to the increased levels of GLP-1, PYY, and PP. It is important to note that it is almost certain that other and likely multiple, pathways are involved in exercise mediated changes in appetite and energy homeostasis in addition to the gut hormones in this study.

Technological advancements that allow experimenters to consistently measure small physiological changes have permitted the field of exercise physiology to progress significantly. One of the areas in which this has made the greatest difference is the study of changes at the genetic or transcriptional level that are propagated by exercise instead of just the translational or activated protein level of regulation. It has been reported that in the MC4RKO mouse, that voluntary exercise changes the level of hypothalamic expression of POMC, AGRP, NPY, CART, the NPY-1R and the melanocortin-3 receptor.[44]

Because of its central involvement in the feeding pathway, the melanocortin system and specifically the melanocortin-4 receptor, is a viable drug target for the reduction of food intake for the treatment of obesity. Additionally, exercise is a complex behavior affecting the entire body that not only increases the body's energy expenditure, but also has positive effects on animals with obese phenotypes that might be acting through the melanocortin pathway. Neurons expressing melanocortin-4 receptors involved in the POMC/AGRP regulatory circuit (Fig. 2) are believed to propagate the signaling cascade resulting the change in feeding behavior. To fully understand the regulation by the melanocortin system, it is necessary for all the downstream neurons/pathways to be identified and characterized. Better understanding of the pathways and how they are positively effected by exercise may allow for the generation of a new generation of drugs designed to mimic specific interactions while avoiding undesirable side effects associated with nonspecific drug actions.

Due to the wide spread expression of the melanocortin-3 and melanocortin-4 receptors in the brain, it is reasonable that the melanocortin system may play a less passive role in behavior that originally believed. New studies utilizing melanocortin-3 receptor null mice have demonstrated that the melanocortin signaling pathway plays a larger role in feeding behavior other than just whether feeding is stimulated or inhibited. Sutton et al demonstrated that the MC3R is involved in meal entrainment with wildtype mice showing increased activity in the time leading up to food access compared to MC3R KO mice which did not exhibit the same anticipatory behaviors.[88]

Conclusion

The obesity epidemic, along with the financial costs and health risks associated with being overweight, has reached a point where it can no longer be ignored. Action must be taken to stem and reverse the trend by whatever means necessary. Shifting the energy balance of the body to create a deficit, promoting weight loss, remains the most practical and non-invasive alternative. Drugs that target the melanocortin-4 receptors located in the feeding center of the brain are one option for reducing food intake, while exercise remains a practical option for increasing energy expenditure.

In order to exploit MC4R agonists as drugs to reduce eating many obstacles still exist that must be overcome. First, because of the high level of homology between the melanocortin receptors and the similarities between their ligands, undesirable interactions might occur unless a highly selective agonist is developed for the MC4R. Second, due to the central location of the neurons that possess the receptors, drugs must be able to pass through the blood brain barrier in order to be effective. Additionally, route of administration must be considered. Because of the location of the neurons that control feeding behavior, central administration of the drug would be ideal, however central administration of drugs to human patients is rarely practical. Instead, options for peripheral or oral administration must be investigated with oral bioavailability and drug stability taken into account. Finally, the long term effects of chronic melanocortin agonist exposure must be studied to be sure that no complications develop.

Exercise is generally considered a benign activity, with the benefits gained from regular physical activity far outweighing any potential detrimental effects. Exercise as a means of weight loss or the prevention of the onset of an obese phenotype has been demonstrated in both diet induced obesity and genetic risk of obesity animal models. Better understanding of the molecular mechanisms of exercise will allow for the design of more comprehensive exercise regimens and potentially new drug targets that could increase the quality of life for overweight or obese individuals. Additionally, there is an increasing body of evidence showing that the benefits gained from regular exercise provides are not limited solely to weight loss.

Regardless of the underlying cause of obesity, the need to be able to shift the energy balance remains unchanged. It will be important to consider treatment plans that will address both the underlying cause of the disease and establish ongoing treatment to prevent relapse. Drugs that decrease hunger through the melanocortin-4 receptor pathway and exercise are two alternatives for the modulation of energy homeostasis and the reduction of body weight.

Acknowledgements

We would like to acknowledge financial support from NIH Grants RO1DK57080, RO1DK64250, RO1DK063974 and an American Diabetes Research Award.

References

1. Spiegelman BM, Flier JS. Obesity and the regulation of energy balance. Cell 2001; 104:531-543.
2. Obesity: Preventing and managing the global epidemic: Report of a WHO consultation. Geneva, Switzerland: World Health Organization; 1999.
3. O'Brien PE, Dixon JB. The extent of the problem of obesity. Am J Surg 2002; 184(6):S4-S8.
4. West DB, Boozer CN, Moody DL et al. Dietary obesity in nine inbred mouse strains. Am J Physiol Regul Integr Comp Physiol 1992; 262(6):R1025-1032.
5. Vaisse C, Clement K, Guy-Grand B et al. A frameshift mutation in human MC4R is associated with a dominant form of obesity. Nat Genet 1998; 20:113-114.
6. Yeo GSH, Farooqi IS, Aminian S et al. A frameshift mutation in MC4R associated with dominantly inherited human obesity. Nat Genet 1998; 20:111-112.
7. Krude H, Biebermann H, Luck W et al. Severe early-onset obesity, adrenal insufficiency and red hair pigmentation caused by POMC mutations in humans. Nat Genet 1998; 19:155-157.
8. Marti A, Corbalan M, Forga L et al. A novel nonsense mutation in the melanocortin-4 receptor associated with obesity in a Spanish population. Int J Obes Relat Metab Disord 2003; 27(3):385-388.
9. Farooqi IS, Keogh JM, Yeo GS et al. Clinical spectrum of obesity and mutations in the melanocortin 4 receptor gene. N Engl J Med 2003; 348(12):1085-1095.

10. Mountjoy KG, Robbins LS, Mortrud MT et al. The cloning of a family of genes that encode the melanocortin receptors. Science 1992; 257(5074):1248-1251.

11. Chhajlani V, Wikberg JE. Molecular cloning and expression of the human melanocyte stimulating hormone receptor cDNA. FEBS Lett 1992; 309(3):417-420.

12. Gantz I.; Konda, Y.; Tashiro, T et al. Molecular cloning of a novel melanocortin receptor. J Biol Chem 1993; 268:8246-8250.

13. Roselli-Rehfuss L.; Mountjoy, K.G.; Robbins, L.S. et al. Identification of a receptor for gamma melanotropin and other proopiomelanocortin peptides in the hypothalamus and limbic system. Proc Natl Acad Sci USA 1993; 90:8856-8860.

14. Gantz I, Miwa H, Konda Y et al. Molecular cloning, expression and gene localization of a fourth melanocortin receptor. J Biol Chem 1993; 268(20):15174-15179.

15. Gantz I, Shimoto Y, Konda Y et al. Molecular cloning, expression and characterization of a fifth melanocortin receptor. Biochem Biophys Res Commun 1994; 200(3):1214-1220.

16. Mountjoy K.G.; Mortrud, M.T.;Low M.J. et al. Localization of the melanocortin-4 receptor (MC4-R) in neuroendocrine and autonomic control circuits in the brain. Mol Endocrinol 1994; 8:1298-1308.

17. Buckley DI, Ramachandran J. Characterization of corticotropin receptors on andrenocortical cells. PNAS 1981; 78(12):7431-7435.

18. Gerst JE, Sole J, Saloman Y. Dual regulation of beta-melanotropin receptor function and adenylate cyclase by calcium and guanosine nucleotides in the M2R melanoma cell line. Mol Pharmacol 1987; 31:81-88.

19. Mertz LM, Catt KJ. Adrenocorticotropin receptors functional expression from rat adrenal mRNA in xenopus laevis oocytes. PNAS 1991; 88(19):8525-8529.

20. Konda Y, Gantz I, DelValle J et al. Interaction of dual intracellular signaling pathways activated by the melanocortin-3 receptor. J Biol Chem 1994; 269(18):13162-13166.

21. Mountjoy KG, Kong PL, Taylor JA et al. Melanocortin receptor-mediated mobilization of intracellular free calcium in HEK293 cells. Physiol Genomics 2001; 5:11-19.

22. Newman EA, Chai B-X, Zhang W et al. Activation of the melanocortin-4 receptor mobilizes intracellular free calcium in immortalized hypothalamic neurons. J Invest Surg 2006; 132:201-207.

23. Al-Majed H, Jones P, Persaud S et al. ACTH stimulates insulin secretion from MIN6 cells and primary mouse and human islets of Langerhans. J Endocrinol. 2004; 180:155-166.

24. Lerner AB, McGuire JS. Effect of alpha- and beta-melanocyte stimulating hormones on the skin colour of man. Nature 1961; 189:176-179.

25. Eberle AN. The melanotropins: Chemistry, physiology and mechanisms of action. Karger: Basel; 1988.

26. Ollmann MM, Wilson BD, Yang YK et al. Antagonism of central melanocortin receptors in vitro and in vivo by agouti-related protein. Science 1997; 278(5335):135-138.

27. Shutter J, Graham M, Kinsey A et al. Hypothalamic expression of ART, a novel gene related to agouti, is up-regulated in obese and diabetic mutant mice. Genes Dev 1997; 11(5):593-602.

28. Graham M, Shutter J, Sarmiento U et al. Overexpression of AGRT leads to obesity in transgenic mice. Nat Genet 1997; 17:273-274.

29. Giraudo SQ, Billington CJ, Levine AS. Feeding effects of hypothalamic injection of melanocortin 4 receptor ligands. Brain Research 1998; 809:302-306.

30. Fan W, Boston BA, Kesterson RA et al. Role of melanocortinergic neurons in feeding and the agouti obesity syndrome. Nature 1997; 385:165-168.

31. Thiele TE, Dijk GV, Yagaloff KA et al. Central infusion of melanocortin agonist MTII in rats assessment of c-Fos expression and taste aversion. Am J Physiol Regulatory Integrative Comp Physiol 1998; 274:248-254.

32. Boston BA, Cone RD. Characterization of melanocortin receptor subtype expression in murine adipose tissues and in the 3T3-L1 cell line. Endocrinology 1996; 137(5):2043-2050.

33. Butler AA, Kesterson RA, Khong K et al. A unique metabolic syndrome causes obesity in the melanocortin-3 receptor-deficient mouse. Endocrinology 2000; 141(9):3518-3521.

34. Chen AS, Marsh DJ, Trumbauer ME et al. Inactivation of the mouse melanocortin-3 receptor results in increased fat mass and reduced lean body mass. Nat Genet 2000; 26:97-102.

35. Kishi T, Aschkenasi CJ, Lee CE et al. Expression of melanocortin 4 receptor mRNA in the central nervous system of the rat. J Comp Neurol 2003; 457(213-235).

36. Liu H, Kishi T, Rosenberry AG et al. Transgenic mice expressing green fluorescent protein under the control of the melanocortin-4 receptor promoter. J Neurosci 2003; 23(18):7143-7154.

37. Van Der Ploeg LH, Martin WJ, Howard AD et al. A role for the melanocortin 4 receptor in sexual function. Proc Natl Acad Sci USA 2002; 99:11381-11386.

38. Huszar D, Lynch CA, Fairchild-Huntress V et al. Targeted disruption of the melanocortin-4 receptor results in obesity in mice. Cell 1997; 88:131-141.

39. Chen W, Kelly MA, Opitz-Araya X et al. Exocrine gland dysfunction in MC5-R deficient mice: Evidence for coordinated regulation of exocrine gland functions by melanocortin peptides. Cell 1997; 91:789-798.
40. Lu D, Willard D, Patel IR et al. Agouti protein is an antagonist of the melanocyte-stimulating-hormone receptor. Nature 1994; 371:799-802.
41. McNulty JC, Jackson PJ, Thompson DA et al. Structures of the agouti signaling protein. J Mol Biol 2005; 346(4):1059-1070.
42. Bultman SJ, Michaud EJ, Woychick RP. Molecular characterization of the mouse agouti locus. Cell 1992; 71:1195-1204.
43. Butler AA, Marks DL, Fan W et al. Melanocortin-4 receptor is required for acute homeostatic responses to increased dietary fat. Nat Neurosci 2001; 4(6):605-611.
44. Haskell-Luevano C, Schaub JW, Andreasen A et al. Voluntary exercise prevents the obese and diabetic metabolic syndrome of the melanocortin-4 receptor knockout mouse. FASEB J 2009; 23(2):642-655.
45. Haskell-Luevano C, Todorovic A, Gridley K et al. The melanocortin pathway: effects of voluntary exercise on the melanocortin-4 receptor knockout mice and ACTH(1-24) ligand SAR at the Melanocortin-2 Receptor. Endocr Res 2004; 30(4):591-597.
46. Irani BG, Xiang Z, Moore MC et al. Voluntary exercise delays monogenetic obesity and overcomes reproductive dysfunction of the melanocortin-4 receptor knockout mouse. Biochem Biophys Res Commun 2005; 326:638-644.
47. Sutton GM, Trevaskis JL, Hulver MW et al. Diet-genotype interactions in the development of the obese, insulin-resistant phenotype of C57BL/6J mice lacking melanocortin-3 or -4 receptors. Endocrinology 2006; 147(5):2183-2196.
48. Haskell-Luevano C, Chen P, Li C et al. Characterization of the neuroanatomical distribution of agouti-related protein immunoreactivity in the rhesus monkey and the rat. Endocrinology 1999; 140(3):1408-1415.
49. Chronwall B, DiMaggio D, Massari V et al. The anatomy of neuropeptide Y containing neurons in the rat brain. Neuroscience 1985; 15:1159-1181.
50. deQuidt M, Emson P. Distribution of Neuropeptide Y-like immunoreactivity in the rat central nervous system. II. Immunohistochemical analysis. Neuroscience 1986; 18:545-618.
51. Allen Y, Adrian T, Allen J et al. Neuropeptide Y distribution in the rat brain. Science 1983; 221:877-879.
52. Broberger C, Visser TJ, Kuhar MJ et al. Neuropeptide Y innervation and neuropeptide-Y-Y1-receptor-expressing neurons in the paraventricular hypothalamic nucleus of the mouse. Neuroendocrinology 1999; 70:295-305.
53. Hahn TM, Breininger JF, Baskin DG et al. Coexpression of Agrp and NPY in fasting-activated hypothalamic neurons. Nat Neurosci 1998; 1(4):271-272.
54. Jacobowitz DM, O'Donohue TL. Alpha-melanocyte stimulation hormone Immunohistochemical identification and mapping in neurons of rat brain. PNAS 1978; 75(12):6300-6304.
55. Wilcox JN, Roberts JL, Chronwall B et al. Localization of proopiomelanocortin mRNA in functional subsets of neurons defined by axonal projections. J Neurosci 1986; 16:89-96.
56. Elias CF, Lee C, Kelly J et al. Leptin activates hypothalamic CART neurons projecting to the spinal cord. Neuron 1998; 21:1375-1385.
57. Couceyro PR, Koylu EO, Kuhar MJ. Further studies on the anatomical distribution of CART by in situ hybridization. J Chem Neuroanat 1997; 12:229-241.
58. Douglass J, McKinzie AA, Couceyro P. PCR differential display identifies a rat brain mRNA that is transcriptionally regulated by cocaine and amphetamine. J Neurosci 1995; 15(3):2471-2481.
59. Low MJ, Simerly RB, Cone RD. Receptors for the melanocortin peptides in the central nervous system. Curr Opin Endocrinol Diabetes 1994; 1:79-88.
60. Cowley MA, Smart JL, Rubinstein M et al. Leptin activates anorexigenic POMC neurons through a neural network in the arcuate nucleus 2001; 411(6836):480-484.
61. Halaas JL, Gajiwala KS, Maffei M et al. Weight-reducing effects of the plasma protein encoded by the obese gene. Science 1995; 269:543-546.
62. Satoh N, Ogawa Y, Katsuura G et al. Satiety effect and the sympathetic activation of leptin are mediated by hypothalamic melanocortin system. Neurosci Lett 1998; 249:107-110.
63. Cheung CC, Clifton DK, Steiner RA. Proopiomelanocortin neurons are direct targets for leptin in the hypothalamus. Endocrinology 1997; 138(10):4489-4492.
64. Niswender K, Baskin D, Schwartz M. Insulin and its evolving partnership with leptin in the hypothalamic control of energy homeostasis. Trends Endocrinol Metab 2004; 15:362-369.
65. Minokoshi Y, Haque M, Shimazu T. Microinjection of leptin into the ventromedial hypothalamus increases glucose uptake in peripheral tissues in rats. Diabetes 1999; 48(2):287-291.

66. Fan W, Dinulescu D, Butler A et al. The central melanocortin system can directly regulate serum insulin levels. Endocrinology 2000; 141:3072-3079.
67. Obici S, Feng Z, Tan J et al. Central melanocortin receptors regulate insulin action. J Clin Invest 2001; 108:1079-1085.
68. Benoit SC, Air EL, Coolen LM et al. The catabolic action of insulin in the brain is mediated by melanocortins. J Neurosci 2002; 22(20):9048-9052.
69. Heisler LK, Cowley MA, Tecott LH et al. Activation of central melanocortin pathways by fenfluramine. Science 2002; 297(5581):609-611.
70. Heisler LK, Jobst EE, Sutton GM et al. Serotonin reciprocally regulates melanocortin neurons to modulate food intake. Neuron 2006; 51(2):239-249.
71. Lam DD, Przydzial MJ, Ridley SH et al. Serotonin 5-HT$_{2C}$ receptor agonist promotes hypophagia via downstream activation of melanocortin 4 receptors. Endocrinology 2008; 149(3):1323-1328.
72. Davidson SR, Burnett M, Hoffman-Goetz L. Training effects in mice after long-term voluntary exercise. Med Sci Sports Exerc 2006; 250-255.
73. Fediuc S, Campbell JE, Riddell MC. Effect of voluntary wheel running on circadian corticosterone release and on HPA axis responsiveness to restraint stress in Sprague-Dawley rats. J Appl Physiol 2006; 100:1867-1875.
74. Flores M.B.; Fernandes, M.F.; Ropelle, E.R. et al. Exercise improves insulin and leptin sensitivity in hypothalamus of wistar rats. Diabetes 2006; 55:2554-2561.
75. Ji LL. Modulation of skeletal muscle antioxidant defense by exercise: Role of redox signaling. Free Radic Biol Med 2008; 44:142-152.
76. Martins C, Morgan LM, Bloom SR et al. Effects of exercise on gut peptides, energy uptake and appetite. J Endocrinol 2007; 193:251-258.
77. Nadel ER. Physiological adaptations to aerobic training. American Scientist 1985; 73:334-343.
78. Noland RC, Thyfault JP, Henes ST et al. Artificial selection for high-capactity endurance running is protective against high-fat diet-induced insulin resistance. Am J Physiol Endocrinol Metab 2007; 293:E31-E41.
79. Patterson CM, Levin BE. Role of exercise in the central regulation of energy homeostasis and in the prevention of obesity. Neuroendocrinology 2008; 87:65-70.
80. Youngstedt SD. Effects of exercise on sleep. Clin Sports Med 2005; 24:355-336.
81. Thompson HJ. Effects of physical activity and exercise on experimentally-induced mammary carcinogenesis. Breast Cancer Res Treat 1997; 46:135-141.
82. Pitts G, Bull L. Exercise, dietary obesity and growth in the rat. Am J Physiol Regul Integr Comp Physiol 1977; 232:38-44.
83. Tsai AC, Rosenberg R, Borer KT. Metabolic alterations induced by voluntary exercise and discontinuation of exercise in hamsters. Am J Clin Nutr 1982; 35:943-949.
84. Yuan Q, Fontenele-Neto JD, Fricker LD. Effect of voluntary exercise on genetically obese Cpe$^{fat/fat}$ mice quantitative proteomics of serum. Obes Res 2004; 12(7):1179-1188.
85. Coutinho AE, Fediuc S, Campbell JE et al. Metabolic effects of voluntary wheel running in young and old Syrian golden hamsters. Physiol Behav 2005; 87:360-367.
86. Barbour KA, Edenfield TM, Blumenthal JA. Exercise as a treatment for depression and other psychiatric disorders. J Cardiopulm Rehabil Prev 2007; 27:359-367.
87. Bono JPD, Adlam D, Paterson DJ et al. Novel quantitative phenotypes of exercise training in mouse models. Am J Physiol Regulatory Integrative Comp Physiol 2005; 290:926-934.
88. Sutton GM, Perez-Tilve D, Nogueiras R et al. The melanocortin-3 receptor is required for entrainment to meal intake. J Neurosci 2008; 28(48):12946-12955.

CHAPTER 5

Melanocortins in Brain Inflammation:
The Role of Melanocortin Receptor Subtypes

Ruta Muceniece* and Maija Dambrova

Abstract

The melanocortins (MC) are released from neurons and paracrine cells in the CNS where they are involved in important physiological functions, including regulation of body temperature and immune responses. MC bind to melanocortin receptors, a class of cell surface G-protein-coupled receptors. Of the five subtypes of MC receptors that have been cloned in mammals, the MC1, MC3, MC4 and MC5 receptors are expressed in brain tissues. Expression of MC receptors in both brain cells and cells of the immune system suggests direct involvement of MC in regulation of inflammatory processes in the brain. The binding of MC to MC receptors induces activation of adenylate cyclase, increase in intracellular cAMP level and, consequently, inhibition of the nuclear transcription factor kappaB (NF-κB) signalling. Inflammatory processes contribute to development of severe CNS diseases, both in acute and chronic conditions. Thus far, the anti-inflammatory effects of MC in the CNS have been mainly studied using peptides that are relatively unselective for individual MC receptor subtypes. Consequently, these studies do not allow identification of specific MC receptor(s) involved in the regulation of inflammatory processes. However, recently synthesized ligands selective for individual MC receptors indicated that both MC4 and MC3 agonists are promising anti-inflammatory agents in treatment of brain inflammation.

Introduction

The melanocyte-stimulating hormones (collectively referred to as melanocortins or MC) are a class of endogenous peptides that were originally found in cells of the intermediate lobe of the pituitary gland. The first scientific report on biological activity of MCs appeared in 1912 when Fuchs et al demonstrated that pituitary extracts darken the skin of frogs.[1] The recent cloning of five MC receptor subtypes prompted localization studies showing expression of MC1, MC3, MC4 and MC5 receptors in the brain.[2-4] Subsequently, it was discovered that MCs are involved in important physiological functions, including regulation of body temperature and immune responses.[3,5] This chapter discusses the role of MCs in regulation of brain inflammation processes with respect to activity of receptor-subtype selective compounds.

Distribution of MC Expressing Neurons and MC Receptors in the Brain

MCs, namely α-, β-, γMSH and ACTH, are generated by posttranslation processing of the precursor pro-opiomelanocortin (POMC) that is cleaved in a tissue-specific manner. In the brain, MCs-expressing neurons are found mainly in the arcuate nucleus of hypothalamus, zona incerta

*Corresponding Author: Ruta Muceniece—Faculty of Medicine, University of Latvia, Sarlotes St. 1a, Riga, LV-1001, Latvia. Email: ruta.muceniece@lu.lv

Melanocortins: Multiple Actions and Therapeutic Potential, edited by Anna Catania.
©2010 Landes Bioscience and Springer Science+Business Media.

and the nucleus of solitary tract in the brain stem. MC-ergic fibers from these neurons project throughout the brain.[1,3,6-8]

By using MSH peptide-specific antibodies, αMSH immunoreactivity is found in all MC-expressing neurons and projecting fibers e.g., forebrain, amygdala, striatum, nucleus accumbens, epithalamus, thalamus, septal area, hypothalamus-preoptic area, midbrain, hindbrain and spinal cord. βMSH immunoreactivity has been detected in the human hypothalamus, but γMSH immunoreactive neurones are demonstrated in two nuclei: the arcuate nucleus and nucleus commissuralis. γMSH-ergic fibers from the arcuate nucleus of hypothalamus innervate the hypothalamus, thalamus, amygdala, forebrain, diencephalon, central gray matter of the midbrain and upper pons, whereas from nucleus commissuralis γMSH immunoreactive fibers project to the medulla oblongata.[1,2,9,10]

The existence of MC specific binding sites in the brain was established by using radioiodinated αMSH and its synthetic analogue, NDP-MSH (Nle[4], D-Phe[7]-αMSH). [2,3,11-13] NDP-MSH binding sites in the brain were found to be distributed more broadly relative to the POMC innervation regions.[2,8,12] Because NDP-αMSH recognizes all the MC receptors, these early studies could not identify specific receptor subtype distribution within the brain. However, the existence of heterogenous receptors was postulated based on differences in binding affinity in different brain regions.[7]

The cloning of five MC receptor subtypes in early 1990s spurred MC-related research significantly.[14-18] Then it became possible to study precise distribution of MC receptors by using corresponding gene cDNA or mRNA, or receptor protein structure data. The studies on distribution of cDNA for all five MC receptor subtypes in human tissue revealed limited distribution of MC1 and MC5 within the brain.[11,12] Whereas MC3 and MC4 were suggested to be the brain receptors.[2,3,19-21]

More detailed distribution studies and comparison with the earlier published distribution of immunoreactivity of the MSH peptides were carried out by using mRNA detection technologies.[12,22-24] As expected from pharmacological profile of MC3 and MC4 receptors,[2,3] the distribution of MC3 mRNA corresponds well with γMSH immunoreactivity.[5,6,24] MC3 mRNA-containing neurons are largely localized in arcuate nucleus and hippocampal formation of forebrain-projecting POMC neurons and in only a few brainstem nuclei.[24]

However, MC3 receptor protein autoradiography studies revealed much wider distribution of the receptor protein compared to that of mRNA. The finding that a large portion of POMC neurons express MC3 receptor led to the proposal of presynaptic localization of MC3 receptor and its role as autoreceptor, regulating the release of MSH peptides from POMC neurons.[3]

MC4 receptor is expressed in the brain much more abundantly than MC3. Neurons that express mRNA for MC4 include more than 100 different discrete brain structures. Overlapping MC3/MC4 mRNA-containing neuron distribution corresponds well with NDP-MSH binding sites.[12,23] However, in several hypothalamic regions MC4 mRNA is abundant and its expression does not overlap with that of MC3 receptor. MC4 mRNA presence in paraventricular nucleus suggests a role for MC4 in neuroendocrine control. The most mRNA for MC4 and MC4 receptor protein are expressed in ventrolateral part of the ventromedial hypothalamic nuclei which is related to neural control of feeding and reproductivity, whereas mRNA for MC3 are expressed in the dorsomedial part.[10,22-25] Also, presence of mRNA for MC4 expressing cells in preoptic, hypothalamic and brainstem nuclei implicated in thermoregulation and fever was found and a role for MC4 in neuroinflammation suggested.[9] MC4 receptors were found not only on neurons but also on glial cells. Indeed, astrocytes also known as astrocytic glial cells, which upon injury of nerve cells and inflammation stimuli become phagocytic, express MC4 receptor protein but not MC3. This fact confirmed the MC4 role in neuroinflammation, stroke therapy and neuroprotection in hypoxia-ischemic brain injury. [6,9,26]

Presence of mRNA for MC1 receptor in mouse brain,[27] murine brain microvascular endothelial cells,[28] human astrocytic cell line A-172,[29] and rat and human periaqueductal gray,[4] demonstrate limited distribution of MC1 in the CNS. The MC1 receptors may play some role in the MCs central effects due to the high MSH peptide binding potency.[30]

Also, mRNA for MC5 receptor were found in human, rat and mouse brain.[3,14,31] However, the role of MC5 in the brain is not clear yet and detailed its distribution within brain structures is not described.

MCR Subtypes and Brain Inflammation

The presence of MC3 and MC4 receptors and, to less extent, MC1 and MC5 receptors in the brain structures suggests that each of them could mediate the anti-inflammatory action of the MCs and other MC receptor active substances. The most convincing evidence about the protective effects against brain injury has been obtained using nonspecific MC receptor agonists.[6] However, these compounds can only show that MC receptors have a role in regulation of inflammatory processes, but do not provide information about receptor subtype. The involvement of specific MC receptor subtypes is deduced from pharmacological studies with receptor subtype selective ligands and animal models. For example, it was concluded that MC1 receptor does not mediate the anti-inflammatory actions of αMSH in the brain because it was shown that αMSH inhibits NF-κB activation in acute brain inflammation even in mice with nonfunctional MC1 receptor.[32] However, since the proportion of MC1 receptor and also MC5 receptor in the brain tissues is relatively small, the contribution of these receptors to overall MC receptor-mediated anti-inflammatory effect might be minor and difficult to trace in vivo.

To date the main candidates in mediation of anti-inflammatory signals within the brain are the MC3 and MC4 receptors. Indeed, it was shown that the MC3/MC4 receptor antagonists HS014 and SHU9119 block αMSH-induced effects on production of inflammatory cytokines within CNS.[33] In an earlier study we showed that the anti-inflammatory effect of βMSH in the acute bacterial lipopolysaccharides (LPS)-induced brain inflammation model was blocked by the MC3/MC4 receptor antagonist HS014.[34] Although HS014 has binding preference for MC4 receptors, its antagonistic selectivity for the MC4 versus MC3 receptor is too low to discriminate between the two receptors in the paradigm used.[34,35]

In the absence of selective antagonists, the peptides with different, non-overlapping affinity profiles for MC receptor subtypes can be used. In such studies, we evaluated the anti-inflammatory effects of low-affinity MC4 receptor peptide ligands in brain inflammation models. The correlation analysis of effect-MC-receptor selectivity indicated the leading MC3 receptor role for the anti-inflammatory effects of peptides.[36] In other studies, the MC3 receptor dependent anti-inflammatory action of the MCs was suggested by use of agonists with a higher selectivity toward MC3 receptor (γ2MSH, MTII) and MC receptor antagonists (more information in the reviews in refs. 37,38). However, thus far there are no MC3 receptor selective synthetic ligands available and this hinders more precise investigations.

The most abundant glial cell population in brain tissues is astrocytes which play an active role in immune responses and tissue repair.[39] Astrocytes do not express MC3 receptor whereas the activation of MC4 receptor in these cells reduces the inflammatory response and prevents apoptosis induced by LPS and interferon (INF-γ).[26] Experiments based on MC receptor agonists and antagonists (e.g., the nonselective antagonist HS024) have led to similar conclusions on involvement of MC4 receptors in regulation of inflammation in the brain. Data showed that αMSH inhibits inducible nitric oxide (NO) synthase (NOS2) activity and expression of the cyclooxygenase-2 (COX2) gene via activation of MC4 receptor in the hypothalamus of male rat;[40] the peptide likewise reduces inflammatory mediator production in glial and neural cells.[6,9] Pharmacological blockade of MC4 receptors prevented the neuroprotective effect of NDP-MSH in a severe model of focal cerebral ischemia, suggesting that MC receptor agonists could produce neuroprotection in different experimental models of ischemic stroke.[41] Consistently, our data show that the MC4 receptor-selective compound THIQ weakly antagonizes LPS-induced NO overproduction in the mice brain after intracisternal administration.[42] A similar, though smaller, effect was exerted by MC3 receptor ligands.[34,43] Recently, lack of protection of another selective MC4 receptor agonist RY767 in rat transient middle cerebral artery occlusion model has been reported.[44]

It should be considered that there is no uniquely selective MC receptor antagonist that can unequivocally indicate which MC receptor subtype is involved in MC receptor-mediated anti-inflammatory effects in vivo. Indeed, the antagonists (SHU119, HS024, HS014) have been shown to be selective towards MC3 or MC4 receptor in the binding assay, but they are nonselective inhibitors of αMSH-stimulated cAMP generation.[35,45] MC receptor agonists (MSH peptides, NDP-MSH) are likewise only partially selective in activation of MC receptor subtypes.[3,11,17,30]

Within brain tissues, compensatory up-regulation of individual MC receptor subtypes likely occurs in response to inflammatory stimuli and/or in physiological conditions. Thus, despite the large number of MC receptor subtype selective substances that have been designed, the relative low selectivity of most of them together with the colocalization of different MC receptor subtypes in the same tissues make difficult a clear-cut definition of which MC receptor subtype is involved in mediation of anti-inflammatory effects.

Main Intracellular Signalling Pathways of MC Receptors

MC receptors are cell surface G-protein coupled receptors (GPCRs) and the main physiological responses of MC are mediated through adenylate cyclase (AC) activation (Fig. 1) to increase levels of cAMP within the cell.[2,5,10,11,19] cAMP target in cells is protein kinase A (PKA). AC is a key enzyme that couples with both the stimulatory and inhibitory G proteins (Gs and Gi), while Gq coupled GPCRs activate phospholipase C (PLC) and trigger the inositol phosphate (IP)/Ca^{2+} cascade. In MC3 and MC4 receptor activation, IP/Ca^{2+} pathway may also be stimulated by cAMP targeted PKA.[46,47] In addition to PKA activation, cAMP regulates the activity of cAMP-gated channels and Rap1-specific guanine nucleotide exchange factors, which facilitate links with mitogen-activated protein kinases (MAPK) cascade. GPCRs can stimulate the MAPK cascade via a few principle pathways: Ras-dependent activation of MAPK via transactivation of receptor tyrosine kinases, Ras-independent MAPK activation via protein kinase C (PKC) at the level of Raf and activation as well as inactivation of MAPK via the cAMP/PKA pathway in dependency on the type of Raf.[48] The recently discovered MC3 and MC4 receptor mediated influences on cell proliferation, differentiation, development, stress responses and apoptosis through MAPK signalling cascades by stimulation of ERK1/2 phosphorylation confirm cross-talk between PKA and MAPK pathways.[6,9,49-51]

It is important to know how activation of AC leads to expression of different genes tht provide start or stop signals for the physiological responses of cells e.g., release of pro-inflammatory or anti-inflammatory agents (Fig. 1). MCs act at least on two transcription factors: cAMP responsible element binding protein (CREB) and NF-κB. CREB in its activated form regulates cell proliferation, differentiation and survival. CREB switches on and off genes responsible for impaired immune responses and long term memory.[3,52]

However, the main mechanism of neuroprotective action of MC has been explained by inhibition of NF-κB translocation to cell nuclei induced by various inflammatory agents.[3,6,10,53] In cytoplasm, NF-κB exists in its resting state complexed to an inhibitory protein of the IκB family.[3,6,54] Phosphorilation of IκB occurs by multi-subunit IκB kinase (IKK) which activation is triggered by multiple pathways, among them from stimulation of cell surface receptors for tumour necrosis factor (TNF-α), LPS and interleukins (IL-1).[54] NF-κB is required for induction of large number of genes that regulate inflammation. Its activation leads to over-expression of several proteins—chemokines, cell adhesion molecules, NOS2, COX2, IL-1 and IL-6, etc.[54] As a consequence of NF-κB inhibition, MC reduce production of IL-1, IL-6, IL-8 and TNF, as well as adhesion molecules ICAM-1 and VCAM-1.[2,5,54,55]

Interactions between cAMP-dependent and NF-κB regulated pathways are complex and depend on cell type. Induction of NF-κB-dependent gene expression is inhibited by elevated

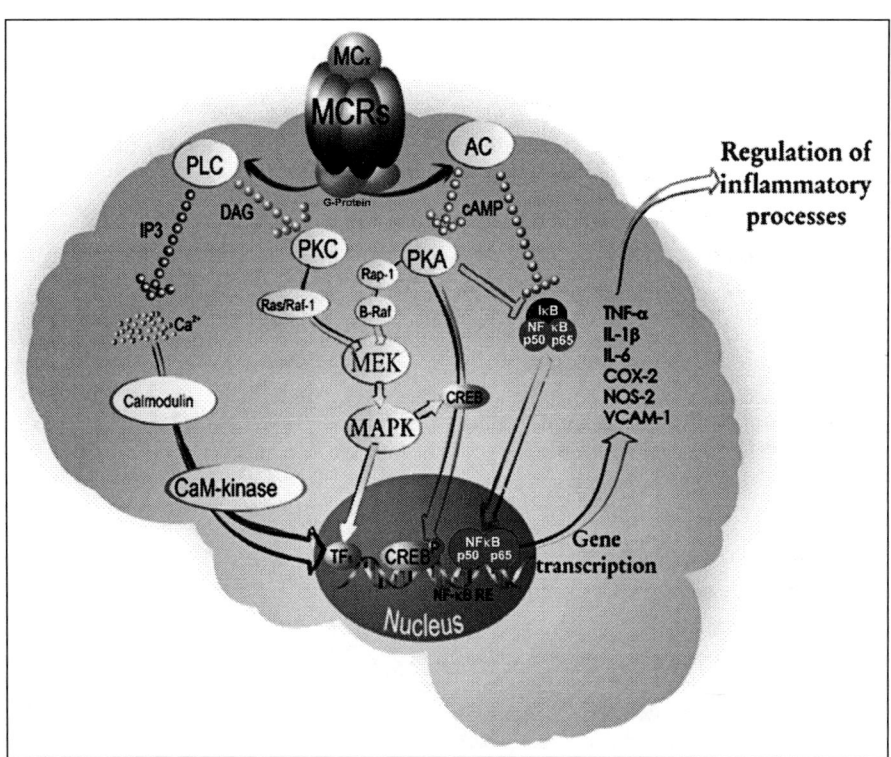

Figure 1. Schematic model for MC receptor signaling. Binding of MC receptor ligands activates adenylate cyclase (AC) and phospholipase C (PLC). Activation of AC leads to the production of cAMP. Then cAMP activates protein kinase A (PKA) leading to the phosphorilation of the cAMP-responsive element-binding protein (CREB) and interaction with mitogen activated protein kinases (MEK/MAPK) cascade, as well as to the inhibition of degradation of inhibitor (IκBα) of the nuclear factor-κB (NF-κB). Thus, MCs inhibit NF-κB translocation to the nucleus and the transcription of various inflammatory genes. Activation of PLC triggers the inositol phosphate (IP)/Ca²⁺ and diacylglycerol (DAG) pathways leading to the activation or inhibition of transcription factors (TF). DAG activates protein kinase C (PKC) and triggers PKC-mediated specific protein (Ras/Raf-1 etc.) phosphorylation in the cell-type specific way.

cAMP and by over-expression of the catalytic subunit of PKA (PKAc).[56] Cellular CREB binding protein (CBP) forms a complex with the phosphorylated NF-κB that is obligatory for its transcriptional activity. At the same time CBP is also involved in regulation of CREB transcriptional activity therefore cAMP-mediated inhibition of NF-κB may be due to competition between activated CREB and NF-κB for a limited CBP binding sites.[57] Also, inhibition of phosphodiesterases that results in elevated cAMP level, significantly reduces IκB phosphorylation and DNA binding activity of NF-κB but enhances DNA binding activity of CREB.[58] However, cAMP and partially PKA independent mechanism for regulating NF-κB nuclear translocation is also suggested.[73] Indeed, PKAc is maintained in an inactive state in NF-κB-IκB-PKAc complex and, when IκB degradates, transcriptional activity of NF-κB is regulated by PKAc subunit through cAMP-independent pathway.[59]

The CREB/CRE transcriptional pathway is activated by MC and regulates the expression of COX2. Dual role of COX2 (excitotoxic and neuroprotective) is described in the dependence on the model systems and stimulus paradigms used. Prostaglandins (PG) PGE-1, PGE-2 and PGI2 released due to the COX-mediated metabolism of arachidonic acid (AA) are shown to be protectants against hypoxia, glutamate-induced neurotoxicity and trauma.[60] Interestingly, the signalling pathway of neuroprotective action of PGE2 is similar to that of MC and is mediated through increase in intracellular cAMP level.[60] In contrast, the anti-inflammatory action of MC may result from inhibition of over-stimulated PG synthesis via inhibition of NF-κB pathway and further to the inhibition of COX2 expression.[9,26,40] Also, MC receptors have recognition sites for protein kinase C (PKC) that links MC receptors to the phospholipase A2 (PLA2) pathway and directly to inhibition of the AA metabolism.[10]

Another controversial endogenous agent in line with PGs is TNF. Under pathological conditions, TNF targets AC in microglia (where MC4 and MC1 receptors are found) that results in reduced cAMP synthesis. Low cAMP level contributes to expression of potentially neurotoxic molecules—IL-12 and IL-1β, NO, chemokines and major histocompatibility complex.[55] MSH peptides in concentration-dependent fashion inhibit production of TNF, IL-6 and NO in LPS and IFN-γ activated microglial cells, probably by increasing cAMP level.[56]

Although MCs may activate diverse signalling pathways (Fig. 1), as key element nowadays is accepted inhibition of NF-κB translocation in nuclei with following decrease of NO over-production by activated NOS2. The anti-inflammatory effects of MCs have a regulatory nature. In line with capacity to reduce all main inflammation markers—cytokine and chemokine production, oxidative stress and inflammatory cell migration—MCs do not change physiological low levels of cytokines and NO if tissue or cells are not activated by proinflammatory stimuli.[34,36,45,56,61]

Potential Therapeutic Applications of MC Receptor Subtype Selective Compounds

It is now clear that inflammation and inflammatory mediators contribute to both acute CNS injury during stroke and cerebral ischemia, brain trauma, epilepsy, as well as chronic CNS diseases, such as multiple sclerosis, Alzheimer's disease, Parkinson's disease.[60,62-64]

Native MC reduce the main aspects of inflammation, such as inflammatory mediator production, oxidative stress and inflammatory cell migration, as it is illustrated by recent review articles describing neuroprotective potential of MC.[6,9,65] The protective effects of MC receptor ligands are expected to find broad therapeutic applications. Therefore, MC receptor active compounds have been continuously synthesized and tested for possible therapeutic applications.[65]

As summarized in Table 1, both native MC peptides and synthetic ligands with differing selectivity for MC receptor subtypes have been tested in CNS inflammation-related experimental models in vivo. The most studied peptide, αMSH, acts as a significant modulator of host reactions including fever and inflammation.[5,6,19,38,66,67] Since αMSH antagonizes pyrogenic and proinflammatory effects of cytokines such as IL-1, IL-6, TNF and IFN-γ, cytokine antagonism is believed to be responsible for at least part of the anti-inflammatory/antipyretic influence of αMSH.[5] The mechanism of action of αMSH is mediated through rapid prevention of IκBα degradation and subsequent modulation of NF-κB-mediated transcription inhibition, as it was shown in glioma cells and in experimental brain inflammation.[3,32,53] Two other native MC peptides, βMSH and γMSH, are studied in models of brain inflammation to much lesser extent. However, in model of LPS-induced brain inflammation model, both βMSH and γMSH were more active inhibitors of NO production than αMSH[34] and in the case of βMSH the protective effect was shown to be NF-κB pathway-dependent and blocked by HS014.[47] These findings suggest that, in addition to αMSH, also βMSH and γMSH peptides may have specific functions in the regulation of brain inflammatory processes.

Centrally administered MC exert anti-pyretic effect by acting through central MC receptors.[66-69] As an additional evidence for MC receptor-mediated central regulation of body temperature serves finding that intracerebroventricular (icv), but not intravenous (iv) administration of SHU9119 exacerbated fever in rats.[67] Both MC3[67] and MC4 receptor[68] have been mentioned as possible mediators of antipyretic activities of MC receptor ligands. It must be noted again that conclusion about specific MC receptor subtype was drawn by using MCR3/4 antagonists SHU9119 and HS014, but this approach in in vivo models has not been predictive enough.

Table 1. The brain inflammation and injury linked effects of MC receptor ligands

Compound	Receptor Activity/Selectivity	Model, Effect	References
αMSH	*MC receptor agonist with binding potency MC1>MC3>MC4>MC5	Anti-pyretic, anti-inflammatory	27,34,65 * 30
βMSH	*MC receptor agonist with binding potency MC1>MC3>MC4>MC5	Anti-inflammatory in LPS induced brain inflammation	34,43 * 30
γ1,2MSH	*MC receptor agonist with binding potency MC1 = MC3 and almost nonbinding to MC5 and MC4	Anti-inflammatory in LPS induced brain inflammation	34, * 30
γ2MSH	*MC receptor agonist with binding potency MC1 = MC3 and almost nonbinding to MC5 and MC4	No effect, ischemic stroke	70, * 30
SHU9119	**MC3/MC4 receptor antagonist	Icv, exacerbates fever in rats	67, ** 35
RY767	MC4 receptor agonist	No effect, rat transient middle cerebral artery occlusion	44
NDP- αMSH	*Nonselective MC receptor agonist with binding potency MC1>MC3≥MC4≥MC5	Brain ischemia, improvement	41,70,71, * 30
THIQ	MC4 receptor agonist (in vitro)	LPS-induced brain inflammation, partial improvement	42
ME10501	MC4 receptor agonist	Spinal cord injury, protective	71,72
Ro27-3225	MC4 receptor agonist	Haemorrhagic shock	71
HS024	***MC4 receptor antagonist unselective in cAMP assay with the order of binding affinity: MC4≫MC3≫MC5>MC1;	Blocks effects of αMSH in LPS induced inflammation in astrocites	40, *** 45
HS014	**MC3/MC4 receptor antagonist with order of the binding affinity: MC4≫MC3>MC1>MC5	Blocks effects of βMSH in LPS induced brain inflammation	43, ** 35

*Schioth et al, 1996
**Schioth et al, 1999
***Kask et al, 1998

In a gerbil model of ischemic stroke, the αMSH analogue NDP-MSH modulated the inflammatory and apoptotic cascades and reduced hippocampus injuries even when delayed up to 9 h after ischemia, with a dose-dependent improvement in subsequent functional recovery.[41,70]

The neurotropic effect of the MC receptor ligands has been suggested also in pathophysiology of spinal cord injury following trauma as peripheral nerve regeneration.[6] In these experimental conditions, the neuroprotective effect was shown for MC4 receptor synthetic agonist ME10501 in a rat model of spinal cord injury.[72,73]

Conclusion

It is clear that MC receptors and their ligands are potent inhibitors of inflammatory processes within the CNS. Therefore, MC receptor agonists are potential drugs for treatment of global cerebral ischemia and reperfusion, focal cerebral ischemia, brain inflammation and traumatic injury. Recognition of the receptor(s) subtypes involved in this protective action would be important for therapeutic development. Unfortunately, most of the in vivo experiments are based on MC-receptor unselective compounds. This prevents unequivocal identification of a specific MC receptor subtype as the most important for treatment of inflammation-related conditions within brain. The anti-neuroinflammatory effects of MC may depend on the localization of MC receptor subtypes in the corresponding brain structure, as well as on the colocalization with other receptor subtypes and cross-talk of signalling pathways.

MC receptors are very promising targets for therapeutical applications in brain inflammatory conditions. Targeting multiple MC receptors with small molecule agonists might provide novel therapeutic strategy for the treatment of acute and chronic disorders of the nervous system.

Acknowledgements

The authors acknowledge Dr. pharm. E. Liepinsh for assistance and preparation of figure.

References

1. Eberle AN. The Melanotropins. Chemistry, Physiology and Mechanism of Action. Basel: Karger Press 1998.
2. Wikberg JE. Melanocortin receptors: perspectives for novel drugs. Eur J Pharmacol 1999; 375:295-310.
3. Wikberg JE, Muceniece R, Mandrika I et al. New aspects on the melanocortins and their receptors. Pharmacol Res 2000; 42:393-420.
4. Xia Y, Wikberg JE, Chhajlani V. Expression of melanocortin 1 receptor in periaqueductal gray matter. Neuroreport 1995; 6:2193-2196.
5. Catania A, Gatti S, Colombo G et al. Targeting melanocortin receptors as a novel strategy to control inflammation. Pharmacol Rev 2004; 56:1-29.
6. Catania A. Neuroprotective actions of melanocortins: a therapeutic opportunity. Trends Neurosci 2008; 31:353-360.
7. Tatro JB, Entwistle ML. Heterogeneity of brain melanocortin receptors suggested by differential ligand binding in situ. Brain Res 1994; 635:148-158.
8. Tatro JB, Reichlin S. Specific receptors for alpha-melanocyte-stimulating hormone are widely distributed in tissues of rodents. Endocrinology 1987; 121:1900-1907.
9. Lasaga M, Debeljuk L, Durand D et al. Role of alpha-melanocyte stimulating hormone and melanocortin 4 receptor in brain inflammation. Peptides 2008; 29:1825-1835.
10. Starowicz K, Przewlocka B. The role of melanocortins and their receptors in inflammatory processes, nerve regeneration and nociception. Life Sci 2003; 73:823-847.
11. Adan RA, Gispen WH. Brain melanocortin receptors: from cloning to function. Peptides 1997; 18:1279-1287.
12. Low M, Simerly RB, Cone RD. Receptors for the melanocortin peptides in the central nervous system. Curr Opin Endocrinol Diabetes 1994; 1:79-88.
13. Tatro JB. Receptor biology of the melanocortins, a family of neuroimmunomodulatory peptides. Neuroimmunomodulation 1996; 3:259-284.
14. Chhajlani V, Muceniece R, Wikberg JE. Molecular cloning of a novel human melanocortin receptor. Biochem Biophys Res Commun 1993; 195:866-873.
15. Chhajlani V, Wikberg JE. Molecular cloning and expression of the human melanocyte stimulating hormone receptor cDNA (FEBS 11553). FEBS Lett 1992; 309:417-420.
16. Gantz I, Konda Y, Tashiro T et al. Molecular cloning of a novel melanocortin receptor. J Biol Chem 1993; 268:8246-8250.
17. Gantz I, Miwa H, Konda Y et al. Molecular cloning, expression and gene localization of a fourth melanocortin receptor. J Biol Chem 1993; 268:15174-15179.
18. Mountjoy KG, Robbins LS, Mortrud MT et al. The cloning of a family of genes that encode the melanocortin receptors. Science 1992; 257:1248-1251.
19. Adan RA, Oosterom J, Toonen RF et al. Molecular pharmacology of neural melanocortin receptors. Receptors Channels 1997; 5:215-223.
20. Chhajlani V. Distribution of cDNA for melanocortin receptor subtypes in human tissues. Biochem Mol Biol Int 1996; 38:73-80.

21. Magenis RE, Smith L, Nadeau JH et al. Mapping of the ACTH, MSH and neural (MC3 and MC4) melanocortin receptors in the mouse and human. Mamm Genome 1994; 5:503-508.
22. Kishi T, Aschkenasi CJ, Lee CE et al. Expression of melanocortin 4 receptor mRNA in the central nervous system of the rat. J Comp Neurol 2003; 457:213-235.
23. Mountjoy KG, Mortrud MT, Low MJ et al. Localization of the melanocortin-4 receptor (MC4-R) in neuroendocrine and autonomic control circuits in the brain. Mol Endocrinol 1994; 8:1298-1308.
24. Roselli-Rehfuss L, Mountjoy KG, Robbins LS et al. Identification of a receptor for gamma melanotropin and other proopiomelanocortin peptides in the hypothalamus and limbic system. Proc Natl Acad Sci USA 1993; 90:8856-8860.
25. Paues J, Mackerlova L, Blomqvist A. Expression of melanocortin-4 receptor by rat parabrachial neurons responsive to immune and aversive stimuli. Neuroscience 2006; 141:287-297.
26. Caruso C, Durand D, Schioth HB et al. Activation of melanocortin 4 receptors reduces the inflammatory response and prevents apoptosis induced by lipopolysaccharide and interferon-gamma in astrocytes. Endocrinology 2007; 148:4918-4926.
27. Rajora N, Boccoli G, Burns D et al. alpha-MSH modulates local and circulating tumor necrosis factor-alpha in experimental brain inflammation. J Neurosci 1997; 17:2181-2186.
28. de AE, Sahm UG, Ahmed AR et al. Identification of a melanocortin receptor expressed by murine brain microvascular endothelial cells in culture. Microvasc Res 1995; 50:25-34.
29. Wong KY, Rajora N, Boccoli G et al. A potential mechanism of local anti-inflammatory action of alpha-melanocyte-stimulating hormone within the brain: modulation of tumor necrosis factor-alpha production by human astrocytic cells. Neuroimmunomodulation 1997; 4:37-41.
30. Schioth HB, Muceniece R, Wikberg JE. Characterisation of the melanocortin 4 receptor by radioligand binding. Pharmacol Toxicol 1996; 79:161-165.
31. Fathi Z, Iben LG, Parker EM. Cloning, expression and tissue distribution of a fifth melanocortin receptor subtype. Neurochem Res 1995; 20:107-113.
32. Ichiyama T, Sakai T, Catania A et al. Systemically administered alpha-melanocyte-stimulating peptides inhibit NF-kappaB activation in experimental brain inflammation. Brain Res 1999; 836:31-37.
33. Cragnolini AB, Perello M, Schioth HB et al. alpha-MSH and gamma-MSH inhibit IL-1beta induced activation of the hypothalamic-pituitary-adrenal axis through central melanocortin receptors. Regul Pept 2004; 122:185-190.
34. Muceniece R, Zvejniece L, Kirjanova O et al. Beta- and gamma-melanocortins inhibit lipopolysaccharide induced nitric oxide production in mice brain. Brain Res 2004; 995:7-13.
35. Schioth HB, Muceniece R, Mutulis F et al. Further pharmacological characterization of the selective melanocortin 4 receptor antagonist HS014: comparison with SHU9119. Neuropeptides 1999; 33:191-196.
36. Muceniece R, Zvejniece L, Liepinsh E et al. The MC3 receptor binding affinity of melanocortins correlates with the nitric oxide production inhibition in mice brain inflammation model. Peptides 2006; 27:1443-1450.
37. Lam CW, Getting SJ. Melanocortin receptor type 3 as a potential target for anti-inflammatory therapy. Curr Drug Targets Inflamm Allergy 2004; 3:311-315.
38. Getting SJ, Perretti M. MC3-R as a novel target for antiinflammatory therapy. Drug News Perspect 2000; 13:19-27.
39. Farina C, Aloisi F, Meinl E. Astrocytes are active players in cerebral innate immunity. Trends Immunol 2007; 28:138-145.
40. Caruso C, Mohn C, Karara AL et al. Alpha-melanocyte-stimulating hormone through melanocortin-4 receptor inhibits nitric oxide synthase and cyclooxygenase expression in the hypothalamus of male rats. Neuroendocrinology 2004; 79:278-286.
41. Giuliani D, Ottani A, Mioni C et al. Neuroprotection in focal cerebral ischemia owing to delayed treatment with melanocortins. Eur J Pharmacol 2007; 570:57-65.
42. Muceniece R, Zvejniece L, Vilskersts R et al. Functional evaluation of THIQ, a melanocortin 4 receptor agonist, in models of food intake and inflammation. Basic Clin Pharmacol Toxicol 2007; 101:416-420.
43. Muceniece R, Zvejniece L, Kirjanova O et al. Beta-MSH inhibits brain inflammation via MC(3)/(4) receptors and impaired NF-kappaB signaling. J Neuroimmunol 2005; 169:13-19.
44. Regan C, Shepherd C, Strack A et al. Lack of protection with a novel, selective melanocortin receptor subtype-4 agonist RY767 in a rat transient middle cerebral artery occlusion stroke model. Pharmacology 2009; 83:38-44.
45. Kask A, Mutulis F, Muceniece R et al. Discovery of a novel superpotent and selective melanocortin-4 receptor antagonist (HS024): evaluation in vitro and in vivo. Endocrinology 1998; 139:5006-5014.
46. Konda Y, Gantz I, DelValle J et al. Interaction of dual intracellular signaling pathways activated by the melanocortin-3 receptor. J Biol Chem 1994; 269:13162-13166.
47. Newman EA, Chai BX, Zhang W et al. Activation of the melanocortin-4 receptor mobilizes intracellular free calcium in immortalized hypothalamic neurons. J Surg Res 2006; 132:201-207.

48. Robinson-White A, Stratakis CA. Protein kinase A signaling: "cross-talk" with other pathways in endocrine cells. Ann NY Acad Sci 2002; 968:256-270.
49. Chai B, Li JY, Zhang W et al. Melanocortin-3 receptor activates MAP kinase via PI3 kinase. Regul Pept 2007; 139:115-121.
50. Chai B, Li JY, Zhang W et al. Melanocortin-4 receptor-mediated inhibition of apoptosis in immortalized hypothalamic neurons via mitogen-activated protein kinase. Peptides 2006; 27:2846-2857.
51. Ho HY, Lee HH, Lai MZ. Overexpression of mitogen-activated protein kinase kinase kinase reversed cAMP inhibition of NF-kappaB in T-cells. Eur J Immunol 1997; 27:222-226.
52. Lonze BE, Ginty DD. Function and regulation of CREB family transcription factors in the nervous system. Neuron 2002; 35:605-623.
53. Ichiyama T, Sakai T, Catania A et al. Inhibition of peripheral NF-kappaB activation by central action of alpha-melanocyte-stimulating hormone. J Neuroimmunol 1999; 99:211-217.
54. Siebenlist U, Franzoso G, Brown K. Structure, regulation and function of NF-kappa B. Annu Rev Cell Biol 1994; 10:405-455.
55. Patrizio M. Tumor necrosis factor reduces cAMP production in rat microglia. Glia 2004; 48:241-249.
56. Delgado R, Carlin A, Airaghi L et al. Melanocortin peptides inhibit production of proinflammatory cytokines and nitric oxide by activated microglia. J Leukoc Biol 1998; 63:740-745.
57. Parry GC, Mackman N. Role of cyclic AMP response element-binding protein in cyclic AMP inhibition of NF-kappaB-mediated transcription. J Immunol 1997; 159:5450-5456.
58. Deree J, Martins JO, Melbostad H et al. Insights into the regulation of TNF-alpha production in human mononuclear cells: the effects of nonspecific phosphodiesterase inhibition. Clinics 2008; 63:321-328.
59. Zhong H, SuYang H, Erdjument-Bromage H et al. The transcriptional activity of NF-kappaB is regulated by the IkappaB-associated PKAc subunit through a cyclic AMP-independent mechanism. Cell 1997; 89:413-424.
60. Kim EJ, Kwon KJ, Park JY et al. Neuroprotective effects of prostaglandin E2 or cAMP against microglial and neuronal free radical mediated toxicity associated with inflammation. J Neurosci Res 2002; 70:97-107.
61. Galimberti D, Baron P, Meda L et al. Alpha-MSH peptides inhibit production of nitric oxide and tumor necrosis factor-alpha by microglial cells activated with beta-amyloid and interferon gamma. Biochem Biophys Res Commun 1999; 263:251-256.
62. Farooqui AA, Horrocks LA, Farooqui T. Modulation of inflammation in brain: a matter of fat. J Neurochem 2007; 101:577-599.
63. Hamby ME, Gragnolati AR, Hewett SJ et al. TGF beta 1 and TNF alpha potentiate nitric oxide production in astrocyte cultures by recruiting distinct subpopulations of cells to express NOS-2. Neurochem Int 2008; 52:962-971.
64. Lucas SM, Rothwell NJ, Gibson RM. The role of inflammation in CNS injury and disease. Br J Pharmacol 2006; 147(Suppl 1):S232-S240.
65. Brzoska T, Luger TA, Maaser C et al. Alpha-melanocyte-stimulating hormone and related tripeptides: biochemistry, antiinflammatory and protective effects in vitro and in vivo and future perspectives for the treatment of immune-mediated inflammatory diseases. Endocr Rev 2008; 29:581-602.
66. Catania A, Lipton JM. Peptide modulation of fever and inflammation within the brain. Ann NY Acad Sci 1998; 856:62-68.
67. Huang QH, Entwistle ML, Alvaro JD et al. Antipyretic role of endogenous melanocortins mediated by central melanocortin receptors during endotoxin-induced fever. J Neurosci 1997; 17:3343-3351.
68. Sinha PS, Schioth HB, Tatro JB. Roles of the melanocortin-4 receptor in antipyretic and hyperthermic actions of centrally administered alpha-MSH. Brain Res 2004; 1001:150-158.
69. Luger TA, Scholzen TE, Brzoska T et al. New insights into the functions of alpha-MSH and related peptides in the immune system. Ann NY Acad Sci 2003; 994:133-140.
70. Giuliani D, Mioni C, Altavilla D et al. Both early and delayed treatment with melanocortin 4 receptor-stimulating melanocortins produces neuroprotection in cerebral ischemia. Endocrinology 2006; 147:1126-1135.
71. Giuliani D, Mioni C, Bazzani C et al. Selective melanocortin MC4 receptor agonists reverse haemorragic shock and prevent multiple organ damage. Br J Pharmacol 2007; 150:595-603.
72. Sharma HS. Neuroprotective effects of neurotrophins and melanocortins in spinal cord injury: an experimental study in the rat using pharmacological and morphological approaches. Ann NY Acad Sci 2005; 1053:407-421.
73. Sharma HS, Lundstedt T, Flardh M et al. Neuroprotective effects of melanocortins in CNS injury. Curr Pharm Des 2007; 13:1929-1941.

CHAPTER 6

Melanocortins and the Cholinergic Anti-Inflammatory Pathway

Daniela Giuliani, Alessandra Ottani, Domenica Altavilla, Carla Bazzani,
Francesco Squadrito and Salvatore Guarini*

Abstract

Experimental evidence indicates that small concentrations of inflammatory molecules produced by damaged tissues activate afferent signals through ascending vagus nerve fibers, that act as the sensory arm of an "inflammatory reflex". The subsequent activation of vagal efferent fibers, which represent the motor arm of the inflammatory reflex, rapidly leads to acetylcholine release in organs of the reticuloendothelial system. Acetylcholine interacts with $\alpha 7$ subunit-containing nicotinic receptors in tissue macrophages and other immune cells and rapidly inhibits the synthesis/release of tumor necrosis factor-α and other inflammatory cytokines. This neural anti-inflammatory response called "cholinergic anti-inflammatory pathway" is fast and integrated through the central nervous system. Preclinical studies are in progress, with the aim to develop therapeutic agents able to activate the cholinergic anti-inflammatory pathway. Melanocortin peptides bearing the adrenocorticotropin/α-melanocyte-stimulating hormone sequences exert a protective and life-saving effect in animals and humans in conditions of circulatory shock. These neuropeptides are likewise protective in other severe hypoxic conditions, such as prolonged respiratory arrest, myocardial ischemia, renal ischemia and ischemic stroke, as well as in experimental heart transplantation. Moreover, experimental evidence indicates that melanocortins reverse circulatory shock, prevent myocardial ischemia/reperfusion damage and exert neuroprotection against ischemic stroke through activation of the cholinergic anti-inflammatory pathway. This action occurs via stimulation of brain melanocortin MC_3/MC_4 receptors. Investigations that determine the molecular mechanisms of the cholinergic anti-inflammatory pathway activation could help design of superselective activators of this pathway.

Introduction

Melanocortins have long been considered to only exert control on endocrine and pigmentary processes. For the first time our Teacher, Professor William Ferrari, in 1955,[1-3] then Professor David De Wied[4] and over the subsequent decades several other independent groups, reported many important extra-hormonal effects of melanocortins.[5-10] In addition to the pituitary gland, production of melanocortins was also documented in a variety of peripheral tissues and within the central nervous system (CNS).[5,9,11] Altered production of these neuropeptides has been recognized among the causes of many morbid conditions including anorexia, hyperfagia, obesity, cachexia, pain, inflammation, sexual dysfunctions, circulatory shock, organ damage induced by ischemia/reperfusion, neurodegeneration.[5,7,9-13] α-Melanocyte-stimulating hormone (α-MSH) is the natural

*Corresponding Author: Salvatore Guarini—Department of Biomedical Sciences,
Section of Pharmacology, University of Modena and Reggio Emilia, Modena, Italy.
Email: salvatore.guarini@unimore.it

Melanocortins: Multiple Actions and Therapeutic Potential, edited by Anna Catania.
©2010 Landes Bioscience and Springer Science+Business Media.

melanocortin peptide able to induce all extra-hormonal effects of melanocortins. Identification and cloning of the five melanocortin receptors (MC_1-MC_5) in the nineties,[14-21] as well as the synthesis of selective agonists and antagonists at MC receptors,[13,16,21] increased the general interest for this family of molecules in view of their possible therapeutic use.[5,7,11,13,22-25]

The protective and resuscitating effects of melanocortins in extreme hypoxic condition appear particularly promising for therapeutic purposes. Adrenocorticotropin (ACTH)/α-MSH sequences, as well as shorter fragments and synthetic analogs, have a life-saving effect in animals and humans in conditions of circulatory shock.[26-34] These neuropeptides are likewise protective in other severe hypoxic conditions, including prolonged respiratory arrest,[35] myocardial ischemia,[36-41] renal ischemia[42-44] and ischemic stroke,[45-49] as well as in experimental heart transplantation.[50]

Preclinical evidence indicates that melanocortins produce their protective and life-saving effects, at least in part, by activating the recently recognized "cholinergic anti-inflammatory pathway", the motor arm of the "inflammatory reflex".[51-53]

The Inflammatory Reflex

In the past, the vagus nerve was only considered a part of the parasympathetic nervous system with precise functions, such as the regulation of heart and gut activities and respiration. However, more recent data have disclosed previously unrecognized functions of the vagus nerve. Electrical stimulation of the vagus nerve is currently approved for treatment of epilepsy and major depression; additional therapeutic uses under investigations include obesity, Alzheimer's disease, chronic pain and some neuropsychiatric disorders.[54,55] The mechanisms underlying the beneficial effects of the vagus nerve therapy are not fully understood.

The CNS modulates local and systemic inflammatory responses to various stressor agents through humoral and neural mechanisms.[56-58] High levels of cytokines and other inflammatory mediators can reach brain areas devoid of blood-brain barrier (dorsal vagal complex including the sensory nuclei of the solitary tract, area postrema and dorsal motor nucleus of the vagus).[59-61] This humoral route for communication between the immune system and the CNS seems to be involved in several processes, including fever, anorexia and activation of hypothalamic-pituitary responses. Knowledge of the humoral route was the base for development of anti-inflammatory drugs including glucocorticoids.[52,62-64]

Efferent vagus nerve signalling contributes to modulation of inflammation. Efferent vagal signalling may facilitate lymphocyte release from the thymus through a nicotinic acetylcholine receptor-mediated mechanism; moreover, clinical studies indicate that nicotine exerts beneficial influences in inflammatory bowel disease.[52] These observations led Tracey and coworkers to hypothesize that the parasympathetic nervous system could modulate the systemic inflammatory response, as an alternative mechanism for rapid cytokine control. They verified this hypothesis in experimental models of endotoxic shock in rats and their investigations led to the identification of the "cholinergic anti-inflammatory pathway", the motor arm of the "inflammatory reflex".[51] Low levels of inflammatory molecules produced in damaged tissues activate afferent signals through ascending vagus nerve fibers (neural inflammation-sensing pathways at low threshold of detection) and this could serve as the sensory arm of the inflammatory reflex.[52,62-64] The subsequent activation of vagus efferent activity, which includes the motor arm of the inflammatory reflex, rapidly leads to acetylcholine release in organs of the reticuloendothelial system (liver, lung, heart, spleen, kidney and gastrointestinal tract). Acetylcholine interacts with α7 subunit-containing nicotinic acetylcholine receptors in tissue macrophages and other immune cells surrounding the cholinergic terminals and rapidly inhibits synthesis/release of tumor necrosis factor-α (TNF-α), interleukin-1 (IL-1) and other cytokines: this neural anti-inflammatory response is fast and integrated within the CNS.[51-53,65] The old observations by Guarini and coworkers,[66,67] that nicotine and dimethylphenylpiperazinium reverse hemorrhagic shock through a peripheral, nicotinic receptor-mediated mechanism, can be explained on the basis of these novel findings.

Based on the observations by Tracey and coworkers, our group identified the cholinergic anti-inflammatory pathway in hemorrhage-shocked rats.[65] Subsequently, several other groups have shown the activity of this cholinergic anti-inflammatory pathway in various experimental conditions characterized by a systemic inflammatory response.[52,53,68-71] Preclinical studies are in progress to verify the role of the cholinergic anti-inflammatory pathway in local and systemic experimental diseases. Indeed, activation of this pathway could be used therapeutically. Vagus nerve control of visceral organs is integrated and regulated through the CNS. Reciprocal neural interconnections among the nucleus tractus solitarius, dorsal motor nucleus of the vagus, nucleus ambiguus, other forebrain structures such as hypothalamus, amygdala and insular cortex, form a brain network that regulates efferent vagal activity and related visceral organ functions.[72] Receptors belonging to this central autonomic network could be targets for activators of the cholinergic anti-inflammatory pathway.

Antishock Effects of Melanocortins

Circulatory shock is a severe pathological condition accompanied by a systemic inflammatory response, with upregulated expression of inflammatory mediators and recruitment of inflammatory cells in several tissues. Activation of nuclear transcription factors including NF-kB triggers an inflammatory cascade with production of cytokines, such as TNF-α, chemokines, cell adhesion molecules, free radicals including nitric oxide and other inflammatory mediators.[31,32,34,51-53,65,73-77] The multiple organ injury that is often associated with shock can be caused by both hypoperfusion and reperfusion during resuscitation.[73,78-80]

The antishock effects of melanocortin peptides ACTH-(4-10), α-MSH, ACTH-(1-17), ACTH-(1-24), discovered in our laboratory, has been subsequently confirmed in several studies. The original investigations were performed in a severe model of hemorrhagic shock, induced by stepwise withdrawal of about 50% of the circulating blood in rats and dogs. This procedure causes death in all animals within 30-35 min.[26,27,81-83] Conversely, intravenous injection of melanocortin peptides rapidly induces a dose-dependent restoration of arterial blood pressure and tissue blood flow. Normalization of arterial and venous pH and base excess, as well as of venous tension of O_2 and CO_2 and of venous oxygen saturation and lactate, also gradually occur.[84] The reversal of hemorrhagic shock induced by melanocortin peptides is associated with marked increase in circulating blood volume. Such increase is the consequence of mobilization of the peripherally pooled residual blood from the liver, spleen and other organs.[28,83,85] Subsequent studies using the same experimental model indicated that melanocortins greatly prolong survival and extend the time-limit for effective blood reinfusion (up to 3-4 hours after shock, versus 10-15 min in saline-treated animals) for complete shock reversal.[29]

These resuscitating effects have been confirmed in the same animal models of hemorrhagic shock,[86] as well as in hemorrhage-shocked/resuscitated hamsters,[87] in hypovolemic shock induced in rabbits by graded occlusion of the inferior vena cava,[88] in a rat model of splanchnic artery occlusion[34] and in a severe model of prolonged respiratory arrest in rats.[35] ACTH-(1-24) has then been successfully used in human conditions of hemorrhagic and cardiogenic shock (intravenous bolus of 5-10 mg), both in anecdotal cases and randomized controlled studies.[33,89-92]

Clinical studies on the effectiveness of melanocortins in circulatory shock are in progress. From a practical point of view, availability of drugs able to retard shock progression toward an irreversible state, extending the time-limit for a successful first aid of civilian and military victims of traumatic accidents, is of great importance.

The antishock effects of melanocortins are adrenal-independent, can be obtained with intracerebroventricular injection of doses much lower than those required by the intravenous route and are mediated by melanocortin MC_4 receptors located in the CNS.[26,30,32,82] Such effects are associated with marked reduction in NF-κB activation and plasma concentrations of inflammatory mediators, including TNF-α, oxygen free radicals and nitric oxide and in intercellular adhesion molecule expression by vascular endothelium.[31,34,75,76,93] This action is consistent with the established anti-inflammatory influence of melanocortins[7,11] and suggests that the ability of these neuropeptides to extend the time-limit for an effective blood reinfusion[29] may be due to blockade of the mechanisms responsible for late organ failure and death.

The antishock effect of melanocortins is prevented by a) bilateral cervical vagotomy, b) the intracerebroventricular injection of the acetylcholine-depleting agent hemicholinium-3 and c) the pharmacological blockade of central (but not peripheral) muscarinic acetylcholine receptors.[94,95] These observations suggest a contribution by CNS cholinergic pathways involving muscarinic receptors. Indeed, cholinomimetic agents, able to cross the blood-brain barrier, likewise reverse hemorrhagic shock, in rats and rabbits.[96-98]

The impressive resuscitating effect of melanocortins in severe shock models, the ineffectiveness of the conventional antishock drugs in the same animal models,[99] as well as the beneficial results obtained in human conditions of hemorrhagic and cardiogenic shock, suggest that melanocortins acting at MC_4 receptors could be innovative and promising resuscitating drugs in conditions of circulatory shock.

Melanocortins Reverse Circulatory Shock through Activation of the Cholinergic Anti-Inflammatory Pathway

Efferent vagus nerve signalling reduces the systemic inflammatory response in endotoxic shock. Indeed, electrical stimulation of efferent vagal fibers during experimental letal endotoxemia blunts hepatic TNF-α synthesis/release, attenuates serum levels of this cytokine and prevents shock development.[51] Moreover, acetylcholine reduces release of several inflammatory cytokines by lipopolysaccharide-stimulated human macrophages and this effect is counteracted by nicotinic receptor antagonists. In hemorrhagic shock, as well as in splanchnic artery occlusion shock, electrical stimulation of efferent vagal fibers rapidly reverses hypotension, prevents hepatic NF-κB activation, blunts hepatic TNF-α synthesis/release, lowers TNF-α serum levels and improves survival in rats.[65,77] These findings suggest that a "cholinergic anti-inflammatory pathway" operates during endotoxic, hemorrhagic and splanchnic artery occlusion shock, to counterbalance development of the inflammatory cascade responsible for vascular derangement and multiple organ failure (Fig. 1). Identification of drugs able to activate this pathway might provide highly effective and innovative approaches for treatment of circulatory shock.

As reviewed above, melanocortin peptides of the ACTH/MSH family exert a prompt and sustained resuscitating effect in conditions of circulatory shock. This effect is adrenal-independent and occurs through inhibition of the systemic inflammatory response.[31,34,75,76,93] Previous investigations on the anti-inflammatory effects of melanocortins showed that systemic administration of α-MSH reduces blood concentrations of IL-1α and TNF-α in a mouse model of lipopolysaccharide-induced systemic inflammation.[100] Furthermore, Lipton and coworkers showed that in a mouse model of peritonitis/endotoxemia induced by cecal ligation and puncture, systemic treatment with α-MSH improves survival.[101] Collectively, these findings indicate that melanocortins counteract the systemic inflammatory response in circulatory shock.

The next question was whether hemorrhagic shock reversal produced by melanocortins depends on activation of the vagus nerve-mediated cholinergic anti-inflammatory pathway.[31] Action potential recordings in hemorrhage-shocked rats treated with nanomolar concentrations of ACTH-(1-24), indicate that neural efferent activity along the vagus nerve markedly increases. This effect is associated with the restoration of cardiovascular and respiratory functions, blunted NF-κB activity and decreased TNF-α in liver and plasma. Bilateral cervical vagotomy, or pharmacological blockade of brain melanocortin MC_4 receptors and muscarinic acetylcholine receptors, or of peripheral nicotinic acetylcholine receptors, prevents the life-saving effect of ACTH-(1-24) and the associated effects on NF-κB activity and TNF-α levels.[31] Blockade of brain MC_4 receptors and muscarinic receptors (a) blunts the stimulating effect of ACTH-(1-24) on efferent vagal activity, (b) reduces, like bilateral cervical vagotomy, the blood volume to be withdrawn in order to induce shock and (c) prevents the compensatory increase in efferent vagal activity normally occurring during bleeding in control shocked animals.[31]

Collectively, these findings indicate that melanocortins suppress the NF-kB-dependent systemic inflammatory response triggered by hemorrhage and reverse shock condition, through activation of the cholinergic anti-inflammatory pathway within the brain (Fig. 1). These results likewise indicate

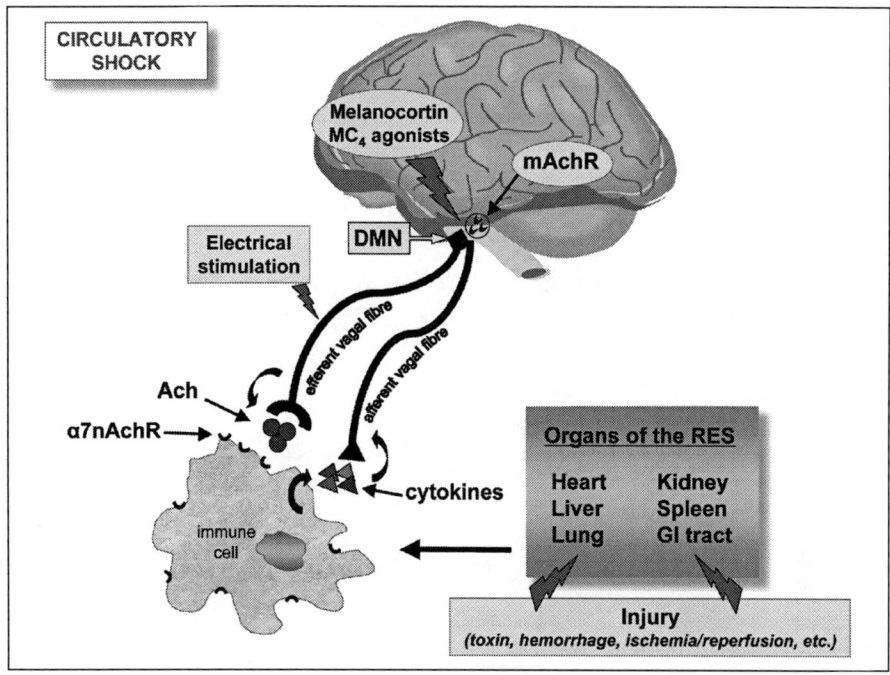

Figure 1. Modulation of the inflammatory response in circulatory shock, through the cholinergic anti-inflammatory pathway. Low levels of inflammatory molecules produced in damaged tissues activate afferent signals through ascending vagus nerve fibers (sensory arm of the inflammatory reflex). Activation of the cholinergic anti-inflammatory pathway (motor arm of the inflammatory reflex, that is impaired during shock) by electrical stimulation of efferent vagal fibers, or by stimulation of brain melanocortin MC_4 receptors (likely in the vagus dorsal motor nucleus: DMN), rapidly leads to acetylcholine (Ach) release in organs of the reticuloendothelial system (RES). Acetylcholine released from efferent vagal terminals interacts with α7 subunit-containing nicotinic acetylcholine receptors (α7nAchR) on tissue macrophages and other immune cells surrounding the cholinergic terminals and inhibits the synthesis/release of inflammatory cytokines, with consequent reduction in cytokine plasma levels and attenuation of the systemic inflammatory response. Acetylcholine interaction with peripheral muscarinic receptors (mAchR) does not play a role in circulatory shock. On the contrary, brain muscarinic receptors also are involved in triggering the cholinergic anti-inflammatory pathway.

that blockade of either brain MC_4 receptors, or brain muscarinic receptors, or efferent vagal transmission, accelerates the evolution of shock. These observations suggest the existence of a melanocortin-dependent antishock pathway. The involvement of brain muscarinic receptors in activation of the cholinergic anti-inflammatory pathway has been subsequently confirmed in experimental endotoxic shock.[102] Blockade of the cholinergic anti-inflammatory pathway activity by the nicotinic acetylcholine receptor antagonist chlorisondamine provides a mechanism for the original observations by Guarini and coworkers,[66,67] that dimethylphenylpiperazinium and surprisingly nicotine (a CNS acting drug) reverse hemorrhagic shock through a peripheral, nicotinic receptor-mediated pathway.

Interestingly, melanocortins exert their well-known anti-inflammatory activity mainly via a central mechanism that leads to reduced pro-inflammatory cytokines and chemokines production and increased release of the anti-inflammatory cytokine IL-10.[11] This mechanism partly overlaps with the cholinergic anti-inflammatory pathway, which modulates the systemic inflammatory response in shock conditions by inhibiting monocyte production and release of pro-inflammatory cytokines, but not of the anti-inflammatory cytokine IL-10.[51]

Protective Effect of Melanocortins in Myocardial Ischemia/Reperfusion

Melanocortins are also highly effective in treatment of animal models of myocardial ischemia. Ischemia rapidly causes profound biochemical and morphological changes and induces an inflammatory reaction in the heart tissue. Reperfusion is associated with severe alterations of cellular metabolism that may lead to further tissue injury. Myocardial reperfusion causes severe arrhythmias, endothelial dysfunction, myocardial stunning, cell death either by necrosis or apoptosis and a high lethality.[36,103,104] It appears that myocardial ischemia triggers apoptosis and reperfusion accelerates the process.[105] Both ischemia and reperfusion induce oxidative and nitrosative stress[36,106-108] as well as early activation of mitogen-activated protein kinases and NF-κB[109,110] in cardiac myocytes. These signal transduction mechanisms may in part contribute to cardiac injury, by causing early increase in expression of heart damaging factors and in part to cardioprotection.[111] A number of innovative pharmacological approaches to myocardial ischemia/reperfusion injury have been investigated, but the results are either conflicting or not confirmed in clinical trials.[105,112-114]

We have shown that melanocortins, including [Nle^4,D-Phe^7]α-MSH (NDP-α-MSH), γ$_1$-MSH and γ$_2$-MSH, injected intravenously during experimental coronary occlusion, exert a protective effect both in rats subjected to transient myocardial ischemia followed by reperfusion—an animal model characterized by high incidence of ventricular tachycardia (VT), ventricular fibrillation (VF) and death—and in rats subjected to permanent coronary artery occlusion.[36,37,39,115] Myocardial ischemia/reperfusion injury also activates the anti-apoptotic, pro-survival cascades of the phosphatidylinositol 3-kinase-Akt and extracellular signal-regulated kinases (ERK 1/2), that appear to make up an universal pro-survival signalling pathway mediating myocardial protection at reperfusion.[111] In the rat model of myocardial ischemia/reperfusion described above, ACTH-(1-24) enhanced ERK 1/2 activation, triggering therefore the pro-survival cascade. In addition, melanocortins reduced histological alterations in the left ventricle, including those involving structural proteins, counteracted the inflammatory response and stimulated anti-apoptotic reactions.[40]

The cardioprotective effect of melanocortins has been confirmed in rat hearts isolated 12 hours after treatment with α-MSH or ACTH-(4-10) and then subjected to a 30-min period of ischemia followed by 120 min of reperfusion.[41,116] In this experimental model, melanocortin treatment results in a reduction in VF, infarct size and activity of the apoptotic protein caspase-3 and in an increase in the expression of the anti-inflammatory protein heme oxygenase-1. Melanocortins have also been shown to be effective in mouse models of myocardial ischemia/reperfusion.[12,38]

The prevention of ventricular arrhythmias in transient myocardial ischemia and the reduction of infarct size in permanent ischemia may be due to the melanocortin ability to inhibit the oxygen free radical discharge and to reduce the inflammatory and apoptotic responses.[12,36,39,40] Indeed, melanocortin peptides have a peculiar, adrenal-independent, anti-inflammatory activity.[7,11,21] An anti-apoptotic activity, has also been demonstrated.[5,22,45]

It appears that the cardioprotective effect of melanocortins could be mediated by brain melanocortin MC$_3$ receptors.[36,37,39,40,115] Indeed, when the selective MC$_3$ agonist γ$_2$-MSH was administered intracerebroventricularly, a dose ten times lower than that needed by the intravenous route provided full protection. This observation could explain the reason why treatment of isolated rat hearts with ACTH-(4-10) given at the time of reperfusion, rather than "in vivo" before heart harvest, failed to improve the post-ischemic recovery.[116] However, the data of Getting and coworkers[38] suggest a minor participation of cardiac MC$_3$ receptors.

Interestingly, melanocortins also cause a significant increase in allograft survival in experimental heart transplantation. Although they do not eventually prevent rejection, treatment was associated with a marked decrease in leukocyte infiltration and in expression of inflammatory molecules involved in allograft rejection.[50] Gene expression profile studies have revealed that melanocortin treatment of recipients preserves transplanted heart function by altering multiple protective pathways.[117]

Thus, melanocortins could be an useful tool for the prevention of cardiac damage, in different conditions of ischemia/reperfusion injury.

Melanocortins Prevent Myocardial Ischemia/Reperfusion-Induced Damage through Activation of the Cholinergic Anti-Inflammatory Pathway

Electrical stimulation of the vagus nerve has been proposed as a novel approach for treatment of myocardial ischemia/reperfusion injury. Indeed, stimulation of the vagus nerve prevented VF and VT in cats after myocardial reperfusion following a 20-min period of coronary occlusion[118] and VF in dogs with a healed myocardial infarction.[119] Moreover, it has been reported that vagus stimulation improves long-term survival after chronic heart failure in rats.[120] These investigations have provided a robust framework for the interpretation of findings by Cheng and coworkers.[121]

The nucleus ambiguus has long been considered the major vagal nucleus controlling the heart activity, whereas the vagus dorsal motor nucleus was thought to play only a marginal role. Recently, Cheng and colleagues[121] provided anatomical evidence for dual vagal cardiac efferent pathways in rats, that could play different roles in control of heart function. The data showed that neurons of the nucleus ambiguus and dorsal motor nucleus of the vagus project axons that converge to the same cardiac ganglia and innervate separate nonoverlapping populations of principal neurons within each cardiac ganglion. These findings, together with functional observations by the same investigators,[122,123] suggest that both brain nuclei play important, though different, roles in controlling cardiac function. During myocardial ischemia and reperfusion, therefore, one of these dual vagal cardiac efferent pathways could be a cholinergic anti-inflammatory pathway, involved in cardioprotection, as it occurs in circulatory shock. Indeed, in conditions of heart failure, a systemic inflammatory response plays a fundamental pathogenetic role.[124]

These observations encouraged further investigations, aimed at determining whether melanocortin peptides activate such vagal efferent pathway(s) in experimental conditions of ischemic heart disease. In rats subjected to coronary artery occlusion (5 min) followed by reperfusion (5 min), electrical stimulation of efferent vagal fibers (5 V, 2 ms, 1-9 Hz, for the whole period of ischemia/reperfusion) has been shown to strongly reduce the incidence of severe arrhythmias and lethality and the increases in free radical blood levels and left ventricle histological alterations and to augment the activation of the anti-apoptotic prosurvival kinase ERK 1/2.[40] Nanomolar amounts of the melanocortins ACTH-(1-24) (agonist at all MC receptors) and γ_2-MSH (selective agonist at MC_3 receptors)—administered in rats during coronary occlusion, intravenously or intracerebroventricularly at a dose 10 times lower—produces the same protective effects of efferent vagal fiber electrical stimulation (Fig. 2).[40] Since bilateral cervical vagotomy blunts the beneficial effect of ACTH-(1-24) and of the selective MC_3 agonist γ_2-MSH, the protective effect of melanocortins likely involves such vagal pathway. Accordingly, blockade of peripheral muscarinic acetylcholine receptors prevents the effects of both electrical stimulation and melanocortins; in the latter case, also central muscarinic receptors seem to be involved.[40]

More recently, the improvement in functional recovery, following vagus nerve electrical stimulation of isolated rat hearts subjected to ischemia/reperfusion injury, has been associated with inhibition of cardiomyocyte adenosine triphosphate depletion; indeed, it is established that rapid depletion of adenosine triphosphate leads cells to death. In the same investigation, the beneficial effect of acetylcholine against depletion of adenosine triphosphate has been also shown in isolated cardiomyocytes subjected to hypoxia/reoxygenation. In both studies, the protective effects seem to be mediated by muscarinic acetylcholine receptors.[125]

Overall, these results indicate a protective, efferent vagal cholinergic pathway operative in conditions of ischemic heart disease, that could be activated by melanocortins (Fig. 2). The melanococortin-induced activation of such a pathway seems to be triggered by stimulation of brain MC_3 receptors,[37,40,115] with involvement of brain and (as main final step) heart muscarinic receptors. Ischemia/reperfusion injury is still considered a major problem in patients with acute coronary occlusion and in patients undergoing surgical operations, such as coronary artery bypass grafting. These patients could benefit by a pharmacological activation of the cholinergic anti-inflammatory pathway. Benefits for patients with ischemic heart diseases by melanocortin-induced triggering

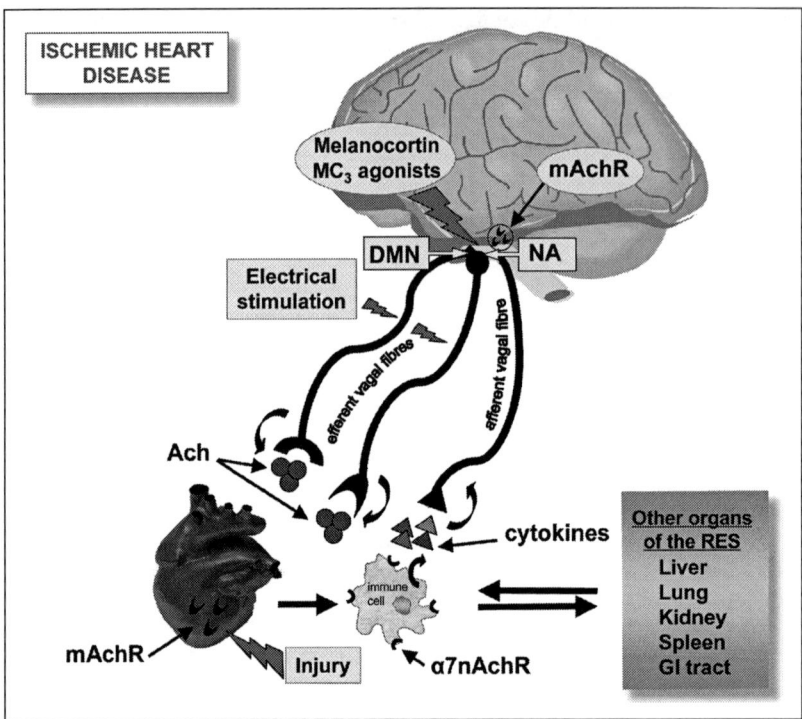

Figure 2. Modulation of the inflammatory response in myocardial ischemia/reperfusion and heart failure, through the cholinergic anti-inflammatory pathway. Low levels of inflammatory molecules produced in damaged tissues activate afferent signals through ascending vagus nerve fibers (sensory arm of the inflammatory reflex). Activation of the cholinergic anti-inflammatory pathway (motor arm of the inflammatory reflex, that is impaired during ischemia/reperfusion) by electrical stimulation of efferent vagal fibers, or by stimulation of brain melanocortin MC$_3$ receptors likely located in the vagus dorsal motor nucleus (DMN) or nucleus ambiguous (NA), rapidly leads to acetylcholine (Ach) release in the heart. Acetylcholine released from efferent vagal terminals interacts with muscarinic acetylcholine receptors (mAchR) on myocardial tissue leading to cardioprotection. Likely, acetylcholine interaction with peripheral nicotinic receptors (α7nAchR) in organs of the reticuloendothelial system (RES) plays a role in myocardial ischemia/reperfusion and heart failure, a condition where also a systemic inflammatory response can occur. Brain muscarinic receptors are also involved in triggering the cholinergic anti-inflammatory pathway.

of the cholinergic anti-inflammatory pathway could be even greater, because of the established ability of melanocortins to increase the anti-inflammatory cytokine IL-10 production.[11] Indeed, modulation of inflammation with IL-10 attenuates left ventricle disfunction and remodeling after acute myocardial infarction in mice.[126]

Neuroprotection by Melanocortins in Ischemic Stroke

Stroke is the third main cause of death and the leading cause of adult disability in developed countries. Within minutes to days after a cerebral vessel occlusion, several pathological pathways are triggered, which may potentially damage brain cells.[25,127] Despite intensive investigations aimed at developing innovative neuroprotective treatments for brain injury, no novel drugs have established clinical effectiveness. Toxic side effects, short therapeutic treatment window, single-mechanism of neuronal damage blockade are the main problems.[127-129] Indeed, information from clinical trials suggests that targeting an array of key pathophysiological mechanisms is essential for an effective and safe management of stroke.[25,127,128,130] At present, the only approved therapy for ischemic stroke is thrombolysis within 3 hours of symptom onset.[25,128,131] However, only 3% of all stroke patients can receive thrombolytic agents, only few of treated patients experience some benefits and a growing body of evidence indicates that these drugs also have deleterious effects.[25,132]

Protective properties of melanocortins in experimental brain ischemia have been reported by Lipton's group. These experiments showed that α-MSH improves recovery of auditory-evoked potentials in a dog model of transient brain stem ischemia.[133] Tatro's group reported that α-MSH reduces brain TNF-α levels in transient global and focal cerebral ischemia in mice.[134] Recently, our research group provided the first clear evidence that melanocortins afford a strong neuroprotection against damage consequent to global or focal cerebral ischemia in gerbils and rats, through the activation of CNS melanocortin MC$_4$ receptors.[45-47,49] Eleven-day intraperitoneal treatment with nanomolar amounts of the melanocortin NDP-α-MSH, but not of the selective MC$_3$ receptor agonist γ$_2$-MSH, protects against impairment in learning and memory caused by transient global brain ischemia in gerbils (induced by occlusion of the common carotid arteries for 10 min).[45,46] This protective and long-lasting (67 days, at least) effect, which is prevented by pharmacological blockade of MC$_4$ receptors, occurs also when treatment starts several hours after ischemia (being 18 hours the approximate time-limit). In transient global brain ischemia in gerbils, functional recovery after stroke is associated with a modulation of the excitotoxic, inflammatory and apoptotic responses in the hippocampus and with a consequent reduction of the morphological damage and an increase in the number of viable neurons. The same melanocortin treatment given for 11 days also protects against impairment in learning and memory, sensory-motor orientation and coordinated limb use in a rat model of focal cerebral ischemia caused by intrastriatal microinjection of endothelin-1.[47] In this severe experimental model, the MC$_4$ receptor-dependent protective effect of NDP-α-MSH is associated with diminished excitotoxic, inflammatory and apoptotic reactions.[49] Other beneficial features involve a significant reduction of the severe morphological damage of the nucleus striatum, including a reduction of neuronal death, demyelination and phagocytic activity. Neuroprotection is also associated with a significant increase in number of small vessels within ischemic areas, relative to saline-treated rats. Of great importance, also in these rat studies NDP-α-MSH showed a broad therapeutic treatment window.[47] Subsequently, Forslin Aronsson and coworkers[135] and Chen and coworkers[48] confirmed the neuroprotective effect of α-MSH in other models of global and focal cerebral ischemia, without investigating MC receptors.

In conclusion, melanocortin agonists at MC$_4$ receptors appear to produce effective neuroprotection with a broad time window and through counteraction of the main ischemia-related mechanisms of brain damage. Furthermore, the antipyretic action of melanocortins is well established[136] and hypothermia might contribute to neuroprotection during cerebral ischemia.[137] Stroke therapy with these neuropeptides, therefore, could take a further advantage by melanocortin-induced hypothermia.[25] No novel drug has so far been shown to possess so many favourable and promising characteristics, at least in experimental stroke models.

Melanocortins Produce Neuroprotection Against Ischemic Stroke by Activating the Cholinergic Anti-Inflammatory Pathway

Observations in animals[138,139] and humans[140,141] indicate that stroke is associated with systemic pathophysiological reactions. Widespread production/activation of inflammatory mediators in the peripheral immune system following focal cerebral ischemia has been reported in mice.[142]

The systemic pathophysiological reactions associated with focal cerebral ischemia and a possible protective involvement of the cholinergic anti-inflammatory pathway, have been investigated in rats.[49] Following intrastriatal microinjection of endothelin-1, the activation of ERK 1/2, c-jun N-terminal kinases and caspase-3, the increase in TNF-α concentration and DNA fragmentation, as well as the increase in TNF-α plasma levels, occur over the ensuing hours in the striatum and liver of control stroke rats. This suggests cerebral and systemic activation of

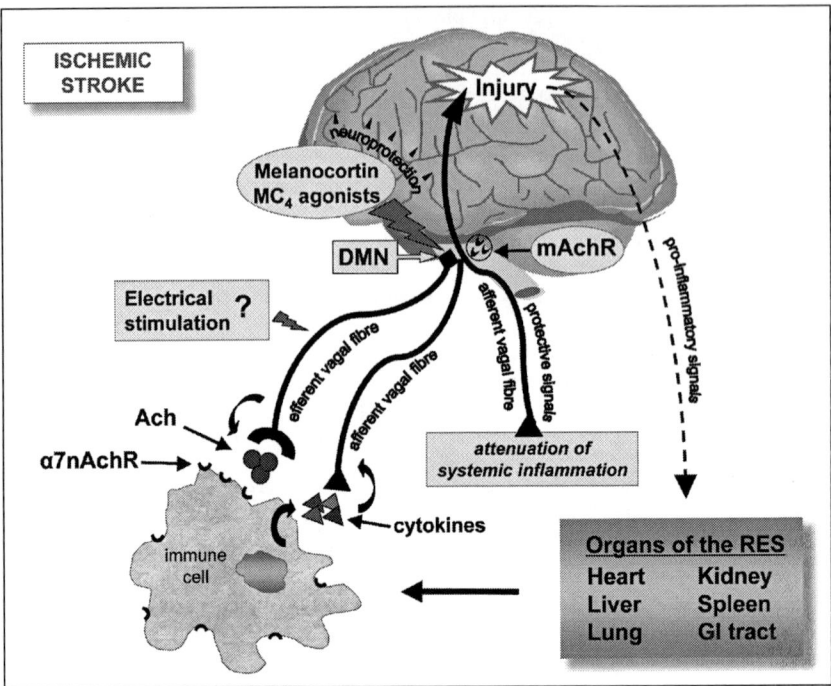

Figure 3. Modulation of the inflammatory response in ischemic stroke, through the cholinergic anti-inflammatory pathway. Low levels of both brain inflammatory molecules spreading outside the blood-brain barrier and inflammatory molecules produced in damaged peripheral tissues, activate afferent signals through ascending vagus nerve fibers (sensory arm of the inflammatory reflex). Brain melanocortin MC_4 receptor agonists, besides to produce strong neuroprotection in the injured brain area, activate the cholinergic anti-inflammatory pathway (motor arm of the inflammatory reflex, that is impaired after stroke), likely by acting on MC_4 receptors in the vagus dorsal motor nucleus (DMN), leading to acetylcholine (Ach) release in organs of the reticuloendothelial system (RES). Acetylcholine released from efferent vagal terminals interacts with α7 subunit-containing nicotinic acetylcholine receptors (α7nAchR) on tissue macrophages and other immune cells surrounding the cholinergic terminals and inhibits the synthesis/release of inflammatory cytokines, with a consequent reduction in cytokine plasma levels and the attenuation of the systemic inflammatory response. Protective signals towards the CNS via the afferent vagal fibers (owing to the activation of the vagus nerve-mediated cholinergic anti-inflammatory pathway) also seem to occur in stroke. It is unknown whether acetylcholine interaction with peripheral muscarinic receptors (mAchR) plays a role in ischemic stroke. Likely, brain muscarinic receptors are also involved in triggering the cholinergic anti-inflammatory pathway. Electrical stimulation has not been assessed in stroke models.

excitotoxic, inflammatory and apoptotic responses. Intraperitoneal treatment with nanomolar doses of NDP-α-MSH 3 to 9 hours after stroke suppresses the excitotoxic, inflammatory and apoptotic cascades at central and peripheral level. Bilateral vagotomy and pharmacological blockade of peripheral nicotinic acetylcholine receptors blunt the neuroprotective effect of NDP-α-MSH.[49] Focal brain ischemia causes, therefore, detrimental effects not only in the brain, but also in the liver. This leads to hypothesize that a protective, melanocortin-activated, vagal cholinergic pathway is likely operative in conditions of ischemic stroke, to modulate cerebral and systemic pathological reactions (Fig. 3). Decreased expression and impaired function of brain muscarinic acetylcholine receptors have been associated with neuron degeneration after ischemic stroke.[143] This suggests that brain muscarinic receptors may be involved in triggering the cholinergic anti-inflammatory pathway much as in circulatoy shock and myocardial ischemia.

However, the vagus nerve-mediated cholinergic anti-inflammatory pathway is an efferent pathway and its activation by melanocortins can only account for the peripheral protective effects observed by Ottani and coworkers.[49] How can we explain why vagotomy and peripheral nicotinic receptor blockade blunt the protective effect of melanocortins against brain damage? It has been reported that lipopolysaccharide-induced systemic inflammation in conjunction with global cerebral ischemia exacerbates brain damage in rats.[144] This suggests that inhibition of systemic responses could result in cerebral protective effects. Moreover, vagal afferents are widely distributed throughout the CNS and vagus nerve stimulation causes synaptic activation at multiple sites in both cerebral hemispheres.[55] Therefore, protective signals towards the CNS owing to the activation of the vagus nerve-mediated cholinergic anti-inflammatory pathway can be hypothesized in stroke (Fig. 3).

Evidence suggests that in conditions of brain ischemia endogenous melanocortins could exert a role in neuroprotection. A) Melanocortin-treated stroke animals learn more rapidly than sham ischemic ones,[45,46] but after the blockade of melanocortin MC_4 receptors there is a worsening in memory recovery, as compared with ischemic control animals.[45,46] B) Melanocortins increase the anti-inflammatory cytokine IL-10 that modulates the inflammatory cascade.[11,21] Interestingly, it has been reported that low plasma concentrations of IL-10 are associated with early worsening of neurological symptoms in stroke patients.[145] C) α-MSH concentrations in plasma are reduced in patients with acute traumatic brain injury. Consistent with a physiological neuroprotective role of melanocortins, patients with the lowest circulating levels have an unfavourable outcome.[11]

Taken together, these observations point to a neuroprotective role of a cholinergic anti-inflammatory pathway, likely activated by melanocortins, that could be physiologically operative in conditions of ischemic stroke and brain injury, to protect against local and systemic damage. This further supports the important role of the cholinergic anti-inflammatory pathway in the defense mechanisms.

Conclusion

MC_3 and MC_4 receptors are the most abundant MC receptor subtypes within the CNS, being brain distribution of MC_4 receptors broader than that of MC_3.[5,7,11,21] MC_3 and MC_4 receptors also occur in the vagus dorsal motor nucleus and ventral division of the nucleus ambiguous[19,146] and these receptors are believed to play an important role in central regulation of certain body functions.[5,147] This supports the hypothesis that central melanocortins activate efferent vagal fiber-mediated cholinergic anti-inflammatory pathway(s) to protect against damage caused by circulatory shock, myocardial ischemia and ischemic stroke and perhaps following other severe inflammatory insults. Such efferent cholinergic pathways could be specific for different pathological conditions; indeed, in circulatory shock and ischemic stroke this pathway seems to be mediated by peripheral nicotinic acetylcholine receptors, whereas in myocardial ischemia peripheral muscarinic acetylcholine receptors appear to be predominantly involved. However, because MC receptors, including MC_3 and MC_4, are also expressed in numerous peripheral tissues,[7,11,15,21] additional protective influences of melanocortins likely occur via interactions with peripheral melanocortin receptors.

The CNS and peripheral organs communicate via neuronal and humoral pathways.[52,53] After brain injury, immunodepression and inflammation in peripheral organs can occur. Indeed, several cerebral injury types have been shown to be associated with intestinal, pulmonary and hepatic inflammation.[5] The abundant distribution of MC_3 and MC_4 receptors within the CNS, together with the preclinically demonstrated ability of melanocortins acting at central MC_3 and MC_4 receptors to prevent central and peripheral detrimental consequences of a brain inflammatory injury due to ischemia and reperfusion, suggest promising perspectives for the clinical use of melanocortins. These brain receptors could be pharmacological targets for the treatment of several central and peripheral disorders, likely through the activation of the efferent vagal anti-inflammatory pathway(s).[31,40,49]

Several instances of ischemia/reperfusion injuries could take advantage of melanocortin-induced activation of the cholinergic anti-inflammatory pathway, also because melanocortins increase the production and release of the potent anti-inflammatory cytokine IL-10 from monocytes through a β_2-adrenergic receptor-dependent mechanism.[11,52] Indeed, it is well established that melanocortins also stimulate adrenergic transmission and therefore they can centrally modulate local and systemic inflammation through both adrenergic and cholinergic pathways.[5,11] Recent data suggest that the splenic nerve, through a complex mechanism involving adrenergic and cholinergic signals, is required for the cholinergic anti-inflammatory pathway activity against systemic inflammation and the spleen could be a primary source of TNF-α.[70,148]

Investigations designed at determining the molecular mechanisms of the cholinergic anti-inflammatory pathway activation could provide further insight into the neural regulation of inflammation and could help design of superselective activators of such a pathway: agonists at individual brain MC receptors could be significant candidates.

Acknowledgements

This work was supported in part by grants from Ministero dell'Istruzione, dell'Università e della Ricerca (MIUR), Roma, Italy.

References

1. Ferrari W, Floris E, Paulesu F. Eosinopenic effect of ACTH injected into the cisterna magna. Boll Soc It Biol Sper 1955; 31:859-862.
2. Ferrari W. Behavioural changes in animals after intracisternal injection with adrenocorticotrophic hormone and melanocyte-stimulating hormone. Nature 1958; 181:925-926.
3. Ferrari W, Gessa GL, Vargiu L. Behavioral effects induced by intracisternally injected ACTH and MSH. Ann NY Acad Sci 1963; 104:330-345.
4. De Wied D. Effect of peptide hormones on behavior. In: Ganon WF, Martini L, eds. Frontiers in Neuroendocrinology, London/New York: Oxford University Press, 1969; 1:97-140.
5. Catania A. Neuroprotective action of melanocortins: a therapeutic opportunity. Trends Neurosci 2008; 31:353-360.
6. Eberle AN. The melanotropins: chemistry, physiology and mechanisms of action. Basel: Karger, 1988.
7. Getting SJ. Targeting melanocortin receptors as potential novel therapeutics. Pharmacol Ther 2006; 111:1-15.
8. O'Donohue TI, Dorsa DM. The opiomelanotropinergic neuronal and endocrine systems. Peptides 1982; 3:353-395.
9. Smith AI, Funder JW. Proopiomelanocortin processing in the pituitary, central nervous system and peripheral tissues. Endocrinol Rev 1988; 9:159-179.
10. Versteeg DHG, Van Bergen P, Adan RAH et al. Melanocortins and cardiovascular regulation. Eur J Pharmacol 1998; 360:1-14.
11. Catania A, Gatti S, Colombo G et al. Targeting melanocortin receptors as a novel strategy to control inflammation. Pharmacol Rev 2004; 56:1-29.
12. Getting SJ, Di Filippo C, D'Amico M et al. The melanocortin peptide HP228 displays protective effects in acute models of inflammation and organ damage. Eur J Pharmacol 2006; 532:138-144.
13. Wikberg JE, Mutulis F. Targeting melanocortin receptors: an approach to treat weight disorders and sexual dysfunction. Nat Rev Drug Discov 2008; 7:307-323.
14. Mountjoy KG, Robbins LS, Mortrud MT et al. The cloning of a family of genes that encode the melanocortin receptors. Science 1992; 257:1248-1251.
15. Mountjoy KG, Wu C-SJ, Dumont LM et al. Melanocortin-4 receptor messenger ribonucleic acid expression in rat cardiorespiratory, musculoskeletal and in tegumentary systems. Endocrinology 2003; 144:5488-5496.
16. Schiöth HB. The physiological role of melanocortin receptors. Vitam Horm 2001; 63:195-232.
17. Schiöth HB, Haitina T, Ling MK et al. Evolutionary conservation of the structural, pharmacological and genomic characteristics of the melanocortin receptor subtypes. Peptides 2005; 26:1886-1900.
18. Tatro JB. Melanotropin receptors in the brain are differentially distributed and recognize both corticotrophin and alpha-melanocyte stimulating hormone. Brain Res 1990; 536:124-132.
19. Tatro JB, Entwistle ML. Distribution of melanocortin receptors in the lower brainstem of the rat. Ann NY Acad Sci 1994; 739:311-314.
20. Tatro JB. Receptor biology of the melanocortins, a family of neuroimmunomodulatory peptides. Neuroimmunomodulation 1996; 3:259-284.

21. Wikberg JES, Muceniece R, Mandrika I et al. New aspects on the melanocortins and their receptors. Pharmacol Res 2000; 42:393-420.
22. Brzoska T, Luger TA, Maser C et al. α-Melanocyte-stimulating hormone and related tripeptides: biochemistry, antiinflammatory and protective effects in Vitro and in Vivo and future perspectives for the treatment of immune-mediated inflammatory diseases. Endocr Rev 2008; 29:581-602.
23. Lasaga M, Debeljuk L, Durand D et al. Role of alpha-melanocyte stimulating hormone and melanocortin 4 receptor in brain inflammation. Peptides 2008; 29:1825-1835.
24. Martin WJ, MacIntyre DE. Melanocortin receptors and erectile function. Eur Urol 2004; 45:706-713.
25. Tatro JB. Melanocortins defend their territory: multifaceted neuroprotection in cerebral ischemia. Endocrinology 2006; 147:1122-1125.
26. Bertolini A, Guarini S, Ferrari W. Adrenal-independent, anti-shock effect of ACTH-(1-24) in rats. Eur J Pharmacol 1986; 122:387-388.
27. Bertolini A, Guarini S, Rompianesi E et al. α-MSH and other ACTH fragments improve cardiovascular function and survival in experimental hemorrhagic shock. Eur J Pharmacol 1986; 130:19-26.
28. Guarini S, Ferrari W, Mottillo G et al. Anti-shock effect of ACTH: haematological changes and influence of splenectomy. Arch In Pharmacodyn 1987; 289:311-318.
29. Guarini S, Tagliavini S, Bazzani C et al. Early treatment with ACTH-(1-24) in a rat model of hemorrhagic shock prolongs survival and extends the time-limit for blood reinfusion to be effective. Crit Care Med 1990; 18:862-865.
30. Guarini S, Bazzani C, Cainazzo MM et al. Evidence that melanocortin 4 receptor mediates hemorrhagic shock reversal caused by melanocortin peptides. J Pharmacol Exp Ther 1999; 291:1023-1027.
31. Guarini S, Cainazzo MM, Giuliani D et al. Adrenocorticotropin reverses hemorrhagic shock in anesthetized rats through the rapid activation of a vagal anti-inflammatory pathway. Cardiovasc Res 2004; 63:357-365.
32. Giuliani D, Mioni C, Bazzani C et al. Selective melanocortin MC$_4$ receptor agonists reverse haemorrhagic shock and prevent multiple organ damage. Br J Pharmacol 2007; 150:595-603.
33. Noera G, Lamarra M, Guarini S et al. Survival rate after early treatment for acute type-A aortic dissection with ACTH-(1-24). Lancet 2001; 358:469-470.
34. Squadrito F, Guarini S, Altavilla D et al. Adrenocorticotropin reverses vascular dysfunction and protects against splanchnic artery occlusion shock. Br J Pharmacol 1999; 128:816-822.
35. Guarini S, Bazzani C, Bertolini A. Resuscitating effect of melanocortin peptides after prolonged respiratory arrest. Br J Pharmacol 1997; 121:1454-1460.
36. Bazzani C, Guarini S, Botticelli AR et al. Protective effect of melanocortin peptides in rat myocardial ischemia. J Pharmacol Exp Ther 2001; 297:1082-1087.
37. Guarini S, Schiöth HB, Mioni C et al. MC$_3$ receptors are involved in the protective effect of melanocortins in myocardial ischaemia/reperfusion-induced arrhythmias. Naunyn-Schmiedeberg's Arch Pharmacol 2002; 366:177-182.
38. Getting SJ, Di Filippo C, Christian HC et al. MC-3 receptor and the inflammatory mechanisms activated in acute myocardial infarct. J Leukoc Biol 2004; 76:845-853.
39. Mioni C, Giuliani D, Cainazzo MM et al. Further evidence that melanocortins prevent myocardial reperfusion injury by activating melanocortin MC$_3$ receptors. Eur J Pharmacol 2003; 477:227-234.
40. Mioni C, Bazzani C, Giuliani D et al. Activation of an efferent cholinergic pathway produces strong protection against myocardial ischemia/reperfusion injury in rats. Crit Care Med 2005; 33:2621-2628.
41. Vecsernyes M, Juhasz B, Der P et al. The administration of α-melanocyte-stimulating hormone protects the ischemic/reperfused myocardium. Eur J Pharmacol 2003; 470:177-183.
42. Chiao H, Kohda Y, McLeroy P et al. Alpha-melanocyte-stimulating hormone protects against renal injury after ischemia in mice and rats. J Clin Invest 1997; 99:1165-1172.
43. Lee YS, Park JJ, Chung KY. Change of melanocortin receptor expression in rat kidney ischemia-reperfusion injury. Transplant Proc 2008; 40:2142-2144.
44. Jo SK, Yun SY, Chang KH et al. α-MSH decreases apoptosis in ischaemic acute renal failure in rats: possibile mechanism of this beneficial effect. Nephrol Dial Transplant 2001; 16:1583-1591.
45. Giuliani D, Mioni C, Altavilla D et al. Both early and delayed treatment with melanocortin 4 receptor-stimulating melanocortins produces neuroprotection in cerebral ischemia. Endocrinology 2006; 147:1126-1135.
46. Giuliani D, Leone S, Mioni C et al. Broad therapeutic treatment window of the [Nle^4, D-Phe^7] α-melanocyte-stimulating hormone for long-lasting protection against ischemic stroke, in Mongolian gerbils. Eur J Pharmacol 2006; 538:48-56.
47. Giuliani D, Ottani A, Mioni C et al. Neuroprotection in focal cerebral ischemia owing to delayed treatment with melanocortins. Eur J Pharmacol 2007; 570:57-65.

48. Chen G, Frøkiær J, Pedersen M et al. Reduction of ischemic stroke in rat brain by alpha melanocyte stimulating hormone. Neuropeptides 2008; 42:331-338.
49. Ottani A, Giuliani D, Mioni C et al. Vagus nerve mediates the protective effects of melanocortins against cerebral and systemic damage after ischemic stroke. J Cereb Blood Flow Metab 2008; doi:10.1038/jcbfm.2008.140.
50. Gatti S, Colombo G, Buffa R et al. α-Melanocyte-stimulating hormone protects the allograft in experimental heart transplantation. Transplantation 2002; 74:1678-1684.
51. Borovikova LV, Ivanova S, Zhang M et al. Vagus nerve stimulation attenuates the systemic inflammatory response to endotoxin. Nature 2000; 405:458-462.
52. Tracey KJ. The inflammatory reflex. Nature 2002; 420:853-859.
53. Tracey KJ. Physiology and immunology of the cholinergic antiinflammatory pathway. J Clin Invest 2007; 117:289-296.
54. Hatton KW, McLarney JT, Pittman T et al. Vagal nerve stimulation: overview and implications for anesthesiologists. Anesth Analg 2006; 103:1241-1249.
55. Wheless JW, Baumgartner J. Vagus nerve stimulation therapy. Drugs Today 2004; 40:501-515.
56. Basedovsky H, Rey DA, Sorkin E et al. Immunoregulatory feedback between interleukin-1 and glucocorticoid hormones. Science 1986; 233:652-654.
57. Hu XX, Goldmuntz EA, Brosnan CF. The effect of norepinephrine on endotoxin-mediated macrophage activation. J Neuroimmunol 1991; 31:35-42.
58. Lipton JM, Catania A. Antiinflammatory action of neuroimmunomodulator α-MSH. Immunol Today 1997; 18:140-145.
59. Goehler LE, Gaykema RP, Hansen MK et al. Vagal immune-to-brain communication: a visceral chemosensory pathway. Auton Neurosci 2000; 85:49-59.
60. Herman GE, Emch GS, Tovar CA et al. c-Fos generation in the dorsal vagal complex after systemic endotoxin is not dependent on the vagus nerve. Am J Physiol Regul Integr Comp Physiol 2001; 208:289-299.
61. Emch GS, Herman GE, Rogers RC. TNF-α activates solitary nucleus neurons responsive to gastric distension. Am J Physiol Gastrointest Liver Physiol 2000; 279:G582-G586.
62. Watkins LR, Maier SF. Implications of immune-to-brain communication for sickness and pain. Proc Natl Acad Sci USA 1999; 96:7710-7713.
63. Stenberg EM. Neural-immune interactions in health and disease. J Clin Invest 1997; 100:2641-2647.
64. Scheimann RI, Cogswell PC, Lofquist AK et al. Role of trancriptional activation of IkBα in mediation of immunosuppression by glucocorticoids. Science 1995; 270:283-286.
65. Guarini S, Altavilla D, Cainazzo MM et al. Efferent vagal fibre stimulation blunts nuclear factor-kB activation and protects against hypovolemic hemorrhagic shock. Circulation 2003, 107:1189-119.
66. Guarini S, Tagliavini S, Bazzani C et al. Nicotine reverses hemorrhagic shock in rats. Naunyn-Schmiedeberg's Arch Pharmacol 1991; 343:427-430.
67. Guarini S, Bazzani C, Tagliavini S et al. Reversal of experimental hemorrhagic shock by dimethylphenylpiperazinium (DMPP). Experientia 1992; 48:663-667.
68. Pavlov VA, Tracey KJ. The cholinergic anti-inflammatory pathway. Brain Behav Immun 2005; 19:493-499.
69. Oke SL, Tracey KJ. From CNI-1493 to the immunological homonculus: physiology of the inflammatory reflex. J Leukoc Biol 2008; 83:512-517.
70. Parrish WR, Gallowitsch-Puerta M, Czura CJ et al. Experimental therapeutic strategies for severe sepsis: mediators and mechanisms. Ann N Y Acad Sci 2008; 1144:210-236.
71. Van der Zanden EP, Boeckxstaens Ge, de Jonge WJ. The vagus nerve as a modulator of intestinal inflammation. Neurogastroenterol Motil 2009; 21:6-17.
72. Loewy AD. Central autonomic pathways. In: Loewy AD, Spyer KM, eds. Central Regulation of Autonomic Functions. Oxford: Oxford University Press, 1990:88-104.
73. Baue AE. Multiple organ failure, multiple organ dysfunction syndrome and systemic inflammatory response syndrome. Why no magic bullets? Arch Surg 1997; 132:703-707.
74. Le Tulzo Y, Shenkar R, Kaneko D et al. Hemorrhage increases cytokine expression in lung mononuclear cells in mice: involvement of catecholamines in nuclear factor-kB regulation and cytokine expression. J Clin Invest 1997; 99:1516-1524.
75. Guarini S, Bazzani C, Mattera Ricigliano G et al. Influence of ACTH-(1-24) on free radical levels in the blood of haemorrhage-shocked rats: direct ex vivo detection by electron spin resonance spectrometry. Br J Pharmacol 1996; 119:29-34.
76. Guarini S, Bini A, Bazzani C et al. Adrenocorticotropin normalizes the blood levels of nitric oxide in haemorrhage-shocked rats. Eur J Pharmacol 1997; 336:15-21.

77. Altavilla D, Guarini S, Bitto A et al. Activation of the cholinergic anti-inflammatory pathway reduces NF-kB activation, blunts TNF-α production and protects against splanchnic artery occlusion shock. Shock 2006; 25:500-506.
78. McDonald MC, Mota-Filipe H, Paul A et al. Calpain inhibitor I reduces the activation of nuclear factor-kB and organ injury/dysfunction in hemorrhagic shock. FASEB J 2001; 15:171-186.
79. Cui X, Wu R, Zhou M et al. Adrenomedullin and its binding protein attenuate the proinflammatory response after hemorrhage. Crit Care Med 2005; 33:391-398.
80. Jarrar D, Chaudry IH, Wang P. Organ dysfunction following hemorrhage and sepsis: mechanisms and therapeutic approaches. Int J Mol Med 1999; 4:575-583.
81. Bertolini A, Guarini S, Ferrari W et al. Adrenocorticotropin reversal of experimental hemorrhagic shock is antagonized by morphine. Life Sci 1986; 39:1271-1280.
82. Guarini S, Vergoni AV, Bertolini A. Anti-shock effect of ACTH-(1-24): comparison between intracerebroventricular and intravenous route of administration. Pharmacol Res Commun 1987; 19:255-260.
83. Guarini S, Tagliavini S, Bazzani C et al. Effect of ACTH-(1-24) on the volume of circulating blood and on regional blood flow in rats bled to hypovolemic shock. Resuscitation 1989; 18:133-134.
84. Bazzani C, Tagliavini S, Bertolini E et al. Influence of ACTH-(1-24) on metabolic acidosis and hypoxemia induced by massive hemorrhage in rats. Resuscitation 1992; 23:113-120.
85. Guarini S, Ferrari W, Bertolini A. Anti-shock effect of ACTH-(1-24): influence of subtotal hepatectomy. Pharmacol Res Commun 1988; 20:395-403.
86. Jochem J. Involvement of proopiomelanocortin-derived peptides in endogenous central istamine-induced reversal of critical haemorrhagic hypotension in rats. J Physiol Pharmacol 2004; 55:57-71.
87. Bertuglia S, Giusti A. Influence of ACTH-(1-24) and plasma hyperviscosity on free radical production and capillary perfusion after hemorrhagic shock. Microcirculation 2004; 11:227-238.
88. Ludbrook J, Ventura S. ACTH-(1-24) blocks the decompensatory phase of the haemodynamic response to acute hypovolaemia in conscious rabbits. Eur J Pharmacol 1995; 275:267-275.
89. Bertolini A, Guarini S, Ferrari W et al. ACTH-(1-24) restores blood pressure in acute hypovolaemia and haemorrhagic shock in humans. Eur J Clin Pharmacol 1987; 32:537-538.
90. Noera G, Pensa P, Guelfi P et al. ACTH-(1-24) and hemorrhagic shock: preliminary clinical results. Resuscitation 1989; 18:145-147.
91. Noera G, Angiello L, Biagi B et al. Haemorrhagic shock in cardiac surgery. Pharmacological treatment with ACTH (1-24). Resuscitation 1991; 22:123-127.
92. Pinelli G, Chesi G, Di Donato C et al. Preliminary data on the use of ACTH-(1-24) in human shock conditions. Resuscitation 1989; 18:149-150.
93. Altavilla D, Cainazzo MM, Squadrito F et al. Tumour necrosis factor-α as a target of melanocortins in haemorrhagic shock, in the anaesthetized rat. Br J Pharmacol 1998; 124:1587-1590.
94. Guarini S, Tagliavini S, Bazzani C et al. Intracerebroventricular injection of hemicolinium-3 prevents the ACTH-induced, but not the physostigmine-induced, reversal of hemorrhagic shock in rats. Pharmacology 1990; 40:85-89.
95. Guarini S, Rompianesi E, Ferrari W et al. Influence of vagotomy and of atropine on the anti-shock effect of adrenocorticotropin. Neuropeptides 1986; 8:19-24.
96. Guarini S, Tagliavini S, Ferrari W et al. Reversal of haemorrhagic shock in rats by cholinomimetic drugs. Br J Pharmacol 1989; 98:218-824.
97. Savić J, Varagić VM, Prokić DJ et al. The life-saving effect of physostigmine in haemorrhagic shock. Resuscitation 1991; 21:57-60.
98. Onat F, Aslan N, Gören Z et al. Reversal of hemorrhagic shock in rats by oxotremorine: the role of muscarinic and nicotinic receptors and AV3V region. Brain Res 1994; 660:261-266.
99. Bazzani C, Balugani A, Bertolini A et al. Comparison of the effects of ACTH-(1-24), methylprednisolone, aprotinin and norepinephrine in a model of hemorrhagic shock in rats. Resuscitation 1993; 25:219-226.
100. Gonindard C, Goigoux C, Hollande E et al. The administration of an α-MSH analogue reduces the serum release of IL-1 α and TNF α induced by the injection of a sublethal dose of lipopolysaccharides in the BALB/c mouse. Pigment Cell Res 1996; 9:148-153.
101. Lipton JM, Ceriani G, Macaluso A et al. Antiinflammatory effects of the neuropeptide α-MSH in acute, chronic and systemic inflammation. Ann NY Acad Sci 1994; 741:137-148.
102. Pavlov VA, Ochani M, Gallowitsch-Puerta M et al. Central muscarinic cholinergic regulation of the systemic inflammatory response during endotoxemia. Proc Natl Acad Sci USA 2006; 103:5219-5223.
103. Vinten-Johansen J. Involvement of neutrophils in the pathogenesis of lethal myocardial reperfusion injury. Cardiovasc Res 2004; 61:481-497.
104. Frangogiannis NG, Smith CW, Entman ML. The inflammatory response in myocardial infarction. Cardiovasc Res 2002; 53:31-47.

105. Eefting F, Rensing B, Wigman J et al. Role of apoptosis in reperfusion injury. Cardiovasc Res 2004; 61:414-426.
106. O'Neill CA, Fu LW, Halliwell B et al. Hydroxyl radical production during myocardial ischemia and reperfusion in cats. Am J Physiol Heart Circ Physiol 1996; 271:H660-H667.
107. Bolli R, Marban E. Molecular and cellular mechanisms of myocardial stunning. Physiol Rev 1999; 79:609-634.
108. Ramasamy R, Hwang YC, Liu Y et al. Metabolic and functional protection by selective inhibition of nitric oxide synthase 2 during ischemia-reperfusion in isolated perfused hearts. Circulation 2004; 109:1668-1673.
109. Li C, Browder W, Kao RL. Early activation of transcription factor NF-kB during ischemia in perfused rat heart. Am J Physiol Heart Circ Physiol 1999; 276:H543-H552.
110. Shimizu N, Yoshiyama M, Omura T et al. Activation of mitogen-activated protein kinases and activator protein-1 in myocardial infarction in rats. Cardiovasc Res 1998; 38:116-124.
111. Hausenloy DJ, Yellon DM. New directions for protecting the heart against ischaemia-reperfusion injury: targeting the reperfusion injury salvage kinase (RISK)-pathway. Cardiovasc Res 2004; 61:448-460.
112. Moukarbel GV, Ayoub CM, Abchee AB. Pharmacological therapy for myocardial reperfusion injury. Curr Opin Pharmacol 2004; 4:147-153.
113. Monassier JP. Reperfusion injury in acute myocardial infarction: from bench to cath lab. Part II: Clinical issues and therapeutic options. Arch Cardiovasc Dis 2008; 101:565-575.
114. Landmesser U, Wollert KC, Drexler H. Potential novel pharmacological therapies for myocardial remodelling. Cardiovasc Res 2009; 81:519-527.
115. Bazzani C, Mioni C, Ferrazza G et al. Involvement of the central nervous system in the protective effect of melanocortins in myocardial ischaemia/reperfusion injury. Resuscitation 2002; 52:109-115.
116. Juhasz B, Der P, Szodoray P et al. Adrenocorticotrope hormone fragment (4-10) attenuates the ischemia/reperfusion-induced cardiac injury in isolated rat hearts. Antioxid Redox Signal 2007; 9:1851-1861.
117. Colombo G, Gatti S, Turcatti F et al. Gene expression profiling reveals multiple protective influences of the peptide α-melanocyte-stimulating hormone in experimental heart transplantation. J Immunol 2005; 175:3391-3401.
118. Zuanetti G, De Ferrari GM, Priori SG et al. Protective effect of vagal stimulation on reperfusion arrhythmias in cats. Circ Res 1987; 61:429-435.
119. Vanoli E, De Ferrari GM, Stramba-Badiale M et al. Vagal stimulation and prevention of sudden death in conscious dog with a healed myocardial infarction. Circ Res 1991; 68:1471-1481.
120. Li M, Zheng C, Sato T et al. Vagal nerve stimulation markedly improves long-term survival after chronic heart failure in rats. Circulation 2004; 109:120-124.
121. Cheng Z, Zhang H, Guo SZ et al. Differential control over postganglionic neurons in rat cardiac ganglia by NA and DmnX neurons: anatomical evidence. Am J Physiol Regul Integr Comp Physiol 2004; 286:R625-R633.
122. Cheng Z, Guo SZ, Lipton AJ et al. Domoic acid lesions in nucleus of the solitary tract: time-dependent recovery of hypoxic ventilatory response and peripheral afferent axonal plasticity. J Neurosci 2002; 22:3215-26.
123. Zhang H, Gozal D, Yu J et al. Attenuation of baroreflex control of the heart rate following domoic acid (DA) lesions in the nucleus ambiguus (NA) of the rat. Soc Neurosci Abstr 2002; 29.
124. Anderson MR. The systemic inflammatory response in heart failure. Prog Ped Card 2000; 11:219-230.
125. Katare RG, Ando M, Kakinuma Y et al. Vagal nerve stimulation prevents reperfusion injury through inhibition of opening of mithocondrial permeability transition pore independent of the bradycardiac effect. J Thorac Cardiovasc Surg 2009; 137:223-231.
126. Krishnamurthy P, Rajasingh J, Lambers E et al. IL-10 inhibits inflammation and attenuates left ventricular remodeling after myocardial infarction via activation of STAT3 and suppression of HuR. Circ Res 2009; 104:e9-e18.
127. Leker RR, Shohami E. Cerebral ischemia and trauma—different etiologies yet similar mechanisms: neuroprotective opportunities. Brain Res Rev 2002; 39:55-73.
128. Gladstone DJ, Black SE, Hakim AM. Toward wisdom from failure: lessons from neuroprotective stroke trials and new therapeutic directions. Stroke 2002; 33:2123-2136.
129. Wise PM, Dubal DB, Rau SW et al. Are estrogens protective or risk factors in brain injury and neurodegeneration? Re-evaluation after the women's health initiative. Endocr Rev 2005; 26:308-312.
130. Rogalewski A, Schneider A, Ringelstein EB et al. Toward a multimodal neuroprotective treatment of stroke. Stroke 2006; 37:1129-1136.
131. Adams HP, Del Zoppo G, Alberts MJ et al. Guidelines for the early management of adults with ischemic stroke. Stroke 2007; 38:1655-711.

132. Yepes M, Roussel BD, Ali C et al. Tissue-type plasminogen activator in the ischemic brain: more than a thrombolytic. Trends Neurosci 2009; 32:48-55.

133. Huh SK, Lipton JM, Batjer HH. The protective effects of α-melanocyte stimulating hormone on canine brain ischemia. Neurosurgery 1997; 40:132-140.

134. Huang Q, Tatro JB. α-Melanocyte stimulating hormone suppresses intracerebral tumor necrosis factor-α and interleukin-1β gene expression following transient cerebral ischemia in mice. Neurosci Lett 2002; 334:186-190.

135. Forslin Aronsson S, Spulber S, Popescu LM et al. α-Melanocyte-stimulating hormone is neuroprotective in rat global cerebral ischemia. Neuropeptides 2006; 40:65-75.

136. Tatro JB, Sinha PS. The central melanocortin system and fever. Ann N Y Acad Sci 2003; 994:246-257.

137. Spulber S, Moldovan M, Oprica M et al. α-MSH decreases core and brain temperature during global cerebral ischemia in rats. Neuroreport 2005; 16:69-72.

138. Gendron A, Teitelbaum J, Cossette C et al. Temporal effects of left versus right middle cerebral artery occlusion on spleen lymphocyte subsets and mitogenic response in Wistar rats. Brain Res 2002; 955:85-97.

139. Prass K, Meisel C, Hoflich C et al. Stroke-induced immunodeficiency promotes spontaneous bacterial infections and is mediated by sympathetic activation reversal by poststroke T helper cell type 1-like immunostimulation. J Exp Med 2003; 198:725-736.

140. Emsley HCA, Smith CJ, Gavin CM et al. An early and sustained peripheral inflammatory response in acute ischaemic stroke: relationships with infection and atherosclerosis. J Neuroimmunol 2003; 139:93-101.

141. Smith CJ, Emsley HCA, Gavin CM et al. Peak plasma interleukin-6 and other peripheral markers of inflammation in the first week of ischaemic stroke correlate with brain infarct volume, stroke severity and long-term outcome. BMC Neurol 2004; 4:2.

142. Offner H, Subramanian S, Parker SM et al. Experimental stroke induces massive, rapid activation of the peripheral immune system. J Cereb Blood Flow Metab 2006; 26:654-665.

143. Zhang G, Zhang L, Logan R et al. Decreased expression and impaired function of muscarinic acetylcholine receptors in the rat hippocampus following transient forebrain ischemia. Neurobiol Dis 2005; 20:805-813.

144. Spencer SJ, Mouihate A, Pittman QJ. Peripheral inflammation exacerbates damage after global ischemia independently of temperature and acute brain inflammation. Stroke 2007; 38:1570-1577.

145. Vila N, Castillo J, Dávalos A et al. Levels of anti-inflammatory cytokines and neurological worsening in acute ischemic stroke. Stroke 2003; 34:671-675.

146. Mountjoy KG, Mortrud MT, Low MJ et al. Localization of the melanocortin-4 receptor (MC4-R) in neuroendocrine and autonomic control circuits in the brain. Mol Endocrinol 1994; 8:1298-1308.

147. Li SJ, Varga K, Archer P et al. Melanocortin antagonists define two distinct pathways of cardiovascular control by α- and γ-melanocyte-stimulating hormones. J Neurosci 1996; 16:5182-5188.

148. Rosas-Ballina M, Ochani M, Parrish WR et al. Splenic nerve is required for cholinergic anti-inflammatory pathway control of TNF in endotoxemia. Proc Natl Acad Sci USA 2008; 105:11008-11013.

Melanocortin Control of Cell Trafficking in Vascular Inflammation

Hetal B. Patel, Giovanna Leoni, Trinidad Montero Melendez, André L.F. Sampaio and Mauro Perretti*

Abstract

Over 20 years of research based upon application of experimental models of inflammation and tissue injury have revealed exquisite controlling functions for melanocortin hormones and, subsequently, their synthetic derivatives. More recent discoveries have shed light on the receptor targets responsible for these effects, leading to what could be the next step-change for this line of research, the development of novel therapeutics for the control of human inflammatory pathologies. Here we review some of this work with particular emphasis on more recent studies that have substantiated the activities of melanocortin peptides to reveal important regulatory functions for their receptors in vascular inflammation and disease models. Moreover, we summarise the drug discovery activities (for what is published knowledge) attempting to capitalise on this wealth of research on melanocortins, though we should not forget the successful employment of ACTH to treat human gouty arthritis. Altogether, this chapter would corroborate and flare the enthusiasm for this line of research, as we are confident that the right times might have arrived to develop novel anti-arthritic and tissue-protective compounds that will be acting by mimicking the way our endogenous melanocortins would act to exert their homeostatic and check-point functions.

Introduction

It is often said that the seminal study of Philip Hench published in 1949 reporting the efficacy of compound E (later characterised and synthesised by Sarett as cortisol), "'... a new day dawned in rheumatology. Therapy was now dated BC (before cortisone) or after (AC)!'".[1] Whereas this is true, it is also true that in the same study Philip Hench and colleagues reported also the therapeutic efficacy of pituitary adrenocorticotrophin (ACTH) when administered in rheumatoid arthritis patients.[2] The effect of ACTH on changing the numbers of circulating leukocytes had already been reported.[3] The clinical efficacy of ACTH was rapidly confirmed in patients suffering of gouty arthritis[4] a therapeutic response attributed to increased endogenous cortisol[2] and, possibly as a consequence, to modulation of circulating white blood cells.[5] The buzz of those frontier years yielded the notion that '... glucocorticoids changed much of the face of therapeutics not only in rheumatological practice but throughout the whole field of medicine'.[1] Whereas this is certainly true even at the end of the first decade of the third millennium, that is 60 years after the discoveries of Hench and colleagues (!), it is surprising how little—or not enough—has been done to capitalise on the clinical observations produced with ACTH. In reality the literature *stores* the data, the problem is to go out to find them. In fact, a mid -90s clinical study in gouty arthritis patients

*Corresponding Author: Mauro Perretti—The William Harvey Research Institute, Barts and the London School of Medicine, Queen Mary University of London, Charterhouse Square, London, EC1M 6BQ, United Kingdom. Email: m.perretti@qmul.ac.uk

Melanocortins: Multiple Actions and Therapeutic Potential, edited by Anna Catania.
©2010 Landes Bioscience and Springer Science+Business Media.

confirmed the efficacy of ACTH also when a controlled design was used, with the hormone affording a therapeutic control of the disease that suggested, to the Authors, the existence of other molecular mechanisms beside the expected adrenal gland activation and the ensuing increase in circulating cortisol.[6] ACTH is still used in US for gouty arthritis, in patients manifesting intolerance to nonsteroidal anti-inflammatory drugs.[7]

So what could be the *alternative mode of action* of ACTH? Nowadays and this book is a testimony to this, our knowledge is much increased and the biosynthetic link between ACTH and melanocyte stimulating hormone (MSH) species is clear.[8] Moreover, alpha-MSH is the prototype of a series of natural and synthetic peptides (melanocortins) endowed with potent biological properties. This Chapter attempts to summarise some of their major effects with particular emphasis on peripheral inflammation. We will also address, though at its infancy, the issue of whether therapeutic exploitation of this line of research could be an effective way for the development of novel anti-inflammatory therapeutics.

Inflammation: Cell Trafficking and Microcirculation

The response that our body sets up to counteract the attacks by xenobiotics and infective agents has the main goal of producing a safe, space limited and temporal controlled reaction, disposing of the agent(s) and with minimal damage to the host tissue in order to assure rapid regain of the homeostasis. A hallmark of this inflammatory response is the movement of white blood cells from the vascular district towards the site of the tissue injury or xenobiotic invasion. This movement of cells is orchestrated by several classes of inflammatory mediators, including adhesion molecules, rapidly acting mediators such as autacoids (e.g., histamine or leukotrienes) and polypeptides such as cytokines and chemokines.[9] The sequential activation of specific processes, promoted by these pro-inflammatory mediators, then occurs are reported in Figure 1.

Whereas the life-saving importance of the inflammatory reactions is out of dispute,[10,11] the appreciation that inflammation does not extinguish by itself has recently emerged. Therefore, in parallel and possibly as a consequence to the increased levels of pro-inflammatory mediators, classes of anti-inflammatory mediators are being discovered. In analogy to the variety of pro-inflammatory mediators, there are short-lived lipids such as lipoxins, proteins and peptides, autacoids such as adenosine and even, as recently reported, adhesion molecules[12] within the umbrella of endogenous anti-inflammation.[13-15] It is important to establish how each of these mediators, part of specific homeostatic circuits, would operate. Appreciation of specific patho-physiological pathways is important to characterise the cellular and tissue-restricted events that each of these checkpoints mediators bring about; similarly, in terms of pharmacology, the investigation of the specific receptor target(s) that mediate the actions at the molecular level of a given anti-inflammatory mediator is of crucial importance. The best approach would be to parallel increment of our knowledge at both levels.

Figure 1 illustrates not only the sequelae of events responsible for the extravasation of the blood borne leucocytes (granulocytes, monocytes and lymphocytes; all of these groups being formed by multiple subgroups) via the processes of cell rolling, adhesion and emigration (also referred to as diapedesis), but it also shows tissue resident cells. The inflammatory vascular response is initiated by mast cells[16] and macrophages,[17] resident cells that play a whistle blower role: release of pro-inflammatory mediators by these cells would activate the vascular endothelium initiating the cascade of molecular and cellular processes required for the inflammatory reaction to begin and progress. However, in line with the notion of the existence of pivotal checkpoints in the body to assure that the inflammatory reaction is confined to the affected tissue and that it is also limited in its time frame, both resident cells and blood borne leucocytes would be targeted by endogenous anti-inflammatory mediators to assure proper activation of the resolution phase and termination of the inflammatory reaction in a safe manner.

ACTH, alpha-MSH and other melanocortin peptides belong to this large family of anti-inflammatory mediators. This is evident from their modulatory effect on cells which play important roles in the initiation, maintenance as well as resolution of the inflammatory reaction;[18,19]

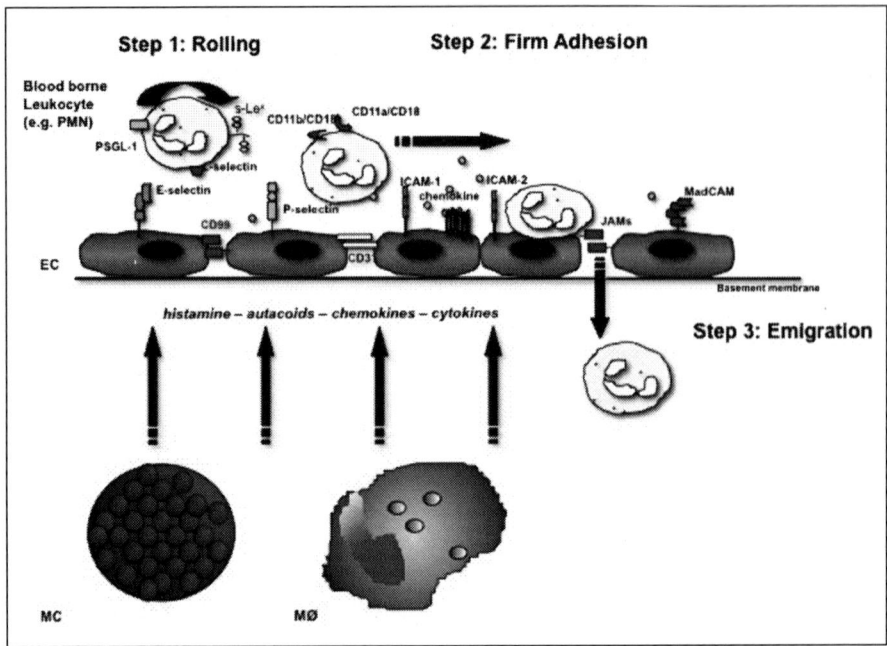

Figure 1. Recruitment of blood borne cells in inflammation. Depicted is a schematic representation of the initial events regulating the extravasation of blood borne leukocyte, with emphasis on their interaction with the endothelial cell (EC) monolayers on the vascular wall. Highlighted are the processes of leukocyte (a neutrophil is shown as an example, PMN) rolling, adhesion and emigration, with the sequential involvement of multiple players, including adhesion molecules and leukocyte activators. The initiating role of tissue resident cells, such as the mast cell (MC) and the macrophages (MØ), is also indicated. Melanocortin peptides can act on their receptors to modulate the re-activity of many cellular players operative in the context of inflamed vessel. Abbreviations: CD: cluster definition; ICAM: inter-cellular adhesion molecule; MadCAM: mucosal addressin cell adhesion molucule; PSGL-1: P-selectin glycoprotein-1.

moreover, the application of models of inflammation to animals which have been nullified for specific components of the melanocortin system, in particular specific receptors responsible for bringing about its homeostatic functions, confirms the checkpoint role of these mediators in the overall complex scenario of inflammation. We will now discuss some of the properties associated with melanocortin biology in the context of experimental and human inflammation.

Melancortins in Experimental Inflammation

The therapeutic effectiveness of natural and synthetic melanocortins as anti-inflammatories has been widely studied in experimental models of vascular inflammation and disease. Local as well as systemic treatment seems to improve, in many cases, disease outcome. Table 1 summarises the use of melanocortin peptides in experimental models of inflammation.

Studies from the late 1980s were the first to suggest that alpha-MSH had anti-inflammatory properties. Pyretic responses are induced upon the release of inflammatory mediators within the brain; treatment with alpha-MSH completely antagonised the effect of endotoxin, tumour necrosis factor (TNF)-α and interleukin (IL)-6 induced febrile responses.[20,21] These intriguing results led to the wider studies of melanocortin peptides in other inflammatory settings including ischaemia reperfusion injury, lipolysaccharide (LPS)-induced inflammation and arthritis.[22-25]

Table 1. *Non-exhaustive list of experimental models of inflammation and tissue injury where the effects of melanocortin receptor agonism has been tested with success*

Model	Species	Stimulus/Procedure	Agonist	Outcome Following Treatment	Reference
Adjuvant-induced arthritis	Rat	CFA containing *Myc. butyricum*	α-MSH	↓ Disease	25
				↓ Histological score	
	Rat		POMC gene therapy	↓ Pain (thermal hypersensitivity response)	90
				↓ Paw swelling	
Carrageenan inflammation	Mouse	Airpouch	HP228	↓ PMN accumulation	53
Colitis	Mouse	DSS *Citrobacter rodentium*	MC1R e/e mutant mice	↑ Weight loss	66
				↓ Survival	
				↑ Histological damage	
				↑ Colonic MPO activity	
Cutaneous vasculitis	Mouse	LPS	α-MSH	↓ Haemorrhagic lesions (clinical/histological score)	59
				↓ E-selectin (ear)	
Endotoxaemia	Rat	LPS	(CKPV)₂ NDP-α-MSH	↓ TNF-α	23
	Mice	LPS	BMS-470539	↓ Systemic TNA-α	24
				↓ Leukocytic infiltration (lung)	

continued on next page

Table 1. *Continued*

Model	Species	Stimulus/Procedure	Agonist	Outcome Following Treatment	Reference
Gouty arthritis	Rat	Monosodium urate crystals	D[Trp^8]-γ-MSH	↓ Arthritic score	91
				↓ Joint PMN accumulation	
				↓ KC	
				↓ IL-1β	
Heart transplantation	Rat	Allograft transplantation	NDP-α-MSH	↑ Allograft survival	30
				↓ Histopathologic score	
				↓ Leukocytic infiltrate	
				↓ Endothelin-1, NOS2, MCP-1, RANTES, ICAM-1, VCAM-1, FasL, IFNγ, IL-1β	
Ischaemia reperfusion (brain)	Mouse	Middle cerebral artery occlusion	α-MSH	↑ α-MSH in bronchoalveolar lavage fluids	92
				↑ Intrabronchial bacterial load	
Ischaemia reperfusion (heart)	Rat	Occlusion	ACTH-(1-24) NDP-α-MSH	↓ Ischemic myocardial tissue	34
				↓ Apoptotic bodies	
				↓ Systemic free radical levels	
				Normal ESR	
	Mouse	Occlusion	HP228	↓ Infarct size	53
	Mouse	Occlusion	MTII	↓ Infarct size	35
				↓ Systemic and local KC, IL-1β	
				↓ Local MPO	
				↓ Lethality	

continued on next page

Table 1. *Continued*

Model	Species	Stimulus/Procedure	Agonist	Outcome Following Treatment	Reference
Ischaemia reperfusion (kidney)	Mouse	Occlusion	α-MSH	↓ Creatinine ↓ Lung and kidney histology score ↓ Lung and kidney MPO ↓ Lung edema ↓ KC, ICAM-1 and TNFα mRNA	22, 93
Ischaemia reperfusion (mesentery)	Mouse	Occlusion	*[1] MC3R null mice *[2] D-Trp⁸-γ-MSH	↑ MPO*[1] ↑ Albumin leakage*[1] ↑ Cell emigration/adhesion*[1] ↑ MCP-1/KC*[1] ↑ Nitrite/nitrate*[1] ↓ V$_{WBC}$*[2] ↓ Cell adhesion/emigration*[2]	31
Ischemic stroke	Rat	Endothelin-1	NDP-α-MSH	↓ JNK ↓ ERK ↓ TNF-α ↓ Caspase 3 ↓ Plasma TNF-α	94

continued on next page

Table 1. *Continued*

Model	Species	Stimulus/Procedure	Agonist	Outcome Following Treatment	Reference
Liver inflammation	Mouse	LPS	α-MSH	↓ Serum alanine aminotransferase	29
				↓ PMN accumulation	
				↓ MPO	
				↓ Serum nitrate/nitrite	
				↓ Liver KC and MCP-1 mRNA	
Lung inflammation	Mouse	Ovalbumin	α-MSH	↓ Eosinophil accumulation	69
				↑ PMN accumulation	
				↑ BAL IL-10	
				↓ BAL IL-4, IL-13	
	Mouse	LPS	D[Trp⁸]-γ-MSH	↓ PMN accumulation	68
				↓ BAL TNF-α	
Peritonitis	Mouse	Monosodium urate crystals	ACTH4-10	↓ PMN accumulation	41,43,44, 53,54,67
			γ₂-MSH	↓ KC	
			MTII	↓ IL-1β	
			α-MSH	↑ HO-1	
			HP228		
			D[Trp⁸]-γ-MSH		

continued on next page

Table 1. *Continued*

Model	Species	Stimulus/Procedure	Agonist	Outcome Following Treatment	Reference
Sepsis-induced acute kidney injury	Mouse	Cecal-ligation and puncture	AP214	↓ Serum creatinine	80
				↓ Tubular damage (kidney)	
				↓ Aspartate aminotransferase (liver)	
				↓ Alanine aminotransferase (liver)	
				↓ Hypotension/bradycardia	
				↓ Serum TNF-α	
				↓ Serum IL-10	

Abbreviations: ERK: extracellular regulated kinase; FasL: FAS ligand; HO-1: heme oxygenase-1; KC: keratinocyte chemoattractant; ICAM-1: intercellular adhesion molecule-1; IL: interleukin; IR: ischaemia-reperfusion; JNK: janus kinase; MCP-1: monocyte chemotactic protein-1; MPO: myeloperoxidase; NOS: nitric oxide synthase; PMN: polymorphonuclear leukocytes; RANTES: regulated upon activation normal T-cell expressed and secreted; TNF: tumour necrosis factor; V_{WBC}: white blood cell velocity; VCAM-1: vascular cell adhesion molecule-1.

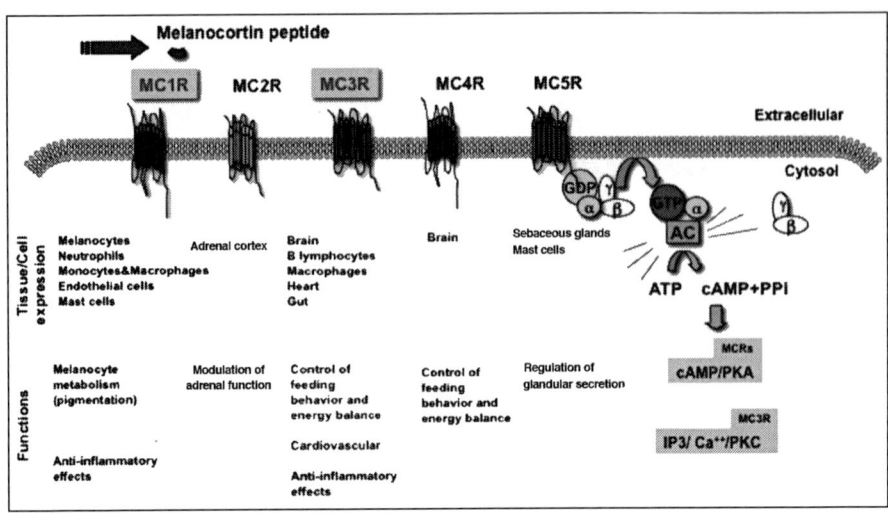

Figure 2. Melanocortin receptors. Schematic representation of MCRs on a hypothetical plasma membrane. Activation of any of these receptors by a melanocortin peptide will cause activation of a stimulatory G protein (Gs) leading to accumulation of intracellular cAMP. In some cell system, MC3R has also been associated with inositol-tri-phosphate (IP3) accumulation. Succinct distribution patterns for each receptor and their main biological functions, are also reported. AC: adenylate cyclase; GDP and GTP: guanine diphosphate and guanine triphosphate; PK, protein kinase. This schematic figures highlights the proposed functional importance of MC1R and MC3R in controlling experimental and human inflammatory disease.

A rapid overview of Table 1 allows the formulation of a number of general comments. (1) Endogenous peptides and synthetic melanocortin compounds inhibit activation of the masterminder nuclear factor κB (NFκB);[26-28] as a consequence, (2) they affect classical markers of inflammation downregulating cytokine (TNF-α, IL-1β) and chemokine (IL-8) levels as well as levels of others pro-inflammatory agents (inducible nitric oxide synthase, nitrites and nitrates).[29-31] Furthermore (3) melanocortins control leucocyte-endothelial interactions by decreasing cell adhesion molecule expression (examples are intercellular adhesion molecule-1 [ICAM-1] and vascular cell adhesion molecule-1 [VCAM-1])[30] thus blocking leukocyte migration to the site of vascular inflammation. The overall outcome (4) is that treatment of animals with alpha-MSH, and more recently other synthetic derivatives, would generally reduce tissue injury and inflammatory responses (see Table 1).

We now need to mention, briefly, that five melanocortin receptors have so far been cloned and their acronym goes from MC1R to MC5R[8] (Fig. 2). Whereas MC2R, expressed on adrenal cells, is the highly specific receptor for ACTH, MC1R is expressed by melanocytes and controls skin pigmentation, so it mediates one of the major physiological functions of alpha-MSH. Recent reviews[18,19,32] and other chapters in this book have elaborated on the distribution patterns of MC3R, MC4R and MC5R, in addition to MC1R.

Ischaemia reperfusion (IR) injury occurs as a consequence of low oxygen state usually due to inadequate blood flow/supply and is followed by a period when blood flow is restored. IR is usually a reversible process unless the period of ischaemia exceeds a critical period of time when diverse molecular and cellular alterations occur and injury becomes irreversible and restoration of blood flow often exacerbating the deleterious effects of ischaemia.[33] The IR phenomenon is common in a variety of vascular-based pathologies including myocardial infarction, stroke and lung injury. Several melanocortins including the pan-receptor agonists ACTH and alpha-MSH and more selective agonists have been exploited in models of IR injury with promising outcomes (Table 1).

For example, pan-agonist ACTH is cardioprotective in myocardial ischaemia reperfusion injury whilst, selective MC3R agonist; [D-Trp$_8$]-γ-MSH is protective of injury occurring during IR in the mesentery.[31,34]

At the molecular level the melanocortins act to suppress pro-inflammatory cytokines/chemokines including IL-1β, TNF-α and KC. Getting et al showed decreases of ~30% systemic and ~60% local IL-1β levels and ~50% both for systemic and local KC levels, following therapeutic intervention with the MC3/4R agonist melatonin (also termed MTII) in a murine model of myocardial ischaemia reperfusion injury.[35] Furthermore cotreatment with MTII and the mixed MC3/4R antagonist SHU9119, but not selective MC4R antagonist HS024, reverted the effects on IL-1β and KC levels suggesting a role for MC3R in these protective actions; this study also observed that MC3R was present on cardiac macrophages but not parenchymal fibroblasts or cardiomyocytes.[35]

The identification of receptor(s) and cells modulated to bring about the attenuating actions of alpha-MSH in renal IR injury is less clear. Chiao et al convincingly showed that alpha-MSH, dosed either at the start of ischaemic phase or during the late (>6 h) reperfusion phase, attenuates renal damage by downregulating expression of KC and endothelial ICAM-1 expression, thus preventing neutrophil trafficking and adhesion to the kidney.[22] In a further study using mice knockout for ICAM-1, which had a 75% reduction in neutrophil infiltration compared to wild type controls, alpha-MSH was able to provide renal protection despite the lack of involvement of neutrophil adhesion and emigration, indicating that its immunoregulatory actions are unlikely effected solely through the neutrophil.[36]

More recently Lee et al have shown that both MC1R and MC3R are expressed in the outer medullary region of the IR-injured kidney and thus speculated that protective effects afforded by alpha-MSH may be through interaction with these receptors.[37] As to whether one or other MCR or even both may command this regulatory effect remains to be deciphered. The recent availability of transgenic mice mutant or void of MCRs will initiate a surge of experiments in the inflammation field and allow for better understanding of the mechanisms behind which the melanocortin peptide activities lie.

Effects of Melanocortins on Inflammatory Cells In Vitro

As summarised, in part, above and displayed in Table 1, there are no doubts that melanocortin peptides exert a regulatory role on the inflammatory process. In this section one would like to convey the reader's attention to the effects of melanocortins on specific inflammatory cells in vitro mimicking the environment common to various pathologies in mouse and human.

Monocytes and Macrophages

Whereas macrophages are tissue resident cells ready to promote the inflammatory reaction, monocytes are recruited to local sites of injury where they sustain inflammation, but then also mature to macrophages with switch towards an anti-inflammatory phenotype, promoting the resolution of acute inflammation.[17,38] The mouse macrophage has been one of the most common cells studied for addressing the biology of melanocortins and their receptors.

LPS-stimulated RAW264.7 murine macrophages respond with induction of nitric oxide (NO) synthase II and NO release and this was inhibited by alpha-MSH.[39] The same study showed that basal as well as TNF-α stimulated RAW264.7 cells were able to release alpha-MSH, supporting the stimulating hypothesis that peripheral expression of melanocortins could occur, a topic promoted by the studies of Blalock and colleagues.[40] Moreover, RAW264.7 cells expressed MC1R, which was then proposed to be the main effector for the actions of alpha-MSH on this cell type. Therefore, the proposed model was that alpha-MSH released by the inflamed macrophage might exert an immunomodulatory function through its self-expression of MC1R.[39]

RAW264.7 cells expressed not only MC1R, but also MC3R; the same pattern was evident in primary peritoneal macrophages.[41] Incubation of macrophages with ACTH led to a time- and concentration-dependent induction of heme oxygenase Type 1 (HO-1).[42] This response was thought to be through MC3R: the more selective MC3R agonist [D-Trp$_8$]-γ-MSH induced HO-1 with similar profiles to ACTH; moreover, ACTH-induced HO-1 expression was also detected in peritoneal macrophage collected from the recessive yellow e/e mouse, which bears a mutated and inactive form of MC1R.[42] Furthermore in the same macrophage [D-Trp$_8$]-γ-MSH induced a typical cAMP response characteristic of the G-protein coupled melanocortin receptors.[43]

Monosodium urate crystal stimulated macrophage treated with long-lasting selective MC3R agonist MTII inhibited IL-1β and KC release in vitro and in vivo.[44] Collectively these data lead one to speculate that MC3R may be the more influential melanocortin receptor above that of the actions of MC1R, in regulating the mouse macrophage in normal and inflamed settings. In contrast, data studying the effects of alpha-MSH on human monocyte and macrophage indicate a predominant role of MC1R as the anti-inflammatory receptor.

LPS-stimulated human THP-1 monocyte/macrophage cells released TNF-α which was inhibited upon treatment with alpha-MSH.[45] When the stimulated cells were incubated with antibody to human MC1R this inhibitory effect was attenuated supporting the hypothesis that MC1R is the primary MCR operational to regulate alpha-MSH functions.[45] Using primary human blood-derived monocytes, Bhardwaj et al reported up-regulated protein expression for MC1R upon endotoxin and mitogen stimulation.[46] In this study the capacity for alpha-MSH to regulate costimulatory molecule expression was also addressed. Monocytes treated with LPS induced phenotypic expression of costimulatory molecules CD80 and CD86 which coincided with higher levels of MC1R expression. After treatment with alpha-MSH, cells exhibited a strong and weak down-regulatory effect on CD86 and CD80, respectively. Collectively, it seems clear that alpha-MSH may modulate human monocyte activation/maturation through MC1R.[46]

In general, whether the effect of alpha-MSH on monocytes and macrophages are through MC1R or MC3R, the broad anti-inflammatory response can be attained by intracellular accumulation of cyclic adenosine monophosphate (cAMP), because of adenylate cyclase activation and the ensuing protein kinase A activation,[18,42] as well as by inhibition of NFκB activation, a nuclear factor which induces transcription of a cohort of inflammatory genes. Manna and Aggarwal quite elegantly used electrophoresis mobility shift assays to show that inflammatory agents LPS, okadaic acid and ceramide induce cAMP-dependent NFκB activation with the effect being reversed in the presence alpha-MSH. This phenomenon is perhaps counter-intuitive in view of the early increases in cAMP that activation of all melanocortin receptors would cause, but was studied not only in human monocytic U937 cells but also in HeLa epithelial, H4 Glioma and Jurkat T-cell lines.[26] Moreover, similar effects of alpha-MSH were noted in LPS/IFN-γ stimulated RAW264.7 cells.[47]

Mast Cells

Mast cells are the resident cells of connective tissue which once activated instigate multiple effects including release of pro-inflammatory mediators, vasodilation and angiogenesis.[16,48,49] The study of the Metcalfe group showed that bone marrow derived murine mast cells express MC1R at the gene and protein level upon phorbol 12-myristoyl-13-acetate (PMA)-stimulation and the receptor was functional since treatment with alpha-MSH led to intracellular accumulation of cAMP.[50] Furthermore, alpha-MSH was also able to downregulate IL-1β, TNF-α and lymphotactin responses of IgE receptor-dependent mast cell activation.[50]

Human mast cells are also responsive to alpha-MSH. Both primary skin mast cells and leukemic mast cell line (HMC-1) express prohormone convertases and the pro-opiomelanocortin gene product. IgE immune complex stimulation of both cell types cause a time-dependent extracellular release of alpha-MSH.[51]

We believe that a great potential exists for further and more detailed analysis of melanocortin peptides actions upon mast cells, in several inflammatory contexts, both in mouse and man, nonetheless these initial studies are strongly indicative that a cell type which sustains multiple functions in early and late phase of inflammation[52] can be a major understudied yet target cell for melanocortins.

Neutrophils

Neutrophils are the first cells to migrate to sites of inflammation where they can release detrimental products to kill the xenobiotic inflammogen, but could also damage the host tissue. A number of in vivo studies have shown inhibitory effects of alpha-MSH on the process of neutrophil migration.[30,53,54]

Some hints to cellular mechanisms have been derived from in vitro studies: alpha-MSH brought about up-regulation of elastase in IL-8-stimulated human HL-60 cells (surrogate for human neutrophils) and subsequently down-regulated CXCR1 and CXCR2, two chemokine receptors that drive neutrophil chemotaxis.[55] In another study with a synthetic molecule (CKPV)$_2$ based on the functionally active lys-pro-val (KPV) C-terminal sequence of alpha-MSH, inhibition of PMA-induced reactive oxygen species (ROS) production from neutrophils was observed.[56] Similarly, alpha-MSH was able to reverse LPS/PMA production of ROS from rat peritoneal neutrophils and effect that appeared to be cyclo-oxygenase dependent manner.[57]

Endothelial Cells

Microvascular endothelial cells are crucially located to promote and control, the initial processes of vascular inflammation, namely leukocyte rolling, adhesion and emigration (Fig. 1), prior to sub-endothelial tissue matrix migration to the site inflammation. Mouse brain and human dermal (both primary and transformed) microvascular endothelial cells are known to express MC1R.[58] Moreover and intriguingly, it is well established that endothelial cells can be source of POMC and its peptides[59] pointing again to the existence of integral peripheral loops (as we have seen it in the macrophage) for activation of this counter-regulatory pathway.

Upon TNF-α or LPS stimulation of human dermal microvascular endothelial cells, alpha-MSH significantly decreased mRNA and protein levels of cell adhesion molecules E-selectin, VCAM-1 and ICAM-1.[59] These properties of alpha-MSH explained the inhibitory effect of this melanocortin on adhesion of leukocytes to endothelial cells in vitro, as seen using static assays; alpha-MSH attenuated T- and B-cell adhesion to dermal endothelial cells promoted by LPS.[59]

Other Cells

The actions of melanocortins have also been implicated in non-acute immunomodulatory functions of fibroblasts, lymphocytes and dendritic cells (DC).

MC1R expressing dermal fibroblasts stimulated with TNF-α and treated with alpha-MSH and KP$_D$V (a modification of the tripeptide KPV) inhibited NFκB activation and ICAM-1 up-regulation.[60] Human peripheral monocyte-derived DC also express MC1R mRNA, with protein levels increasing upon maturation. In mature DCs, costimulatory molecule CD86 was significantly downregulated in the presence of alpha-MSH, whilst only a slight decrease in CD40 was observed.[61] Thus, melanocortin peptides may play a role in the signals required for antigen presentation.

In line with these results, in vivo studies have shown that alpha-MSH induces tolerance in a hapten-specific manner. Hapten dinitro-fluorobenzene (DNFB) pulsed-bone marrow derived DC treated with alpha-MSH were injected into naïve mice. After further challenging with DNFB, ear swelling was significantly reduced compared to pulsed DC untreated with the melanocortin.[62] Furthermore, after resensitisation to study hapten-specific tolerance induction, ear swelling remained suppressed confirming that tolerance had been reached.[62]

Finally, Cooper et al noted an immunosuppressive response in streptodornase-induced, but not anti-CD3 induced, lymphocyte proliferation.[63] The model suggested is that alpha-MSH activate MC1R-expressing monocytes and MC1R- or MC3R-expressing B-lymphocytes and that this is independent of the nonMC1R expressing T-lymphocyte status.[63]

In summary, the portfolio of anti-inflammatory properties of alpha-MSH, ACTH and other natural and synthetic melanocortin peptides, is quite substantial. Many data in experimental animals have been produced and in some cases are corroborated by clinical data, example being the use of ACTH in human gouty arthritis and the anti-inflammatory actions of ACTH, alpha-MSH and other peptides in models where the experimental inflammatory response is elicited by monosodium urate crystals (Table 1). Furthermore, major cell players in the innate immune response are targeted by melanocortin peptides, with some interesting data on cells of the adaptive immune arm also emerging in the most recent years.

In the near future, we should expect further a clearer understanding of the melanocortin receptors through which these POMC cleavage products may be functioning. This will be brought about by the more recent availability of MCR transgenic mice and the ever-expanding synthetic melanocortin analogues being generated.

Lessons from Melanocortin Knockout Mice

The role played by melanocortin peptides in modulating the host inflammatory response is beyond doubt. The availability of mice with nonfunctional MC1 receptor, the recessive yellow e/e mice[64] or the generation of MC3R knockout, by homologous recombination replacing the entire MC3R coding region with a neomycin-resistance cassette,[65] has given an important contribution to the identification of the specific target that could be exploited for drug discovery, in relation to a specific experimental or human pathology. Figure 2 reminds us of some pharmacological and tissue-distribution characteristics of MCRs, including established physiological functions.

In experimental colitis, using two distinct models, an important regulatory role emerged by testing the profile of disease in the recessive yellow e/e mouse. This mouse colony bears a mutated and inactive, MC1R[64] and the animals have a characteristic altered coat colour, despite being on a C57/Black6 background, without clear defects in the immune system. Induction of dodecyl sodium sulphate-induced colitis in the recessive yellow e/e mice resulted in marked epithelial disintegration with multiple ulcerations, increase in immune cell infiltrates and oedema formation.[66] Such an effect for endogenous MC1R was not restricted to this specific model of colitis because upon induction of the experimental disease by administration of *C. rodentium* (mimicking human enteropathogenic *E. coli* infection), the recessive yellow e/e mice displayed again significantly higher responses, including increased colonic hyperplasia and mucosal oedema.[66]

Our own studies have focussed predominantly on acute inflammation, monitoring leukocyte trafficking as a hallmark of the host response and tissue injury, as the one observed after an IR procedure. In crystal-induced peritonitis, a time-dependent accumulation of neutrophils could be monitored and this occurred with a similar profile in wild type and recessive yellow e/e mice.[67] The lack of involvement of endogenous MC1R did not hamper the pharmacological testing of MCR pan- or selective agonists. Treatment of mice with alpha-MSH as well as with the more selective MC3R agonist (D[Trp$_8$]-γ-MSH) displayed an anti-inflammatory action that was intact in recessive yellow e/e mice.[43,67] The crucial role for endogenous MC3R in bringing about these anti-inflammatory properties (inhibition of migrated leukocytes was paralleled by reduction in exudate cytokine and chemokine levels) was assessed because these effects were lost in MC3R knockout animals.[54]

In the ovalbumin-induced airway inflammation model, melanocortin peptides including alpha-MSH and D[Trp$_8$]-γ-MSH, were active in attenuating the extent of allergic inflammation, reducing eosinophil and lymphocyte accumulation.[68] These effects were again maintained in the MC1R recessive yellow e/e mice, but there are no data available for the MC3R knockout mouse as yet. Nonetheless, these findings are supported by a previous study where treatment of mice with α-MSH attenauted airway inflammation, inhibiting the influx of eosinophil and IL-4 and IL-13 levels in bronchoalveolar lavage fluids, as well as reducing peribronchial inflammatory cell infiltrate.[69]

Recently, in a model of mesenteric IR, the early vascular events operative in inflammation could be monitored, comparing responses in wild type, MC1R recessive yellow e/e and MC3R knockout mice. Intravital microscopy of the mesenteric microcirculation allowed us to reveal a marked augmentation of the extent of white blood cell adhesion and emigration in MC3R knockout animals, whereas the MC1R mutant colony yielded no different responses when compared to wild type mice.[31] An interesting, though not fully detailed, observation was the fact that indication for a higher degree of cell adhesion and emigration emerged in MC3R knockout mice even when subjected to the sham procedure: it is highly likely that endogenous MC3R acts an important check point to keep the microvasculature in an anti-inflammatory status, at least in the mesenteric vascular bed.

Treatment of mice with D[Trp$_8$]-γ-MSH produced marked attenuation (>60%) of leukocyte adhesion and emigration, a pharmacological action that was absent in MC3R knockout mice. Altogether these data reveal the existence of a tonic inhibitory signal provided by MC3R in the mesenteric microcirculation of the mouse, able to down-regulate cell trafficking and local genera-tion of inflammatory mediators.[31]

Whereas it is clear that mice knockout for specific MCR are powerful tools for dissecting the functions of these genes in many tissues and disease conditions,[70,71] it is unfortunate that not many studies have been performed with them, applying models of innate and adaptive immunity. Nonetheless, a recent study made use of the MC3R knockout mouse, at an age (>6 weeks) where defects in body weight are evident, reporting reduced expression in markers of inflammation (e.g., monocyte chemotactic protein-1 mRNA) in the absence of application of specific inflammogens.[72] These data are in clear contrast to the majority of the literature on melanocortin peptides and the phenotype observed in the mesenteric microcirculation of MC3R knockout animals, discussed above.[31] Further studies are required to understand the potential fine tuning role that MC3R may sustain and that seems to be subverted in obesity.

Finally, mice knockout for MC5R have also been generated[73] but, again, poorly studied in the context of inflammation. This transgenic colony allowed the identification of an important physi-ological role for MC5R in production and secretion of the major products in multiple exocrine glands (e.g., sebaceous preputial, lacrimal and Harderian grands). MC5R knockout mice have in fact, altered lipid production in various exocrine tissues leading to the defects in maintaining thermoregulation when wet, but no effects on body weight have been noted.[73] Furthermore, MC5R might play an important role in ocular immunity,[74] since its gene deletion is associated with greater damage to the mouse retinal structures in a model of experimental autoimmune uveo-retinitis. Given the wide distribution of MC5R mRNA in peripheral tissues and cells, it is unfortunate that MC5R knockout mice have not been studied in models of inflammation.

Drug Discovery Melanocortin Peptide Pharmacology

As discussed above and in other sections of this book, the discovery in the 1990s of the mel-anocortin receptors and the identification of their biological effects, has raised the interest of pharmaceutical companies in the development of new drugs to target these receptors, potentially, for several medical applications, including pain modulation, obesity, anorexia, inflammation and erectile dysfunction. Surprisingly, despite the growing body of evidence and the traditional use of ACTH for the treatment of gout,[7] most of the programs targeting the generation of new melanocortin agonist/antagonists have focused on the activity of these molecules on food intake and sexual dysfunction. Very few investigators and pharmaceutical companies have attempted to exploit melanocortin receptors, especially MC1R and MC3R, as targets for the development of new anti-inflammatory and immune modulator medicines. As summarised in this chapter, there is a wealth of experimental data supporting inhibitory functions for MC1R and MC3R agonism; furthermore, the recent identification of a possible role for MC5R in inflammation should awake interest in the development of potent and selective MC5R agonists. Targeting of MC1R and MC3R would come with both advantages and disadvantages; but the main obstacle of targeting MC1R relates to its role in skin pigmentation. However, alpha-MSH derivatives have been developed in order to improve the potency, selectivity and safety profile.

The tri-peptides KPV (or alpha-MSH$_{11-13}$ as said above) and KPT [Lys-Pro-Thr; IL-1$\beta_{193-195}$] have emerged as leading candidates due to their ability to conserve anti-inflammatory proper-ties without activation of skin pigmentation.[62] Furthermore, their low molecular weight makes them useful for local delivery; secondly, their low cost production would be favourable for large scale-production. One potential problem could derive from unfavourable pharmacokinetics. Indeed, other approaches have kept alpha-MSH as the basis, but have aimed at increasing its short half-life: alpha-MSH-transferrin[75] and NDP-α-MSH ([Nle$_4$, [D-Phe$_7$] alpha-MSH), also known as MT-I,[76] have been developed for this purpose. The chemical immobilization of small peptides has also been studied as possible delivery systems: peptide GKPV attached to Novagel polystyrene beads and displayed inhibitory effects on HBL human melanoma cells.[77] The alpha-MSH-derived synthetic peptide $(CKPV)_2$ is a dimer produced by inserting a Cys-Cys linker between two units of KPV.[56]

A different strategy has been the one of N-terminal "capping" of the tetrapeptide His-Phe-Arg-Trp (alpha-MSH_{6-9}),[78] which corresponds to the minimal sequence that binds all MCR except MC2R. Furthermore, N-terminal fatty acylation of the tetrapeptide can be used to modulate its potency and selectivity.[79] Along similar lines HP228 [(Ac-Nle_4, Gln_5, [D-Phe_7], [D-Trp_9]) alpha-MSH], a pan-agonist with some degree of preferential activation for MC1R, displays inhibitory properties on leukocyte migration and in a model of myocardial ischaemia in mice.[53] Peptide AP214[80] is also tissue protective and it contains six lysine residues at the amino acid terminus of alpha-MSH.

Cyclic peptides such as MT-II (Ac-Nle4-c[Asp_5,D-Phe_7,Lys_{10}] alpha-MSH) and SHU-9119 (Ac-Nle4-c[Asp_5,D-Nal(2')$_7$,Lys_{10}] alpha-MSH)[81] have been used as a prototype for new analogues that can exert potent anti-inflammatory activity,[44,82-84] longer half life and agonist activity toward specific receptors.

Gamma-MSH has been used as the starting point for the development of specific agonists to activate MC3R-dependent anti-inflammatory pathway. Addition of Trp in position 8 of the γ-MSH molecule increases the potency of the native peptide towards the MC3R.[85] In vitro and in vivo data demonstrates [D-Trp_8]-γ-MSH as a selective agonist for MC3R and that it retains its anti-inflammatory properties in mice lacking functional MC1R (recessive yellow e/e mice). Recently, we reported that [D-Trp_8]-γ-MSH looses its anti-inflammatory activity in mice deficient of the MC3R, reinforcing not only specificity of this compound but, also, the relevance of this receptor as a trigger of the endogenous anti-inflammatory loop centred on MC3R, at least in rodents.[43] With respect to MC3R, a new cyclic peptide cyclo-(Nle-Arg-[D-Phe]-Arg-Trp-Glu)-NH_2 has been recently described with selective agonistic activity to this receptor.[86]

Novel compounds directed to the MC3R can come from R and D programs relating to obesity, as several compounds already in the pipeline of pharmaceutical companies demonstrate agonist activity towards MC3R and MC4R. The main problem with the use of such compounds in inflammatory disorders would be their inherent effects on food intake, however a further analysis of compound libraries and/or the screening programs could allow the identification of molecules retaining MC3R (or MC3/MC4R) agonist activity, but being unable to cross the blood brain barrier (a condition sine qua non for development of novel anti-obesity MC4R agonists), so selecting compounds endowed solely with peripheral anti-inflammatory activities.

Small nonpeptide molecules represent—clearly—another important approach to the development of therapeutics modelled on MCR biology. Usually, though not often, small molecules would have the advantage of longer half-life than their peptide counterparts. BMS-470539 a tyrosine-based molecule developed by Bristol Meyers[24,87] acts through MC1R to produce anti-inflammatory responses, both in vitro and in vivo. EL13, developed by Melacure Therapeutics AB and with affinity for MC1R,[88] is another low molecular weight compound successfully tested in DNFB-induced paw oedema. Furthermore, neuroprotective effects in experimental spinal cord injury model were shown by the small molecule ME10501,[89] a compound with high affinity at MC4 receptors.

Currently, two compounds are under clinical trial assessment. Action Pharma A/S compound AP214 is being tested for postsurgical organ failure, whereas bremelanotide (Palatin Technologies, Inc.) could become a new indication for organ protection, attenuating ischemia reperfusion injury.

Conclusion

A large portfolio of experimental systems has indicated melanocortin agonists as potential therapeutics for the treatment of several inflammatory disorders, including peritonitis, rheumatoid arthritis or inflammatory bowel disease. The wishful success of AP214 and bremelanotide trials would stimulate future drug discovery programs based on potent and selective agonists towards MC1R, MC3R—and possibly MC5R—so to open opportunities for the development of new medicines for inflammatory conditions, exploiting in this manner the endogenous anti-inflammatory pathway centred on this fascinating group of receptor and peptides.

Acknowledgements

Work in our laboratory on this line of research is funded by the Arthritis Research Campaign UK (grants 17299 and 18049), the British Heart Foundation (studentship FS/05/078/19406) and the William Harvey Research Foundation.

References

1. Hart F. Corticosteroid therapy in the rheumatic disorders. In: Huskisson E, ed. Anti-rheumatic drugs New York: Praeger, 1983;497-508.
2. Hench PS, Kendall EC, Slocumb CH et al. The effect of the adrenal cortex (17-hydroxy-11-dehydrocortisone: compound E) and of pituitary adrenocorticotropic hormone on rheumatoid arthritis; preliminary report. Proc Staff Meet Mayo Clin 1949; 24:181-197.
3. Dougherty TF, White A. Influence of hormones on lymphoid tissue structure and function. The role of the pituitary adrenotrophic hormone in the regulation of the lymphocytes and other cellular elements of the blood. Endocrinology 1944; 35:1-14.
4. Gutman AB, Yu TF. Effects of ACTH in gout. Am J Med 1950; 9:24-30.
5. Saunders RH, Adams E. Changes in circulating leukocytes following administration of adrenal cortex extract and adrenocorticotropic hormone (ACTH) in infectious mononucleosis and chronic lymphatic leukaemia. Blood 1950; 5:732-738.
6. Ritter J, Kerr LD, Valeriano-Marcet J et al. ACTH revisited: effective treatment for acute crystal induced synovitis in patients with multiple medical problems. J Rheumatol 1994; 21:696-699.
7. Schlesinger N. Overview of the management of acute gout and the role of adrenocorticotropic hormone. Drugs 2008; 68:407-415.
8. Gantz I, Fong TM. The melanocortin system. Am J Physiol Endocrinol Metab 2003; 284:E468-474.
9. Ley K, Laudanna C, Cybulsky MI et al. Getting to the site of inflammation: the leukocyte adhesion cascade updated. Nat Rev Immunol 2007; 7:678-689.
10. Nathan C. Points of control in inflammation. Nature 2002; 420:846-852.
11. Nathan C. Neutrophils and immunity: challenges and opportunities. Nat Rev Immunol 2006; 6:173-182.
12. Choi EY et al. Del-1, an endogenous leukocyte-endothelial adhesion inhibitor, limits inflammatory cell recruitment. Science 2008; 322:1101-1104.
13. Perretti M. Endogenous mediators that inhibit the leukocyte-endothelium interaction. Trends in Pharmacological Sciences 1997; 18:418-425.
14. Serhan CN et al. Resolution of inflammation: state of the art, definitions and terms. FASEB J 2007; 21:325-332.
15. Serhan CN, Savill J. Resolution of inflammation: the beginning programs the end. Nat Immunol 2005; 6:1191-1197.
16. Kubes P, Granger DN. Leukocyte-endothelial cell interactions evoked by mast cells. Cardiovasc Res 1996; 32:699-708.
17. Gordon S, Taylor PR. Monocyte and macrophage heterogeneity. Nat Rev Immunol 2005; 5:953-964.
18. Getting SJ. Targeting melanocortin receptors as potential novel therapeutics. Pharmacol Ther 2006; 111:1-15.
19. Catania A, Gatti S, Colombo G et al. Targeting melanocortin receptors as a novel strategy to control inflammation. Pharmacol Rev 2004; 56:1-29.
20. Lipton JM. Modulation of host defense by the neuropeptide alpha-MSH. Yale J Biol Med 1990; 63:173-182.
21. Lipton JM, Macaluso A, Hiltz ME et al. Central administration of the peptide alpha-MSH inhibits inflammation in the skin. Peptides 1991; 12:795-798.
22. Chiao H et al. Alpha-melanocyte-stimulating hormone protects against renal injury after ischemia in mice and rats. J Clin Invest 1997; 99:1165-1172.
23. Gatti S et al. Inhibitory effects of the peptide (CKPV)2 on endotoxin-induced host reactions. J Surg Res 2006; 131:209-214.
24. Kang L et al. A selective small molecule agonist of the melanocortin-1 receptor inhibits lipopolysaccharide-induced cytokine accumulation and leukocyte infiltration in mice. J Leukoc Biol 2006; 80:897-904.

25. Ceriani G et al. The neuropeptide alpha-melanocyte-stimulating hormone inhibits experimental arthritis in rats. Neuroimmunomodulation 1994; 1:28-32.
26. Manna SK, Aggarwal BB. Alpha-melanocyte-stimulating hormone inhibits the nuclear transcription factor NF-kappa B activation induced by various inflammatory agents. J Immunol 1998; 161:2873-2880.
27. Ichiyama T et al. Alpha-melanocyte-stimulating hormone inhibits NF-kappaB activation and IkappaBalpha degradation in human glioma cells and in experimental brain inflammation. Exp Neurol 1999; 157:359-365.
28. Lipton JM et al. Mechanisms of antiinflammatory action of alpha-MSH peptides. In vivo and in vitro evidence. Ann N Y Acad Sci 1999; 885:173-182.
29. Chiao H et al. Alpha-melanocyte-stimulating hormone reduces endotoxin-induced liver inflammation. J Clin Invest 1996; 97:2038-2044.
30. Gatti S et al. Alpha-melanocyte-stimulating hormone protects the allograft in experimental heart transplantation. Transplantation 2002; 74:1678-1684.
31. Leoni G et al. Inflamed phenotype of the mesenteric microcirculation of melanocortin type 3 receptor-null mice after ischemia-reperfusion. FASEB J 2008; 22:4228-4238.
32. Catania A, Airaghi L, Colombo G et al. Alpha-melanocyte-stimulating hormone in normal human physiology and disease states. Trends Endocrinol Metab 2000; 11:304-308.
33. Bilenko MV. Ischemia and Reperfusion of Various Organs: Injury Mechanisms, Methods of Prevention and Treatment Nova Science Publishers, 2000.
34. Bazzani C et al. Protective effect of melanocortin peptides in rat myocardial ischemia. J Pharmacol Exp Ther 2001; 297:1082-1087.
35. Getting SJ et al. MC-3 receptor and the inflammatory mechanisms activated in acute myocardial infarct. J Leukoc Biol 2004; 76:845-853.
36. Chiao H et al. Alpha-melanocyte-stimulating hormone inhibits renal injury in the absence of neutrophils. Kidney Int 1998; 54:765-774.
37. Lee YS, Park JJ, Chung KY. Change of melanocortin receptor expression in rat kidney ischemia-reperfusion injury. Transplant Proc 2008; 40:2142-2144.
38. Gordon S. Alternative activation of macrophages. Nat Rev Immunol 2003; 3:23-35.
39. Star RA et al. Evidence of autocrine modulation of macrophage nitric oxide synthase by alpha-melanocyte-stimulating hormone. Proc Natl Acad Sci USA 1995; 92:8016-8020.
40. Blalock JE. Proopiomelanocortin-derived peptides in the immune system. Clinical Endocrinology 1985; 22:823-827.
41. Getting SJ et al. POMC gene-derived peptides activate melanocortin type 3 receptor on murine macrophages, suppress cytokine release and inhibit neutrophil migration in acute experimental inflammation. J Immunol 1999; 162:7446-7453.
42. Lam CW, Getting SJ, Perretti M. In vitro and in vivo induction of heme oxygenase 1 in mouse macrophages following melanocortin receptor activation. J Immunol 2005; 174:2297-2304.
43. Getting SJ et al. [D-Trp8]-gamma-melanocyte-stimulating hormone exhibits anti-inflammatory efficacy in mice bearing a nonfunctional MC1R (recessive yellow e/e mouse). Mol Pharmacol 2006; 70:1850-1855.
44. Getting SJ, Allcock GH, Flower R et al. Natural and synthetic agonists of the melanocortin receptor type 3 possess anti-inflammatory properties. J Leukoc Biol 2001; 69:98-104.
45. Taherzadeh S et al. Alpha-MSH and its receptors in regulation of tumor necrosis factor-alpha production by human monocyte/macrophages. Am J Physiol 1999; 276:R1289-1294.
46. Bhardwaj R et al. Evidence for the differential expression of the functional alpha-melanocyte-stimulating hormone receptor MC-1 on human monocytes. J Immunol 1997; 158:3378-3384.
47. Mandrika I, Muceniece R, Wikberg JE. Effects of melanocortin peptides on lipopolysaccharide/interferon-gamma-induced NF-kappaB DNA binding and nitric oxide production in macrophage-like RAW 264.7 cells: evidence for dual mechanisms of action. Biochem Pharmacol 2001; 61:613-621.
48. Woolley DE. The mast cell in inflammatory arthritis. N Engl J Med 2003; 348:1709-1711.
49. Galli SJ et al. Mast cells as "tunable" effector and immunoregulatory cells: recent advances. Annu Rev Immunol 2005; 23:749-786.
50. Adachi S, Nakano T, Vliagoftis H et al. Receptor-mediated modulation of murine mast cell function by alpha-melanocyte stimulating hormone. J Immunol 1999; 163:3363-3368.
51. Artuc M et al. Human mast cells in the neurohormonal network: expression of POMC, detection of precursor proteases and evidence for IgE-dependent secretion of alpha-MSH. J Invest Dermatol 2006; 126:1976-1981.
52. Oliani SM et al. Fluctuation of annexin-A1 positive mast cells in chronic granulomatous inflammation. Inflamm Res 2008; 57:450-456.
53. Getting SJ, Di Filippo C, D'Amico M et al. The melanocortin peptide HP228 displays protective effects in acute models of inflammation and organ damage. Eur J Pharmacol 2006; 532:138-144.

54. Getting SJ et al. Melanocortin 3 receptors control crystal-induced inflammation. FASEB J 2006; 20:2234-2241.
55. Manna SK, Sarkar A, Sreenivasan Y. Alpha-melanocyte-stimulating hormone down-regulates CXC receptors through activation of neutrophil elastase. Eur J Immunol 2006; 36:754-769.
56. Capsoni F et al. The synthetic melanocortin (CKPV)2 exerts broad anti-inflammatory effects in human neutrophils. Peptides 2007; 28:2016-2022.
57. Oktar BK, Yuksel M, Alican I. The role of cyclooxygenase inhibition in the effect of alpha-melanocyte-stimulating hormone on reactive oxygen species production by rat peritoneal neutrophils. Prostaglandins Leukot Essent Fatty Acids 2004; 71:1-5.
58. Hartmeyer M et al. Human dermal microvascular endothelial cells express the melanocortin receptor type 1 and produce increased levels of IL-8 upon stimulation with alpha-melanocyte-stimulating hormone. J Immunol 1997; 159:1930-1937.
59. Scholzen TE et al. Alpha-melanocyte stimulating hormone prevents lipopolysaccharide-induced vasculitis by down-regulating endothelial cell adhesion molecule expression. Endocrinology 2003; 144:360-370.
60. Hill RP, MacNeil S, Haycock JW. Melanocyte stimulating hormone peptides inhibit TNF-alpha signaling in human dermal fibroblast cells. Peptides 2006; 27:421-430.
61. Becher E et al. Human peripheral blood-derived dendritic cells express functional melanocortin receptor MC-1R. Ann N Y Acad Sci 1999; 885:188-195.
62. Brzoska T et al. Alpha-melanocyte-stimulating hormone and related tripeptides: biochemistry, anti-inflammatory and protective effects in vitro and in vivo and future perspectives for the treatment of immune-mediated inflammatory diseases. Endocr Rev 2008; 29:581-602.
63. Cooper A et al. Alpha-melanocyte-stimulating hormone suppresses antigen-induced lymphocyte proliferation in humans independently of melanocortin 1 receptor gene status. J Immunol 2005; 175:4806-4813.
64. Robbins LS et al. Pigmentation phenotypes of variant extension locus alleles result from point mutations that alter MSH receptor function. Cell 1993; 72:827-834.
65. Chen AS et al. Inactivation of the mouse melanocortin-3 receptor results in increased fat mass and reduced lean body mass. Nat Genet 2000; 26:97-102.
66. Maaser C et al. Crucial role of the melanocortin receptor MC1R in experimental colitis. Gut 2006; 55:1415-1422.
67. Getting SJ et al. Redundancy of a functional melanocortin 1 receptor in the anti-inflammatory actions of melanocortin peptides: studies in the recessive yellow (e/e) mouse suggest an important role for melanocortin 3 receptor. J Immunol 2003; 170:3323-3330.
68. Getting SJ et al. A role for MC3R in modulating lung inflammation. Pulm Pharmacol Ther 2008; 21:866-873.
69. Raap U et al. Alpha-melanocyte-stimulating hormone inhibits allergic airway inflammation. J Immunol 2003; 171:353-359.
70. Huszar D et al. Targeted disruption of the melanocortin-4 receptor results in obesity in mice. Cell 1997; 88:131-141.
71. Butler AA et al. A unique metabolic syndrome causes obesity in the melanocortin-3 receptor-deficient mouse. Endocrinology 2000; 141:3518-3521.
72. Ellacott KL, Murphy JG, Marks DL et al. Obesity-induced inflammation in white adipose tissue is attenuated by loss of melanocortin-3 receptor signaling. Endocrinology 2007; 148:6186-6194.
73. Chen W et al. Exocrine gland dysfunction in MC5-R-deficient mice: evidence for coordinated regulation of exocrine gland function by melanocortin peptides. Cell 1997; 91:789-798.
74. Taylor AW, Kitaichi N, Biros D. Melanocortin 5 receptor and ocular immunity. Cell Mol Biol (Noisy-le-grand) 2006; 52:53-59.
75. Matsubara M, Albone E, Gorman JH et al. Alpha-melanocyte stimulating hormone fused transferrin: A novel adjunct to reperfusion therapy for acute MI. Journal of Cardiac Failure 2007; 13:S92.
76. Giuliani D et al. Both early and delayed treatment with melanocortin 4 receptor-stimulating melano-cortins produces neuroprotection in cerebral ischemia. Endocrinology 2006; 147:1126-1135.
77. Kelly JM et al. Immobilized alpha-melanocyte stimulating hormone 10-13 (GKPV) inhibits tumor necrosis factor-alpha stimulated NF-kappaB activity. Peptides 2006; 27:431-437.
78. Holder JR et al. Characterization of aliphatic, cyclic and aromatic N-terminally "capped" His-D-Phe-Arg-Trp-NH2 tetrapeptides at the melanocortin receptors. Eur J Pharmacol 2003; 462:41-52.
79. Todorovic A et al. N-terminal fatty acylated His-dPhe-Arg-Trp-NH(2) tetrapeptides: influence of fatty acid chain length on potency and selectivity at the mouse melanocortin receptors and human melano-cytes. J Med Chem 2005; 48:3328-3336.
80. Doi K et al. AP214, an analogue of alpha-melanocyte-stimulating hormone, ameliorates sepsis-induced acute kidney injury and mortality. Kidney Int 2008; 73:1266-1274.

81. Fan W et al. Role of melanocortinergic neurones in feeding and the agouti obesity syndrome. Nature 1997; 385:165-168.
82. Getting SJ, Schioth HB, Perretti M. Dissection of the anti-inflammatory effect of the core and C-terminal (KPV) alpha-melanocyte-stimulating hormone peptides. J Pharmacol Exp Ther 2003; 306:631-637.
83. Grieco P et al. Design and synthesis of highly potent and selective melanotropin analogues of SHU9119 modified at position 6. Biochem Biophys Res Commun 2002; 292:1075-1080.
84. Grieco P et al. Extensive structure-activity studies of lactam derivatives of MT-II, SHU-9119: their activity and selectivity at human melanocortin receptors 3, 4 and 5. J Pept Res 2003; 62:199-206.
85. Grieco P et al. D-Amino acid scan of gamma-melanocyte-stimulating hormone: importance of Trp(8) on human MC3 receptor selectivity. J Med Chem 2000; 43:4998-5002.
86. Mayorov AV et al. Development of cyclic gamma-MSH analogues with selective hMC3R agonist and hMC3R/hMC5R antagonist activities. J Med Chem 2006; 49:1946-1952.
87. Herpin TF et al. Discovery of tyrosine-based potent and selective melanocortin-1 receptor small-molecule agonists with anti-inflammatory properties. J Med Chem 2003; 46:1123-1126.
88. Skottner A et al. Anti-inflammatory potential of melanocortin receptor-directed drugs. Ann N Y Acad Sci 2003; 994:84-89.
89. Sharma HS et al. Neuroprotective effects of melanocortins in experimental spinal cord injury. An experimental study in the rat using topical application of compounds with varying affinity to melanocortin receptors. J Neural Transm 2006; 113:463-476.
90. Chuang IC et al. Intramuscular electroporation with the pro-opiomelanocortin gene in rat adjuvant arthritis. Arthritis Res Ther 2004; 6:R7-R14.
91. Getting SJ, Christian HC, Flower RJ et al. Activation of melanocortin type 3 receptor as a molecular mechanism for adrenocorticotropic hormone efficacy in gouty arthritis. Arthritis Rheum 2002; 46:2765-2775.
92. Schulte-Herbruggen O et al. Alpha-MSH promotes spontaneous post-ischemic pneumonia in mice via melanocortin-receptor-1. Exp Neurol 2008; 210:731-739.
93. Deng J, Hu X, Yuen PS et al. Alpha-melanocyte-stimulating hormone inhibits lung injury after renal ischemia/reperfusion. Am J Respir Crit Care Med 2004; 169:749-756.
94. Ottani A et al. Vagus nerve mediates the protective effects of melanocortins against cerebral and systemic damage after ischemic stroke. J Cereb Blood Flow Metab 2008.

CHAPTER 8

Terminal Signal:
Anti-Inflammatory Effects of α-Melanocyte-Stimulating Hormone Related Peptides Beyond the Pharmacophore

Thomas Brzoska,* Markus Böhm, Andreas Lügering, Karin Loser and Thomas A. Luger

Abstract

During the last two decades a significant number of investigations has established the fact that α-Melanocyte-stimulating hormone (α-MSH) is a potent anti-inflammatory mediator. The anti-inflammatory effects of α-MSH can be elicited via melanocortin receptors (MC-Rs) broadly expressed in a number of tissues ranging from the central nervous system to cells of the immune system and on resident somatic cells of peripheral tissues. α-MSH affects various pathways regulating inflammatory responses such as NF-κB activation, expression of adhesion molecules, inflammatory cytokines, chemokine receptors, T-cell proliferation and activity and inflammatory cell migration. In vivo α-MSH has been shown to be anti-inflammatory as well in animal models of fever, irritant and allergic contact dermatitis, cutaneous vasculitis, fibrosis, in ocular, gastrointestinal, brain and allergic airway inflammation and arthritis. A broad range of effects of α-MSH exerted beyond the field of inflammation, its pigmentory capacity being only the most visible aspect, has been one of the major impediments limiting the use of α-MSH in human inflammatory disorders. Interestingly KPV, C-terminal tripeptide of α-MSH, which lacks the entire sequence motif required for binding to any of the known MC-Rs, retains almost all of the anti-inflammatory capacity of the full hormone, but in its activities display a lack of any pigmentory action. While the exact signaling mechanism utilized by KPV and related peptides currently is unknown it has been demonstrated already that significant similarities between anti-inflammatory signaling of α-MSH and those short peptides exist. These α-MSH related tripeptides thus may be useful alternatives for anti-inflammatory peptide therapy. KdPT, a derivative of KPV corresponding to IL-1$\beta_{193-195}$, currently is emerging as another tripeptide with potent anti-inflammatory effects. A more limited spectrum of biologic activities, potentially advantageous physicochemical, pharmacokinetic and pharmacodynamic properties as well as the expectation of low costs for pharmaceutical production make these agents interesting candidates for the treatment of immune-mediated inflammatory skin and bowel diseases, allergic asthma and arthritis.

Introduction

α-Melanocyte-stimulating hormone (α-MSH) which initially was characterized as a pigment-inducing (melanotropic) peptide is meanwhile known to exert a wide range of biologic activities far beyond pigmentation. The anti-inflammatory effects of α-MSH in particular have

*Corresponding Author: Thomas Brzoska—Department of Dermatology, University of Münster, Von Esmarch-Str. 58, D-48149 Münster, Germany. Email: brzoska@uni-muenster.de

Melanocortins: Multiple Actions and Therapeutic Potential, edited by Anna Catania.
©2010 Landes Bioscience and Springer Science+Business Media.

α-MSH	Ac-SYSMEHFRWGKPV-NH$_2$
α-MSH(6-9)	Ac-HFRW-NH$_2$
α-MSH(11-13)	Ac-KPV-NH$_2$
IL-1β(193-195)	H-KPT-OH

Figure 1. Peptide sequences of the melanocortins, the central melanotropic pharmacophore of α-MSH and the α-MSH-related C-terminal tripeptides.

received attention during the last years due to efforts to harness the potent anti-inflammatory in vivo effects of α-MSH and related peptides for the treatment of human inflammatory disorders.[1-3] The mediation of α-MSH effects relies on interaction with a family of five G-protein coupled so called melanocortin receptors, MC-1R to MC-5R. As the core peptide α-MSH$_{6-9}$ (Histidine-Phenylalanine-Arginine-Tryptophane, HFRW) has been identified as the pharmacophore responsible for binding of α-MSH to its family of receptors peptidic, peptidomimetic and nonpeptidic variants of this motif have been synthesized and investigated in a range of in vitro and in vivo models. Beyond this core motif the C-terminal tripeptide of α-MSH (Lysine-Proline-Valine, KPV, α-MSH$_{11-13}$) has been found to retain most if not all of the anti-inflammatory capacities of α-MSH. This tripeptide and peptides of similar composition recently also received growing attention, as they might prove to be exceptionally useful in the therapy of inflammatory diseases, not only due to their anti-inflammatory properties but also to a lack of some α-MSH effects which in a therapeutic setting might cause unwanted side effects. It has, for example, been shown in frog and lizard skin bioassays[4] that these tripeptides do not exert any significant melanotropic effect.

The sequence of α-MSH is contained within ACTH and the sequences of α-, β-, γ-MSH and ACTH all have the core amino acid sequence HFRW in common (Fig. 1). The small C-terminus derived peptides include the N-acetylated and C-amidated tripeptide KPV as well as several stereoisomers, i.e., dKPV, KPdV, KdPV and dKPdV. A structurally related derivate is KdPT (Lysine-D-Proline-Threonine), which in its all-L-form is part of the sequence of IL-1β(IL-1β$_{193-195}$). This tripeptide recently has been shown to possess potent anti-inflammatory effects in many aspects resembling those of KPV or α-MSH. This chapter summarizes our current knowledge on the immunomodulatory spectrum of those α-MSH related tripeptides and derivatives.

α-MSH Related Peptides and Melanocortin Receptors—Mediation of Anti-Inflammatory Effects?

The melanocortins α-, β-, γ-MSH as well as ACTH bind to melanocortin receptors, a family of five cell surface receptors which is part of the superfamily of G-protein coupled receptors with seven transmembranal domains.[5,6] Five MC-R subtypes with differential affinities for the different natural ligands have been cloned. Shortened α-MSH fragments containing the core peptide HFRW are capable of binding to MC-1R, MC-3R, MC-4R and MC-5R albeit with less MC-R subtype specificity than the full length natural melanocortins.[7] Ligand stimulation of all MC-Rs leads to activation of an adenylate cyclase resulting in increased intracellular levels of cAMP. In addition, other signaling events, especially calcium fluxes[8] but also activation of mitogen-activated protein kinases[9] may occur. The exact outcome of ligand binding to the MC-Rs in terms of signaling events appears to depend on the cell type studied. Expression analysis has shown that MC-Rs, in particular MC-1R,[10-15] are expressed in a considerable number of tissues and cells. The majority of anti-inflammatory effects of α-MSH in vitro have been linked to the MC-1R.

While the presence of the C-terminal amino acids clearly is important for the binding of α-MSH to its receptors[16] it is still controversial whether tripeptides like KPV and its stereoisomers alone bind to MC-Rs and whether they thus utilize identical signaling pathways. In several studies using frozen rat brain tissue, murine B16 melanoma cells or RAW 264.7 macrophages, KPV apparently did not compete with binding of radiolabeled α-MSH or NDP-MSH.[17-19] In the latter cell line KPV also failed to increase cAMP levels while, on the other hand, intracellular induction of cAMP has been observed in murine microglial cells.[20] In addition, α-MSH, KPV, KPdV and ACTH elicit intracellular calcium fluxes in human keratinocytes expressing the MC-1R with similar potency. In Chinese hamster ovary cells stably transfected with the MC-1R α-MSH and KPV also elevated intracellular calcium.[8] Other more functional in vitro and in vivo studies in the murine system failed to show an involvement of MC-1R, MC-3R and MC-4R in the anti-inflammatory mechanism of KPV and rather suggested an inhibition of IL-1β functions by this peptide.[21] Interestingly, the addition of tyrosine to the tripeptide KPV, either at the C- or the N-terminus yields tetrapeptides (Ac-Tyr-Lys-Pro-Val-NH$_2$ and Ac-Lys-Pro-Val-Tyr-NH$_2$) which bind to MC-1R weakly and also induce cAMP formation.[22]

Some of the anti-inflammatory effects of α-MSH have been observed at extremely low— in some assays femtomolar—concentrations. Considering the ligand binding affinities for MC-1R only very little receptor occupancy can be expected at such concentrations, indicating that the anti-inflammatory signals mediated by α-MSH are processed not only by MC-Rs but also through additional effector pathways. Data showing that α-MSH, as well as KPV, strongly antagonise hyperalgesia induced by IL-1β in rats are clearly in line with this notion.[23] Moreover, additional studies demonstrated that α-MSH as well as KPV significantly reduces surface binding of radiolabeled IL-1β to the T-cell subclone EL4-6.1.[24] Further support for a nonMC-R-mediated effector pathway involved in the anti-inflammatory action of α-MSH comes from animal studies employing signal-deficient MC-1R mice (recessive yellow e/e mice).[21,25]

An ex vivo study, using peripheral blood mononuclear cells from patients with different variants of MC-1R, also indicated that some effects of α-MSH are independent of receptor status.[13] While the investigated receptor variants are known to compromise signaling through the MC-1R via alterations in adenylate cyclase activity other receptor mediated signaling pathways, such as the aforementioned signaling through calcium influx, may be unchanged. Moreover, some effects of α-MSH and consequently of related peptides capable of binding to the MC-Rs, even if weakly, may require the presence of not only one type of MC-R, namely MC-1R but rather of two, MC-1R and MC-3R. The possible direct antagonistic interaction with IL-1β signaling also has to be taken into consideration when assessing the different effects of α-MSH or the related KPV-like tripeptides in different kinds of cells. In the context of these prevailing uncertainties it is interesting that only recently an observation has been made which may greatly change ideas of pathways through which the effects of KPV or related tripeptides are mediated. In a recent study[26] it was shown that KPV in nanomolar concentrations is capable of suppressing activation of the transcription factor NF-κB by IL-1β in the immortalized colonic carcinoma cell line Caco2-BBE as well as by TNFα in the human T-cell lymphoma cell line Jurkat. While both cell lines express several subtypes of MC-Rs treatment with neither KPV nor α-MSH induced cAMP formation in either cell line. In another immortalized colonic carcinoma cell line, HT29-CL.19A KPV had no effect on IL-1β induced NF-κB activation. Interestingly, it is known that this cell line in contrast to the two aforementioned cell lines does not express the peptide transporter PepT1. Further investigations using radiolabeled KPV revealed that the tripeptide is a substrate for the peptide transporter. Meanwhile it also has been shown that KdPT also is a substrate for this peptide transporter (unpublished data), which generally is capable of moving a broad variety of di- and tripeptides from outside the cell into its interior. Thus the short peptides derived from the C-terminus of α-MSH and their derivatives have—at least in cells expressing PepT1—direct access to intracellular targets. This may be an important part in the puzzle of our understanding the underlying effects in peptide hormone mediated effects. In vivo thus different signaling mechanisms for the full lengths mediators and for shortened peptides released by e.g., protease digestion may exist in parallel and may have additive, subtractive or entirely different effects.

Anti-Inflammatory Effects of α-MSH Related Tripeptides In Vitro and Vivo

Most of the studies evaluating the anti-inflammatory effects of α-MSH-related tripeptides have concentrated on the L-form of KPV. Only a limited number of studies employed other stereoisomers with D-enantiomers of single or all amino acids. KPV was shown to suppress production of TNF-α, IL-6 and NO induced by proinflammatory stressors in astrocytes and microglia.[20,27,28] Suppression of LPS/IFNγ induced NO production by RAW 264.7 cells was similarly effective as with full-length α-MSH.[29] In the same study it was also found that cyclic KPV derivatives (using either the α- or ε-amino group of lysine for cyclisation with the carboxy-group of L-or D-valine) were significantly weaker in their anti-inflammatory activity.

Moreover, the study showed a lack of cAMP formation upon stimulation with KPV, pointing to a MC-1R independent mechanism of KPV activity in this setting. KPV potently blocked activation of NF-κB by TNFα in human keratinocytes and monocytic cells[30,31] displaying a potency comparable to that of α-MSH. In human keratinocytes α-MSH, KPV and KPdV effectively inhibited TNF-α induced NF-κB activation in human keratinocytes. In this study KPV was about 100times less potent than α-MSH while KPdV was about 100times more potent,[30] with maximum inhibition of NF-κB activation at concentrations of 10^{-7} M, 10^{-9} M and 10^{-11} M, respectively. The stereoisomer KdPV was capable of suppressing LPS-induced NF-κB activation in rat alveolar cells with an EC_{50} of 5.5 μg/mL, corresponding to ~1.5×10^{-5} M.[32] Interestingly, these in vitro findings are in some contrast to a previous study in which KdPV was found to lack antipyretic activity in vivo.[33] When tested in a murine picryl chloride model of irritant dermatitis over a dose range of 20 μg to 80 μg per animal KdPV failed to exert any significant anti-inflammatory effect on ear swelling. This lack of effect might be attributable to the dose range tested which—assuming a low effectiveness for KdPV as found in the in vitro experiments on rat alveolar cells—may reconcile these different data sets. However, both lines of evidence seem to indicate that the L-configuration of proline is important for the anti-inflammatory effects mediated by KPV and its stereoisomers at least in the models employed. Finally, KPV was also shown to directly induce IL-10 in human monocytes in the absence of any other, pro-inflammatory stimulus.[34]

However, it is important to note that apart from the already mentioned lack of pigmentary induction by KPV additionally other modulatory effects of α-MSH are not replicated by KPV. Specifically, the cytoprotective effect of α-MSH observed in UVB-induced apoptosis in normal human melanocytes[35] was not observed for KPV. This may either suggest some kind of cell type specificity and/or an indispensable role for MC-1R signaling in the modulatory effect of α-MSH in this system.

While the number of in vivo studies involving KPV or its stereoisomers and derivatives still is quite limited, comprising only a few animal models of inflammation, those studies that were conducted reveal a promising anti-inflammatory activity. Upon intracerebroventricular or intravenous administration to rabbits made hyperthermic by systemic adminstration of IL-1 containing leukocytic pyrogen KPV has antipyretic effects.[36,37] These studies using truncated forms of α-MSH revealed that the antipyretic message sequence of this peptide hormone resides in its C-terminal amino tripeptide KPV as $\alpha\text{-MSH}_{1-10}$ had no effect on fever. The antipyretic activity of KPV was higher upon central than upon peripheral administration and overall lower than the antipyretic effect of full-length α-MSH.[36] Interestingly, $\alpha\text{-MSH}_{10-13}$ as well as $\alpha\text{-MSH}_{9-13}$, i.e., Gly-Lys-Pro-Val and Trp-Gly-Lys-Pro-Val, turned out to have significantly less anti-inflammatory capacity in this setting while $\alpha\text{-MSH}_{8-13}$, i.e., Arg-Trp-Gly-Lys-Pro-Val, was more potent than KPV. Of these $\alpha\text{-MSH}_{9-13}$ and $\alpha\text{-MSH}_{8-13}$ were found not to bind to MC-Rs, despite the fact that they carry increasing portions of the classical pharmacophore.[22]

In accordance with the effect of KPV on NF-κB activation in vitro the peptide suppressed activation of this transcription factor in the brain of LPS-treated mice in vivo.[38] In mouse models of skin inflammation including irritant and allergic contact dermatitis, KPV exerted anti-inflammatory effects as well.[33,39-43] As for α-MSH a single i.v. injection of a low dose of KPV or KdPT (1.5 µg) around the time of sensitisation with a hapten is sufficient to suppress contact hypersensitivity reactions and to induce hapten specific tolerance (unpublished data). Earlier studies on the hyperalgesic effect of IL-1β revealed that KPT and KdPT can counter the hyperalgesia induced by IL-1β[44] suggesting an IL-1 antagonism of KdPT as a possible anti-inflammatory effector mechanism as already speculated for KPV. The analgesic effect of KdPT in its strongest was comparable to that of indomethacine yet did not result in any gastric lesions.[44] In this context again differences in the effects of these peptides were found. Interestingly, the antialgesic effects of KdPV in an acidic-acid induced abdominal constriction test were inhibited by the opioid antagonist naloxone while the effects of KPT or KdPT were not[45] KdPT on the other hand did not antagonize the hyperalgesic effects of PGE_2 and being not effective in the hot plate test appears not to mediate its signals via central nervous system pathways.[23] That descending neurogenic pathways are also of less importance for the anti-inflammatory mechanism of KPV than for full-length α-MSH was shown in mice with experimentally-induced hind paw inflammation. KPV administered intraperitoneally had marked anti-inflammatory activity even in animals with spinal cord transection.[41]

Experiments on inhibition of crystal-induced peritonitis of mice[21] shed additional light on the potent anti-inflammatory effects of KPV and the underlying signaling mechanism. In these experiments α-MSH, KPV and the α-MSH core peptide HFRW significantly reduced accumulation of polymorphonuclear leukocytes in the peritoneal cavity. Interestingly, the selective MC-1R agonistic peptide MS05 did not have any anti-inflammatory effect in this model while the MC-3/4R agonist Melanotan II (MTII) turned out to be about as effective as α-MSH or KPV. As described previously for RAW264.7 macrophages KPV failed to increase cAMP levels, indicating that KPV signaling is independent of MC-Rs and especially of MC-1R. The latter is supported by the fact that in mice with nonfunctional MC-1R KPV likewise had anti-inflammatory effects.

Recently, it was demonstrated in an additional setting that KPV and the IL-1β derived tripeptide KdPT both have potent anti-inflammatory effects in vivo.[46,47] In mice with dextrane sulphate-induced experimental inflammatory colitis (dextrane sulphate sodium = DSS) treatment with KPV or KdPT greatly reduced several signs of colitis. The tripeptide-treated animals recovered earlier and showed significantly less ulceration, less leukocyte infiltrations, submucosal edema and epithelial denudations than the control animals. Interestingly, KdPT was significantly more effective in its anti-inflammatory effect than KPV.[46,47] For KPV it was shown that doses as low as 100 ng per day administered intravenously were already effective. On molecular level it was observed that the activity of myeloperoxidase (MPO) was reduced significantly as well. In another, more immunologic model of colitis KPV was also found to be effective. In the CD45RB[hi] transfer colitis model KPV was found to be effective even when administration started only 26 days after the colitogenic CD45RB[hi] CD4+-T-cells were injected. In both models the anti-inflammatory effects of KPV were quite pronounced and moreover set in rather quickly. In another report on oral application of KPV in DSS-colitis[26] the tripeptide was also shown to be highly effective. In this study KPV was added to the drinking water at 100 µM concentration and the animals were allowed to consume the water ad lib. Intestinal inflammation induced by DSS or by trinitrobenzene sulfonic acid (TNBS) was reduced significantly by KPV. In the DSS model intestinal levels of IL-6 and IL-12 mRNA were also reduced, while in the TNBS model additionally a reduction of IFNγ and TNFα mRNA was observed. Interestingly, KPV also had an effect on DSS-induced colitis in mice with a defect in MC-1R signaling.[48] In these mice, which due to a single base pair deletion in the gene for the MC-1R express only a nonfunctional form of the receptor, a more pronounced form of colitis was observed as compared to wildtype C57BL/6 animals. Using these e⁻/e⁻-mice (also named recessive yellow) it was shown that KPV did not significantly reverse weight loss in treated animals compared to controls. However, while all PBS-treated mice died within nine days of the first DSS-contact while all animals treated with KPV survived during this observation period.

Therapeutic Potential of α-MSH-Related Tripeptides in Human Immune-Mediated Inflammatory Diseases

α-MSH has been investigated in terms of its commercial potential since many years. A significant number of patents have been filed claiming effects of natural MSH-peptides and a multitude of ligands for the melanocortin receptors optimized for MC-R subtype affinity and selectivity has been designed. Among these patents and compounds many have the anti-inflammatory effects of α-MSH as subject and target MC-1R. Commercial success, however, until now essentially has proved elusive, aside from afamelanotide (which is identical to Nle^4-d-Phe^7-α-MSH and currently under development for erythropoietic protoporphyria)[49] or the in certain cycles more or less flagrant abuse of cyclic derivatives like melanotan I and melanotan II.[50]

The natural, full sequence α-MSH would display its full hormonal spectrum of biologic effects some of which will always be unwelcome, which ones depending on the general setting for a given therapeutic situation: a drug to treat inflammation displaying an additional unwarranted tendency towards patchy pigmentation certainly will suffer from acceptance problems in the general population. Thus limiting the width of the spectrum of effects of α-MSH-like anti-inflammatory drugs is necessary. The most trodden way towards this goal lies in making the MSH-like compound more specific for a single MC-R of choice in accordance with contemporary paradigms or in reducing or altering the signaling sequence until some hormonal effects begin to vanish. Moreover, α-MSH is not very stable in biologic environments and becomes degraded rather quickly. The half life of full-length α-MSH administered intravenously is only a few minutes and accordingly the duration of the antipyretic effect of α-MSH is limited to about 1.5 hrs.[51] This is probably due to the fact that α-MSH is readily degraded by a number of proteases. Among these are several serum proteases including aminopeptidase, angiotensin-converting enzyme, alpha-chymotrypsin, neutral endopeptidase 24.11 (NEP), prolyl endopeptidase and trypsin.[52-56] Expression of NEP on the cell surface of many cell types may directly limit the effects of α-MSH on cellular level.[56,57]

While its in vivo half-life yet may suffice for achieving some therapeutic efficacy, especially when one considers that proteolytic digestion may yield still active fragments, α-MSH also is not sufficiently stable in order to give a drug formulation a sufficient shelf-life or to guarantee easy handling. Stability issues as such can be overcome by changing the amino acid sequence and introducing nonnatural amino acids or by altogether leaving behind the amino acid make up, moving towards structurally related but nonnatural small molecular weight compounds. Early on full length variations of α-MSH—optimized with hindsight to efficacy or stability—showed promise, but mostly still communicated the entire range of effects of α-MSH, often with a higher degree of effectiveness or efficacy for one or several of these effects. Indeed, attempts have been successful to create protease-stable α-MSH analogues such as NDP-MSH but with increased potency on pigmentation while interestingly lacking a definitive effect on experimental fever when injected intravenously.[56] A major advantage of KPV and its stereoisomers indeed appears to be the lack of melanotropic effect—which is mostly based on the central message sequence of α-MSH[58]—while most of the anti-inflammatory effects are found to be retained in those peptides. The so far only study on KdPT effects on pigmentation revealed that in homeostatic situations no effects of KdPT on melanogenesis in hair follicles are observed.[59] Only under inflammatory conditions, i.e., upon stimulation with IFNγ increased pigmentation was observed. Whether this can be replicated in vivo or occurs in nonscalp skin is unknown.

Quite a few of the efforts to generate optimized ligands for MC-1R—mainly for the treatment of inflammatory disorders—ended unsuccessfully, often due to a lack of in vivo efficacy of the optimized ligands. In other cases the artificial ligand turned out to possess more or less potent effects in prophylactic settings, but did not affect pro-inflammatory mediators in therapeutic settings.[60] This may point to still unresolved flaws in the paradigm of α-MSH signaling through the Melanocortin receptors and/or additional pathways. The recent identification of a pathway allowing signaling inside the cell certainly will explain some of these failures.

Another issue to keep in mind is the pharmaceutical acceptability of the new ligands, which not only need to be sufficiently stable in vivo but also either have to be capable of permeating the skin in epicutaneous applications or to become systemically available in systemic, preferably oral use while at the same time avoiding the introduction of new and unwarranted or even inacceptable kinds of toxicity. Currently no data exist on the precise pharmacokinetics of KPV and related tripeptides in blood and it is even unknown as to whether such tripeptides are endogenously produced from α-MSH, ACTH, POMC or other precursors. However, when the observed minimal side effects after systemic administration of α-MSH analogues in man are examined in this context the rapid degradation of α-MSH in serum may be related to these findings. Intravenous injection of the superpotent α-MSH analogue NDP-MSH into humans for evaluation of its effect on skin pigmentation yielded little side effects. Adverse effects were minimal at doses of up to 0.16 mg/kg and comprised occasional gastrointestinal upset and facial flushing.[61-64] Considering the well known and rather broad spectrum of adverse effects observed for almost all conventional immunosuppressive therapies (e.g., azathioprine, cyclophosphamide, cyclosporine, methotrexate and mycophenolate mofetil) including modern biologics and also for many anti-inflammatory drugs, the safety profile of α-MSH and related peptides thus far appears to be high with an even more preferable profile expected for shorter peptides.

Considering these facts and the results obtained with pharmacophore-like ligands with high receptor selectivity and affinity yet lacking effect it may be worthwhile to further investigate the anti-inflammatory tripeptides derived from or related to the C-terminus of α-MSH. KPV, its stereoisomers, as well as KdPT are attractive future candidates for pharmaceutical companies that wish to exploit these peptides for the treatment of human inflammatory diseases. These peptides are small in size and can without much further modification permeate the skin and become bioavailable after peroral administration as well. Their composition—mostly natural amino acids and similarity to sequences found in proteins of the human body—allows expecting a moderate degree of toxicity. Introduction of d-enantiomers moreover provides a direct and easy way to enhanced stability against proteolysis. The molecular pathways so-far found to be involved with the anti-inflammatory activity of KPV are very similar to those utilized by α-MSH. A major component of these effector pathways is inhibition of inflammation by reduction of NF-κB activation, resulting in reduced expression of cytokines, chemokines and cell adhesion molecules. Moreover, suppression of TNF-α production and in several systems concomitant induction of IL-10 plays an important role. In many immune-mediated inflammatory diseases ranging from skin diseases such as eczema or psoriasis, to allergic diseases like allergic rhinitis or allergic asthma but also including inflammatory bowel disease, rheumatoid arthritis and others these effector pathways of inflammation are central to the pathogenesis of those diseases. The modern immunosuppressive biologics targeting single mediators in those pathways, as for example in anti-TNF-α therapy, have emerged as novel and powerful treatment for such diseases.[65] Yet the use of these compounds due to their intended effect of mostly complete abrogation of effects of single, central inflammatory mediators come with some strings attached, especially with a view on long-term therapy as often required for the diseases targeted, since this kind of strategy opens doors for opportunistic diseases ranging from infections to cancer. The risk for such side effects should be clearly less for the α-MSH like tripeptides, as they do not abrogate completely any given mediator (as far as tested) but rather mitigate the expression of a flurry of inflammatory effectors and this only in inflammatory conditions.

In this respect it may therefore be of interest that α-MSH and KPV recently were found to possess antimicrobial activity against *S. aureus* and *C. albicans*.[66] This antimicrobial activity of α-MSH peptides results from at least two different effects: an increase in bacterial cAMP content on the one hand and an in vitro increase in killing of both pathogens by human neutrophils.

Conclusion

In summary, α-MSH and related tripeptides have been shown to possess promising anti-inflammatory effects. α-MSH-related tripeptides already display only a limited part of the spectrum of hormone activities attributed to the full length α-MSH. They are small and in comparison to other modern biologics inexpensive molecules suitable for large scale pharmaceutical production, avoiding the traps and costs of biotechnological procedures. The low molecular weight of α-MSH-related tripeptides provides advantages especially for local therapy of inflammatory disorders and based on what is known with regard to toxicology of α-MSH or NDP-MSH can be expected to display a beneficial toxicity profile. The authors are thus confident that α-MSH-related tripeptides or compounds derived from them are promising new tools for the treatment of immune-mediated inflammatory diseases.

References

1. Lipton JM, Catania A. Anti-inflammatory actions of the neuroimmunomodulator alpha-MSH. Immunol Today 1997; 18:140-145.
2. Getting SJ. Targeting melanocortin receptors as potential novel therapeutics. Pharmacol Ther 2006; 111:1-15.
3. Luger TA, Scholzen TE, Brzoska T et al. New insights into the functions of alpha-MSH and related peptides in the immune system. Ann N Y Acad Sci 2003; 994:133-140.
4. Haskell-Luevano C, Sawyer TK, Hendrata S et al. Truncation studies of alpha-melanotropin peptides identify tripeptide analogues exhibiting prolonged agonist bioactivity. Peptides 1996; 17:995-1002.
5. Mountjoy KG, Robbins LS, Mortrud MT et al. The cloning of a family of genes that encode the melanocortin receptors. Science 1992; 257:1248-1251.
6. Cone RD, Lu D, Koppula S et al. The melanocortin receptors: agonists, antagonists and the hormonal control of pigmentation. Recent Prog Horm Res 1996; 51:287-318.
7. Schiöth HB, Muceniece R, Larsson M et al. Binding of cyclic and linear MSH core peptides to the melanocortin receptor subtypes. J Pharmacol 1997; 319:369-373.
8. Elliott RJ, Szabo M, Wagner MJ et al. Alpha-Melanocyte-stimulating hormone, MSH 11-13 KPV and adrenocorticotropic hormone signalling in human keratinocyte cells. J Invest Dermatol 2004; 122:1010-1019.
9. Englaro W, Rezzonico R, Durand-Clement M et al. Mitogen-activated protein kinase pathway and AP-1 are activated during cAMP-induced melanogenesis in B-16 melanoma cells. J Biol Chem 1995; 270:24315-24320.
10. Böhm M, Luger TA, Tobin DJ et al. Melanocortin receptor ligands: new horizons for skin biology and clinical dermatology. J Invest Dermatol 2006; 126:1966-1975.
11. Colombo G, Buffa R, Bardella MT et al. Anti-inflammatory effects of alpha-melanocyte-stimulating hormone in celiac intestinal mucosa. Neuroimmunomodulation 2002; 10:208-216.
12. Bhardwaj R, Becher E, Mahnke K et al. Evidence for the differential expression of the functional alpha-melanocyte-stimulating hormone receptor MC-1 on human monocytes. J Immunol 1997; 158:3378-3384.
13. Cooper A, Robinson SJ, Pickard C et al. Alpha-melanocyte-stimulating hormone suppresses antigen-induced lymphocyte proliferation in humans independently of melanocortin 1 receptor gene status. J Immunol 2005; 175:4806-4813.
14. Andersen GN, Hagglund M, Nagaeva O et al. Quantitative measurement of the levels of melanocortin receptor subtype 1, 2, 3 and 5 and pro-opiomelanocortin peptide gene expression in subsets of human peripheral blood leucocytes. Scand J Immunol 2005; 61:279-284.
15. Catania A, Rajora N, Capsoni F et al. The neuropeptide alpha-MSH has specific receptors on neutrophils and reduces chemotaxis in vitro. Peptides 1996; 17:675-679.
16. Schiöth HB, Mutulis F, Muceniece R et al. Selective properties of C- and N-terminals and core residues of the melanocyte-stimulating hormone on binding to the human melanocortin receptor subtypes. Eur J Pharmacol 1998; 349:359-366.
17. Tatro JB, Entwistle ML. Heterogeneity of brain melanocortin receptors suggested by differential ligand binding in situ. Brain Res 1994; 635:148-158.
18. Lyson K, Ceriani G, Takashima A et al. Binding of anti-inflammatory alpha-melanocyte-stimulating-hormone peptides and proinflammatory cytokines to receptors on melanoma cells. Neuroimmunomodulation 1994; 1:121-126.
19. Mandrika I, Muceniece R, Wikberg JE. Effects of melanocortin peptides on lipopolysaccharide/interferon-gamma-induced NF-kappaB DNA binding and nitric oxide production in macrophage-like RAW 264.7 cells: evidence for dual mechanisms of action. Biochem Pharmacol 2001; 161:613-621.

20. Delgado R, Carlin A, Airaghi L et al. Melanocortin peptides inhibit production of proinflammatory cytokines and nitric oxide by activated microglia. J Leukoc Biol 1998; 63:740-745.

21. Getting SJ, Schiöth HB, Perretti M. Dissection of the anti-inflammatory effect of the core and C-terminal (KPV) alpha-melanocyte-stimulating hormone peptides. J Pharmacol Exp Ther 2003; 306:631-637.

22. Schiöth HB, Muceniece R, Mutule I et al. New melanocortin 1 receptor binding motif based on the C-terminal sequence of alpha-melanocyte-stimulating hormone. Basic Clin Pharmacol Toxicol 2006; 99:287-293.

23. Poole S, Bristow AF, Lorenzetti BB et al. Peripheral analgesic activities of peptides related to alpha-melanocyte stimulating hormone and interleukin-1 beta 193-195. Br J Pharmacol 1992; 106:489-492.

24. Mugridge KG, Perretti M, Ghiara P et al. Alpha-melanocyte-stimulating hormone reduces interleukin-1 beta effects on rat stomach preparations possibly through interference with a type I receptor. Eur J Pharmacol 1991; 197:151-155.

25. Ichiyama T, Sakai T, Catania A et al. Inhibition of peripheral NF-kappaB activation by central action of alpha-melanocyte-stimulating hormone. J Neuroimmunol 1999; 99:211-217.

26. Dalmasso G, Charrier-Hisamuddin L, Thu Nguyen HT et al. PepT1-mediated tripeptide KPV uptake reduces intestinal inflammation. Gastroenterology 2008; 134:166-178.

27. Wong KY, Rajora N, Boccoli G et al. A potential mechanism of local anti-inflammatory action of alpha-melanocyte-stimulating hormone within the brain: modulation of tumor necrosis factor-alpha production by human astrocytic cells. Neuroimmunomodulation 1997; 4:37-41.

28. Galimberti D, Baron P, Meda L et al. Alpha-MSH peptides inhibit production of nitric oxide and tumor necrosis factor-alpha by microglial cells activated with beta-amyloid and interferon gamma. Biochem Biophys Res Commun 1999; 263:251-256.

29. Muceniece R, Krigere L, Suli-Vargha H et al. Effects of alpha-melanotropin C-terminal tripeptide analogues on macrophage NO production. Peptides 2003; 24:701-707.

30. Moustafa M, Szabo M, Ghanem GE et al. Inhibition of tumor necrosis factor-alpha stimulated NFkappaB/p65 in human keratinocytes by alpha-melanocyte stimulating hormone and adrenocorticotropic hormone peptides. J Invest Dermatol 2002; 119:1244-1253.

31. Barcellini W, Colombo G, La Maestra L et al. Alpha-melanocyte-stimulating hormone peptides inhibit HIV-1 expression in chronically infected promonocytic U1 cells and in acutely infected monocytes. J Leukoc Biol 2000; 68:693-699.

32. Haddad JJ, Lauterbach R, Saade NE et al. Alpha-melanocyte-related tripeptide, Lys-d-Pro-Val, ameliorates endotoxin-induced nuclear factor kappaB translocation and activation: evidence for involvement of an interleukin-1beta193-195 receptor antagonism in the alveolar epithelium. Biochem J 2001; 355:29-38.

33. Hiltz ME, Catania A, Lipton JM. Anti-inflammatory activity of alpha-MSH(11-13) analogs: influences of alteration in stereochemistry. Peptides 1991; 12:767-771.

34. Bhardwaj RS, Schwarz A, Becher E et al. Pro-opiomelanocortin-derived peptides induce IL-10 production in human monocytes. J Immunol 1996; 156:2517-2521.

35. Böhm M, Wolff I, Scholzen TE et al. Alpha-Melanocyte-stimulating hormone protects from ultraviolet radiation-induced apoptosis and DNA damage. J Biol Chem 2005; 280:5795-5802.

36. Richards DB, Lipton JM. Effect of alpha-MSH 11-13 (lysine-proline-valine) on fever in the rabbit. Peptides 1984; 5:815-817.

37. Deeter LB, Martin LW, Lipton JM. Antipyretic properties of centrally administered alpha-MSH fragments in the rabbit. Peptides 1989b; 9:1285-1288.

38. Ichiyama T, Sakai T, Catania A et al. Systemically administered alpha-melanocyte-stimulating peptides inhibit NF-kappaB activation in experimental brain inflammation. Brain Res 1999; 836:31-37.

39. Hiltz ME, Lipton JM. Alpha-MSH peptides inhibit acute inflammation and contact sensitivity. Peptides 1990; 11:979-982.

40. Hiltz ME, Catania A, Lipton JM. Alpha-MSH peptides inhibit acute inflammation induced in mice by rIL-1 beta, rIL-6, rTNF-alpha and endogenous pyrogen but not that caused by LTB4, PAF and rIL-8. Cytokine 1992; 4:320-328.

41. Macaluso A, McCoy D, Ceriani G et al. Antiinflammatory influences of alpha-MSH molecules: central neurogenic and peripheral actions. J Neurosci 1994; 14:2377-2382.

42. Ceriani G, Macaluso A, Catania A et al. Central neurogenic antiinflammatory action of alpha-MSH: modulation of peripheral inflammation induced by cytokines and other mediators of inflammation. Neuroendocrinology 1994; 59:138-143.

43. Hiltz ME, Lipton JM. Antiinflammatory activity of a COOH-terminal fragment of the neuropeptide alpha-MSH. FASEB J 1989; 3:2282-2284.

44. Ferreira SH, Lorenzetti BB, Bristow AF et al. Interleukin-1β as a potent hyperalgesic agent antagonized by a tripeptide analogue. Nature 1988; 334:698-700.

45. Oluyomi AO, Poole S, Smith TW et al. Antinociceptive activity of peptides related to interleukin-1 beta-(193-195), Lys-Pro-Thr. Eur J Pharmacol 1994; 258:131-138.
46. Maaser C, Kannengiesser K, Lügering A et al. Successful treatment of murine colitis with the tripeptide KPV. Gastroenterology 2005; 128:A-2001.
47. Maser C, Bettenworth D, Lügering A et al. Therapeutischer Einsatz des Tripeptids K(D)PT im murinen DSS-Modell. Z Gastroenterol 2006; 44:724.
48. Kannengiesser K, Maaser C, Heidemann J et al. Melanocortin-derived tripeptide KPV has anti-inflammatory potential in murine models of inflammatory bowel disease. Inflamm Bowel Dis 2008; 14:324-331.
49. Harms J, Lautenschlager S, Minder CE et al. An alpha-melanocyte-stimulating hormone analogue in erythropoietic protoporphyria. N Engl J Med 2009; 360(3):306-307.
50. Evans-Brown M, Dawson RT, Chandler M et al. Use of melanotan I and II in the general population. BMJ 2009; 338:424-425.
51. Lipton JM. Modulation of host defense by the neuropeptide alpha-MSH. Yale J Biol Med 1990; 63:173-182.
52. Potaman VN, Alfeeva LY, Kamensky AA et al. Degradation of ACTH/MSH(4-10) and its synthetic analog semax by rat serum enzymes: an inhibitor study. Peptides 1993; 14:491-495.
53. Castrucci AM, Hadley ME, Sawyer TK et al. Enzymological studies of melanotropins. Comp Biochem Physiol 1984; 78:519-524.
54. Marks N, Stern F, Kastin AJ. Biodegradation of alpha-MSH and derived peptides by rat brain extracts and by rat and human serum. Brain Res Bull 1976; 1:591-593.
55. Trochard MC, Vaudry H, Leboulenger F et al. The degradation of radioiodinated alpha MSH in vitro: effect of some inhibitors of proteolytic enzymes. C R Seances Soc Biol Fil 1976; 170:1103-1109.
56. Deschodt-Lanckman M, Vanneste Y, Loir B et al. Degradation of alpha-melanocyte stimulating hormone (alpha-MSH) by CALLA/endopeptidase 24.11 expressed by human melanoma cells in culture. Int J Cancer 1990; 46:1124-1130.
57. Aberdam E, Auberger P, Ortonne JP et al. Neprilysin, a novel target for ultraviolet B regulation of melanogenesis via melanocortins. J Invest Dermatol 2000; 115:381-387.
58. Hruby VJ, Wilkes BC, Hadley ME et al. Alpha-Melanotropin: the minimal active sequence in the frog skin bioassay. J Med Chem 1987; 30:2126-2130.
59. Meyer KC, Brzoska T, Abels C et al. The alpha-melanocyte stimulating hormone-related tripeptide K(D)PT stimulates human hair follicle pigmentation in situ under proinflammatory conditions. Br J Dermatol 2008; 160:433-437.
60. Kang L, McIntyre KW, Gillooly KM et al. A selective small molecule agonist of the melanocortin-1 receptor inhibits lipopolysaccharide-induced cytokine accumulation and leukocyte infiltration in mice. J Leukoc Biol 2006; 80:897-904.
61. Ugwu SO, Blanchard J, Dorr RT et al. Skin pigmentation and pharmacokinetics of melanotan-I in humans. Bioph Drug 1997; 18:259-269.
62. Dorr RT, Dvorakova K, Brooks C et al. Increased eumelanin expression and tanning is induced by a superpotent melanotropin [Nle4-D-Phe7]-alpha-MSH in humans. Photochem Photobiol 2000; 72:526-532.
63. Dorr RT, Ertl G, Levine N et al. Effects of a superpotent melanotropic peptide in combination with solar UV radiation on tanning of the skin in human volunteers. Arch Dermatol 2004; 140:827-835.
64. Hadley ME, Dorr RT. Melanocortin peptide therapeutics: historical milestones, clinical studies and commercialization. Peptides 2006; 27:921-930.
65. Baugh JA, Bucala R. Mechanisms for modulating TNF alpha in immune and inflammatory disease. Curr Opin Drug Discov Devel 2001; 4:635-650.
66. Cutuli M, Cristiani S, Lipton JM et al. Antimicrobial effects of alpha-MSH peptides. J Leukoc Biol 2000; 67:233-239.

CHAPTER 9

Protective Effects of Melanocortins in Systemic Host Reactions

Stefano Gatti,* Caterina Lonati, Andrea Sordi and Anna Catania

Abstract

Systemic inflammatory reactions are pivotal in many disorders and have important secondary influences in many more. Although inflammation is initially useful to limit infection, it can also be detrimental and cause organ failure. Modulation of systemic reactions is important to restrict mediator release and limit cell activation that could cause harmful consequences. Experiments in which different models and treatments were used show that melanocortins reduce host responses such as fever, shock, reperfusion injury and allograft rejection. Melanocortin-derived peptides could be an effective treatment to prevent organ failure caused by excessive production of pro-inflammatory mediators. The degree of the modulatory effect exerted by melanocortins should be sufficient to reduce severity of systemic inflammation without impairing the host defense mechanisms.

Introduction

Despite different etiologies, disorders such as sepsis syndrome, septic shock, acute respiratory distress syndrome (ARDS), autoimmune vasculitis and several other conditions are collectively classified as "systemic inflammation". Development of systemic inflammation is promoted by interactions between host cells and external agents such as bacteria or endotoxins in infectious disorders, or endogenous molecules in cancer and autoimmunity. The term acute phase response (APR) indicates the host reaction that occurs during systemic inflammation. APR begins in the circulation or at inflammatory sites where monocytes, macrophages and, to a lesser extent, neutrophils, produce and release inflammatory cytokines such as interleukin (IL)-1, IL-6 and tumor necrosis factor α (TNF)-α. Upon cytokine stimulation, the central nervous system (CNS), the autonomic nervous system (ANS) and the adrenal glands, establish a rapid and intense protective/reactive response. In the CNS, cytokines induce a cascade of events causing the appearance of the three hallmarks of the APR: fever, leukocytosis and increase in acute phase proteins (APPs). In addition, there is activation of a variety of behavioral responses, mostly mediated by the hypothalamic—pituitary—adrenal and hypothalamic—pituitary—gonadal axes, including lethargy, anorexia and adipsia. The systemic inflammatory response is initially useful to limit infection but it can also be detrimental and cause organ failure. Modulation of the systemic reactions is, therefore, important to restrict mediator release and cell activation that could cause harmful consequences.

As extensively discussed in other sections of this book, melanocortins and their receptors are part of a major modulatory system that reduces host responses to infectious, circulatory, or immune-mediated challenge.

*Corresponding Author: Stefano Gatti—Centro di Ricerche Chirurgiche Precliniche, Fondazione IRCCS, Ca' Granda, Ospedale Maggiore Policlinico, Via F. Sforza 35, 20122 Milano, Italy.
Email: stefano.gatti@unimi.it

Melanocortins: Multiple Actions and Therapeutic Potential, edited by Anna Catania.
©2010 Landes Bioscience and Springer Science+Business Media.

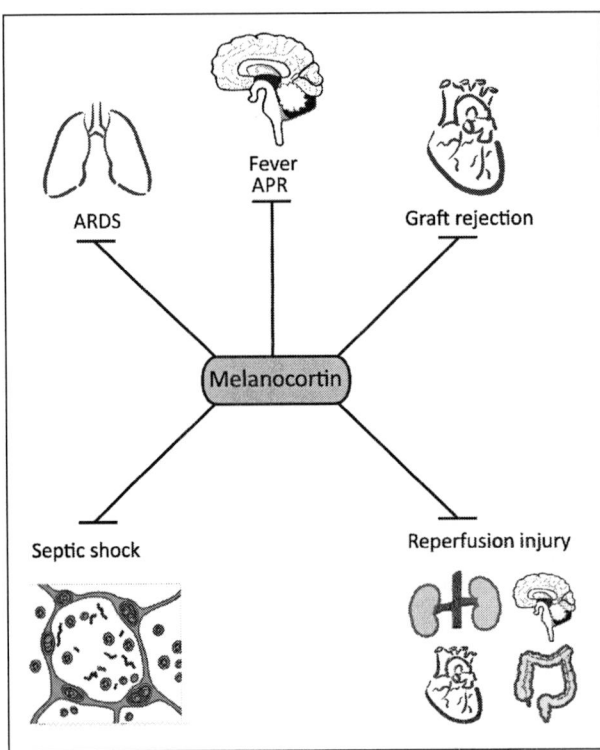

Figure 1. Melanocortins and their receptors are part of a major modulatory system that reduces host responses to infectious, circulatory, or immune-mediated challenge. These modulatory peptides reduce systemic inflammatory reactions such as fever, acute phase response, allograft rejection, reperfusion injury, septic shock and acute lung injury.

This chapter reviews the effects of α-melanocyte stimulating hormone (α-MSH) and related melanocortins in modulation of systemic host reactions of different origin (Fig. 1).

Fever

The febrile reaction is a typical consequence of release of inflammatory mediators within the brain. The traditional view holds that fever occurs via actions of cytokines such as TNF, IL-1, IL-6 and interferons on CNS temperature controls. These endogenous pyrogens produced by host cells in response to exogenous pyrogens cause production of cyclooxygenase (COX)-2-dependent prostaglandin $(PG)E_2$ in the ventromedial preoptic area (VMPO). However, this concept was challenged when specific blockade of either IL-1 or TNF activity did not diminish the febrile response to LPS, to other microbial products or to natural infections in animals and in humans. Evidence indicated that, during infection, fever could occur independently of IL-1 or TNF activity. The cytokine-like property of Toll-like receptor (TLR) signal transduction provides a basis by which any microbial product can cause fever by engaging its specific TLR on the vascular network supplying the thermoregulatory center in the anterior hypothalamus. Because fever induced by IL-1, TNF-α, IL-6 or TLR ligands requires production of PGE_2 and activation of hypothalamic PGE_2 receptors, it appears that there is a common pathway for fever induction by endogenous or exogenous pyrogens. Indeed, fever is caused by COX2-dependent PGE_2 production by either cytokine- or toll-like receptor activation.[1,2] The latter mechanism likely occurs during infectious fever whereas cytokine-dependent fever accompanies autoimmune or malignant disorders.

Endogenous melanocortins act centrally as physiological modulators of fever, recruited during the febrile response to restrain its intensity. The conception that α-MSH is important to control of fever stems from the initial observation that the molecule has antipyretic properties.[3] α-MSH inhibits fever caused by endotoxin, endogenous pyrogen and individual cytokines.[4-12] This effect was discovered in a screening for fever-reducing activity of a large number of peptides administered centrally to rabbits made febrile by injection of endogenous pyrogen, which was produced by incubating white blood cells from a donor rabbit with bacterial lipopolysaccharide.[3] α-MSH reduced fever when given centrally in doses that had no effect on normal body temperature.[13] Neither central nor intravenous injections of antipyretic doses of α-MSH in rabbits exposed to cold had any effect on their temperature.[14] Therefore, like the classical antipyretic drugs, the peptide does not simply inhibit central pathways for heat production and conservation. ACTH(1-24) and ACTH(1-39), which contain the amino acid sequence of α-MSH and recognize the same melanocortin receptors, were likewise very potent in reducing fever. Reduction of fever by central or peripheral administration of ACTH in adrenalectomized rabbits indicates that the molecule is antipyretic per se and does not require adrenal mediation.[15] When it is administered centrally, the antipyretic potency of α-MSH in reducing a standard fever caused by endogenous pyrogen is very great: more than 25,000-fold greater on a molar basis than that of acetaminophen,[16] with intravenous administration the potency of α-MSH is about 20,000 times that of acetaminophen. The superpotent α-MSH analog (Nle⁴,D-Phe⁷)-α-MSH, was approximately 10 times more potent than α-MSH in reducing fever when given centrally.[9] Fevers caused by endotoxin[17-20] and the cytokines IL-1,[21,22] IL-6[6] and TNF[6] but not those caused by IFN γ[23] and PGE₂[5] were inhibited by α-MSH. The antipyretic message sequence of α-MSH(1-13) resides in the C-terminal tripeptide Lys-Pro-Val.[24] Although this tripeptide was not as potent as the 1-13 amino acid sequence, it reduced fever when given centrally or peripherally; both acetylated and non-acetylated forms of the tripeptide were effective. N-terminal and intermediate amino acid sequences of α-MSH have no antipyretic activity. Adding amino acids to the C-terminal tripeptide sequence can either reduce or enhance antipyretic potency.[25] Addition of glycine to form α-MSH(10-13) slightly decreased potency; the 9-13 fragment was almost devoid of antipyretic activity whereas the potency of the α-MSH(8-13) sequence was approximately 10-fold greater than that of α-MSH(11-13).[25]

The great potency of α-MSH and its presence within the brain suggested that this peptide could be an endogenous modulator of fever. To test this idea, α-MSH concentration was measured in aliquots of tissue from brains of febrile and afebrile rabbits. During fever, α-MSH within the septal region increased two- to three-fold whereas there was no significant change in any other region sampled.[26] This observation was subsequently confirmed in research that showed an increase in septal concentration of α-MSH during fever, but no change in animals with comparably high body temperature induced by exposure to a hot environment.[27] These observations indicate that the increase in septal concentration of α-MSH is specific to fever and not caused by nonspecific stress or elevation of brain or body temperature. These findings were interpreted to be compatible with an α-MSH-specific septal modulation of hypothalamic fever controls. Experiments with push-pull perfusion of the septal region indicated that α-MSH is released in a pulsatile fashion during endogenous pyrogen-induced fever; such release did not occur when rabbits were afebrile.[28] α-MSH release was not dependent on body temperature and the pulses appeared to result from a direct action of cytokines because some occurred before there was any rise in body temperature. Such pulsatile release is common in neuroendocrine systems and the peptide released with each pulse would have a certain duration of action, perhaps modulating fever and other host responses. Consistent with this idea, injections of α-MSH into septal sites reduced fever in rabbits.[29,30]

The importance of central α-MSH to control of fever was supported by results of experiments on inactivation of the naturally-occurring peptide. After injections of an antiserum highly specific for α-MSH into the third cerebral ventricle, the febrile response to intravenous administration of endogenous pyrogen was increased in amplitude and was greatly prolonged.[31] Treatment with α-MSH antiserum did not alter normal body temperature nor did injections of normal rabbit serum alter fever. Thus, binding and inactivation of naturally occurring central α-MSH greatly augments fever but does not affect normal thermoregulation. These observations support the idea that endogenous central α-MSH is important for fever control, but that it has no role in control of normal temperature. It is notable that rats treated as neonates with injections of monosodium glutamate, which selectively destroys α-MSH-containing cells in the arcuate nucleus, developed greater increases in temperature after central injections of IL-1[32,33] or PGE[33] than did control animals. α-MSH content of the medial basal hypothalamus and lateral septum of monosodium glutamate-treated rats was reduced relative to control animals.[32]

Subsequently, cloning of melanocortin receptors (MCR) promoted research aimed at determining the MCR subtypes involved in the antipyretic effects of melanocortins.[34] These studies have focused on the potential roles of the MC3R and the MC4R that are prominently distributed in autonomic sites in the hypothalamus and brain stem.[35] Intracerebroventricular injection of a synthetic MC3R/MC4R antagonist, SHU-9119 in endotoxin-challenged rats prevented antipyretic influences of α-MSH. Neither α-MSH nor SHU-9119, alone or in combination, altered body temperatures in afebrile rats. In LPS-treated rats, intracerebroventricular injection of SHU-9119 significantly increased fever, whereas intravenous injection of the same dose of SHU-9119 had no effect. Neither intracerebroventricular nor intravenous SHU-9119 affected LPS-stimulated plasma ACTH or corticosterone levels. These results indicate that endogenous central melanocortins exert an antipyretic influence during fever by acting on MCRs located within the brain, independent of any modulation of the activity of the pituitary-adrenal axis.[34]

Endotoxemia and Septic Shock

The complex Toll-like receptor signaling plays a crucial role in the innate system as a first line of defense against pathogens.[36] However, a sustained inflammatory response can result in tissue damage.[37] A continuum exists from minor systemic reactions associated with a self-limited infection to severe multiorgan dysfunction that marks severe sepsis. Indeed, sepsis occurs as a clinical syndrome when infection is associated with the systemic inflammatory response. Apoptosis, mitochondrial dysfunction, sepsis-related immunosuppression, late mediators of systemic inflammation, control mechanisms for coagulation and reprogramming of immune response genes all have critical roles in the development of sepsis. Counteraction of these events could improve patient outcome.

Initial experiments on α-MSH in modulation of host reactions demonstrated that the peptide reduces the acute phase response to endotoxin.[38] Subsequently, it became clear that α-MSH given centrally or peripherally modulates many aspects of the host response to endotoxemia[39] and improves survival in models of septic shock.[40,41] Treatment with α-MSH increased survival in murine septic peritonitis induced by cecal ligation and puncture.[41] In untreated animals survival at 24 h was approximately 10%. Survival rose to 50% in animals treated with α-MSH alone and to 80% when the peptide was associated with the antibiotic gentamicin. Gentamicin alone increased survival by only 40%.

In a model of acute hepatitis accompanying endotoxemia, hepatic inflammation was induced by administering endotoxin to mice pretreated with *Corynebacterium parvum*.[42] α-MSH treatment clearly prevented liver inflammation. The peptide inhibited systemic NO production, hepatic neutrophil infiltration and decreased hepatic mRNA abundance for TNF-α and the neutrophil and monocyte chemokines (KC/IL-8 and MCP-1). Therefore, α-MSH prevents endotoxin-induced hepatic inflammation by inhibiting production of chemoattractant chemokines which then modulate infiltration of inflammatory cells.[42] These effects on the liver can account for the marked reduction in acute phase proteins observed during melanocortin treatment of endotoxemic animals.

The Shwartzman reaction is a potentially lethal generalized thrombo-haemorrhagic hypersensitivity response that occurs after sequential injections of LPS.[43] Persistent expression of vascular adhesion molecules contributes to enhanced diapedesis and activation of leukocytes, which subsequently leads to hemorrhagic vascular damage. In murine LPS-induced cutaneous vasculitis, a single injection of α-MSH significantly suppressed the deleterious vascular damage and hemorrhage by inhibiting the sustained expression of vascular E-selectin and vascular cell adhesion molecule

(VCAM)-1.[44] These observations indicate that α-MSH may have therapeutic potential for the treatment of vasculitis associated with gram negative infections.

In addition to the natural molecules, certain synthetic melanocortins have been used successfully in models of endotoxemia/septic shock. A heptapeptide analog of α-MSH (HP-228) protected rats against effects of endotoxin.[40] LPS increased iNOS activity in aortic segments and HP-228 pretreatment markedly reduced this response. Further, the rate of conversion of arginine to citrulline in lung homogenates from HP-228-treated rats was significantly reduced.[40]

The synthetic peptide (CKPV)$_2$, based on the C-terminal sequence of α-MSH, is a promising candidate to treat inflammation. Indeed, (CKPV)$_2$ modulates broad cAMP-dependent, anti-inflammatory pathways in human neutrophils[45] and reduces TNF-α production by mononuclear cells.[46] In a rat model of endotoxin-induced peritonitis (CKPV)$_2$ significantly inhibited concentrations of TNF-α and nitric oxide both in plasma and in the peritoneal fluid.[46]

The beneficial effects of melanocortins in endotoxin-induced host reactions are not surprising in view of the capacity of these peptides to inhibit NF-κB activation induced by LPS and other stimuli.[47-49] Indeed, NF-κB induces transcription of most of the molecules responsible for systemic inflammation including cytokines, chemokines, growth factors and iNOS. Therefore, reduction of NF-κB activation by melanocortins exerts protective influences during endotoxemia.

Acute Respiratory Distress Syndrome (ARDS)

Acute lung injury (ALI) and acute respiratory distress syndrome (ARDS) are severe complications of pneumonia, sepsis, trauma and inhaled irritants. Clinically, acute lung injury is characterized by production of proinflammatory mediators, massive neutrophil influx into the lung and damage to lung epithelium. Activation of leukocytes and release of proinflammatory mediators from multiple cell sources cause both local and distant tissue injury. The outcome of ALI/ARDS is determined by the ability of the injured lung to repopulate the alveolar epithelium with functional cells. However, prognosis for survival is poor and, if resolution occurs, there is evolution to severe lung fibrosis in a substantial proportion of cases. Effective therapies for this dire disease are still needed.

Early research on lung injury induced by endotracheal instillation of endotoxin in rats showed that treatment with α-MSH greatly reduces leukocyte concentration in the bronchoalveolar lavage fluid.[41] These salutary effects of α-MSH were recently confirmed and extended in lung injury caused by intratracheal instillation of bleomycin.[50] This model is currently used to investigate cellular and subcellular processes leading to lung fibrosis. However, as signs of lung damage occur immediately after bleomycin instillation, this model is also very helpful to explore early stages of lung injury.[51] Research on bleomycin instillation in rats showed that acute lung injury is associated with endogenous production of α-MSH: the peptide increased in the circulation and was expressed in lung infiltrating cells. Treatment with α-MSH greatly improved the clinical and molecular picture of bleomycin-induced injury. Three main gene categories, stress response, fluid homeostasis and inflammation, known to contribute to development of acute lung injury were modulated by peptide treatment. Further, α-MSH treatment caused significant reduction in bleomycin-induced interstitial edema. This effect was marked by improved histological picture and virtually normal wet to dry weight ratio. This observation is very important in that impaired alveolar fluid clearance is associated with worse survival in patients with acute lung injury.[52]

Ischemia and Reperfusion Injury

Tissue damage that occurs during blood reperfusion after an ischemic period is a serious problem in many vascular disorders and reperfusion procedures. Such damage is caused by migration of inflammatory cells when the blood flow is restored and is the consequence of marked upregulation of endothelial adhesion molecules that occurs during ischemia. α-MSH treatment reduced ischemia and reperfusion injury in heart,[53-55] brain,[56,57] kidney[58-62] and gut.[63]

Both ACTH and NDP-α-MSH reduced consequences of short-term coronary ischemia followed by reperfusion and the damage induced by a permanent coronary occlusion in rats.[55]

Ischemia was produced by ligature of the left anterior descending coronary artery. Postischemic reperfusion induced ventricular tachycardia, in all saline-treated rats and ventricular fibrillation and death in a high percentage of animals. In rats treated with intravenous ACTH(1-24) there was a significantly dose-dependent reduction in the incidence of arrhythmias and lethality. Treatment with ACTH(1-24) almost completely abolished increase in blood free radical concentration induced by ischemia and reperfusion. In rats subjected to permanent coronary occlusion, the amount of healthy myocardial tissue in NDP-α-MSH treated animals was significantly greater than in control rats.[55] The protective effect of ACTH(1-24) against the occurrence of ventricular tachycardia, ventricular fibrillation and lethality was not affected by adrenalectomy. Use of specific melanocortin receptor antagonists suggests that MC3R subtype mediates the protective effect of ACTH(1-24) in myocardial ischemia/reperfusion-induced arrhythmias.[53]

Related research indicated that the protective effects of ACTH(1-24) in these same models of reperfusion injury also occurs when small concentrations of the peptide are injected into the brain.[54] Treatment with ACTH(1-24) by the intracerebroventricular route reduced the incidence of ventricular tachycardia, ventricular fibrillation, fall in mean arterial blood pressure and lethality produced by five min ligature of the left anterior descending coronary artery. Complete (100%) protection occurred with an intracerebroventricular dose 10 times less than that needed by the intravenous route. Therefore, the protective effect of melanocortin peptides against myocardial injury caused by ischemia and reperfusion can occur through an action within the brain.[54] This observation reinforces the idea that damage in peripheral tissues can be reduced by marshaling the anti-inflammatory influence of α-MSH and related peptides within the brain.[64]

Several investigations indicate that α-MSH protects against renal injury after ischemia in mice and rats.[58,59,61,62,65] Influences of α-MSH were explored in a model of bilateral renal ischemia in mice.[58] α-MSH significantly reduced ischemia-induced renal damage, measured by changes in renal histology and plasma blood urea nitrogen and creatinine. Further, the peptide significantly decreased tubule necrosis, neutrophil plugging and capillary congestion. Even when treatment was delayed 6 h after ischemia, α-MSH significantly inhibited renal damage. Peptide treatment was associated with reduction in ischemia-induced increases in mRNA for the murine neutrophil chemokine KC/IL-8. α-MSH also inhibited induction of mRNA for the adhesion molecule ICAM-1, which is known to be critical in renal ischemic injury. The peptide inhibited nitration of kidney proteins and induction of NOS2.[58]

Mesenteric ischemia and reperfusion injury to the intestine is a common and often devastating clinical occurrence for which there are few therapeutic options. α-MSH had protective influences in the postischemic small intestine.[63] The research analyzed the effects of the peptide on intestinal transit, histology, myeloperoxidase activity and NF-κB activation after 45 min of superior mesenteric artery occlusion and/or 6 h of reperfusion. Rats subjected to ischemia and reperfusion exhibited markedly depressed intestinal transit, histological evidence of severe injury to the ileum, increased myeloperoxidase activity in ileal cytoplasmic extracts and biphasic activation of NF-κB in ileal nuclear extracts. In contrast, rats treated with α-MSH before ischemia and reperfusion had intestinal transit and histological injury scores comparable to those of sham-operated controls. In addition, the α-MSH-treated rats demonstrated less ischemia and reperfusion induced activation of intestinal NF-κB and myeloperoxidase activity after prolonged reperfusion. There are indications, therefore, that α-MSH limits postischemic injury to the rat small intestine.[63]

Organ Transplantation

Acute rejection is a significant obstacle to successful organ transplantation and its prevention is crucial for favorable clinical outcome. Although immunosuppressive molecules can reduce rejection, they are associated with serious side effects such as organ toxicity, increased viral infection and cancer.[66] Because most of these harmful effects are dose-dependent, reduction of immunosuppressive drug treatment necessary to prevent rejection is a major clinical target. As intragraft inflammation is known to promote and accelerate rejection,[67] use of anti-inflammatory compounds that enhance effectiveness of immunosuppressive agents could be a successful strategy.

Research on experimental heart transplantation showed that treatment with α-MSH prolongs survival and improves allograft histopathology in the highly MHC mismatched transplantation model Brown Norway into Lewis rats.[68] Such beneficial effects were associated with reduced intragraft expression of cytokines, chemokines and adhesion molecules.[68] Subsequent research based on gene expression profiling, revealed multiple protective influences exerted by α-MSH that could account for the reduced damage in transplantated heart grafts.[69] Indeed, peptide treatment caused substantial up-regulation of several salutary molecules including signal transduction mediators, metalloproteinases, serine proteases, energy pathway mediators and ion channels. Concurrent down-regulation of growth factors, cytokines, chemokines, oxidative stress mediators and ribosomal proteins likely contributes to preserve myocardium from injury. Consistent with the idea that α-MSH protects organs from reperfusion injury, peptide treatment also prevented antigen-independent damage in syngenic transplantation. In addition, α-MSH treatment exerted remarkable protective effects on a number of calcium regulatory proteins that were severely reduced by heart transplantation.[70]

Conclusion

Preclinical evidence indicates that melanocortins are key modulators of host reactions including systemic inflammation. Experiments in which different models and treatments were used show that melanocortins modulate fever, vasculitis, reperfusion injury and other host responses. Melanocortin treatment reduces but does not abolishes inflammatory mediator production. Therefore, the degree of the modulatory effect should be sufficient to reduce severity of systemic inflammation without impairing the host defense mechanisms.

References

1. Dinarello CA. Infection, fever and exogenous and endogenous pyrogens: some concepts have changed. J Endotoxin Res 2004; 10:201-222.
2. Steiner AA, Chakravarty S, Rudaya AY et al. Bacterial lipopolysaccharide fever is initiated via Toll-like receptor 4 on hematopoietic cells. Blood 2006; 107:4000-4002.
3. Lipton JM, Glyn JR, Zimmer JA. Hypothermic and antipyretic effects of centrally administered ACTH(1-24) and α-melanotropin. Fed Proc 1981; 40:2760-2762.
4. Tatro JB, Sinha PS. The central melanocortin system and fever. Ann N Y Acad Sci 2003; 994:246-257.
5. Davidson J, Milton AS, Rotondo D. Alpha-melanocyte-stimulating hormone suppresses fever and increases in plasma levels of prostaglandin E2 in the rabbit. J Physiol 1992; 451:491-502.
6. Martin LW, Catania A, Hiltz ME et al. Neuropeptide alpha-MSH antagonizes IL-6- and TNF-induced fever. Peptides 1991; 12:297-299.
7. Martin LW, Deeter LB, Lipton JM. Acute-phase response to endogenous pyrogen in rabbit: effects of age and route of administration. Am J Physiol 1989; 257:R189-193.
8. Shih ST, Lipton JM. Intravenous alpha-MSH reduces fever in the squirrel monkey. Peptides 1985; 6:685-687.
9. Holdeman M, Lipton JM. Antipyretic activity of a potent alpha-MSH analog. Peptides 1985; 6:273-275.
10. Murphy MT, Lipton JM. Peripheral administration of alpha-MSH reduces fever in older and younger rabbits. Peptides 1982; 3:775-779.
11. Murphy MT, Richards DB, Lipton JM. Antipyretic potency of centrally administered alpha-melanocyte stimulating hormone. Science 1983; 221:192-193.
12. Catania A, Lipton JM. Peptide modulation of fever and inflammation within the brain. Ann N Y Acad Sci 1998; 856:62-68.
13. Glyn JR, Lipton JM. Hypothermic and antipyretic effects of centrally administered ACTH(1-24) and α-melanotropin. Peptides 1981; 2:177-187.
14. Richards DB, Lipton JM. Antipyretic doses of α-MSH do not alter afebrile body temperature in the cold. J Thermal Biol 1984; 9:299-301.
15. Zimmer JA, Lipton JM. Central and peripheral injections of ACTH (1-24) reduce fever in adrenalectomized rabbits. Peptides 1981; 2:419-423.
16. Murphy MT, Richards DB, Lipton JM. Antipyretic potency of centrally administered α-melanocyte stimulating hormone. Science 1983; 221:192-193.

17. Martin LW, Lipton JM. Acute phase response to endotoxin: rise in plasma α-MSH and effects of α-MSH injection. Am J Physiol 1990; 259:R768-R772.
18. Goelst K, Mitchell D, Laburn H. Effects of alpha-melanocyte stimulating hormone on fever caused by endotoxin in rabbits. J Physiol 1991; 441:469-476.
19. Huang QH, Hruby VJ, Tatro JB. Systemic α-MSH suppresses LPS fever via central melanocortin receptors independently of its suppression of corticosterone and IL-6 release. Am J Physiol 1998; 275:R524-530.
20. Villar M, Perassi N, Celis ME. Central and peripheral actions of α-MSH in the thermoregulation of rats. Peptides 1991; 12:1441-1443.
21. Robertson BA, Gahring LC, Daynes RA. Neuropeptide regulation of interleukin-1 activities. Capacity of α-melanocyte stimulating hormone to inhibit interleukin-1 inducible responses in vivo and in vitro exhibits target cell selectivity. Inflammation 1986; 10:371-385.
22. Daynes RA, Robertson BA, Cho BH et al. Alpha-melanocyte-stimulating hormone exhibits target cell selectivity in its capacity to affect interleukin 1-inducible responses in vivo and in vitro. J Immunol 1987; 139:103-109.
23. Hori T, Nakashima T, Take S et al. Immune cytokines and regulation of body temperature, food intake and cellular immunity. Brain Res Bull 1991; 27:309-313.
24. Richards DB, Lipton JM. Effect of α-MSH(11-13) (lysine-proline-valine) on fever in the rabbit. Peptides 1984; 5:815-817.
25. Deeter LB, Martin LW, Lipton JM. Antipyretic properties of centrally administered α-MSH fragments in the rabbit. Peptides 1989; 9:1285-1288.
26. Samson WK, Lipton JM, Zimmer JA. The effect of fever on central α-MSH concentrations in the rabbit. Peptides 1981; 2:419-423.
27. Holdeman M, Khorram O, Samson WK et al. Fever specific changes in MSH and CRF concentrations. Am J Physiol 1985; 248:R125-R129.
28. Bell RC, Lipton JM. Pulsatile release of antipyretic neuropeptide α-MSH from septum of rabbit during fever. Am J Physiol 1987; 252:R1152-R1157.
29. Glyn-Ballinger JR, Bernardini GL, Lipton JM. α-MSH injected into the septal region reduces fever in rabbits. Peptides 1983; 4:199-203.
30. Feng JD, Dao T, Lipton JM. Effects of preoptic microinjections of alpha-MSH on fever and normal temperature control in rabbits. Brain Res Bull 1987; 18:473-477.
31. Shih ST, Khorram O, Lipton JM et al. Central administration of α-MSH antiserum augments fever in the rabbit. Am J Physiol 1986; 250:R803-R806.
32. Opp MR, Obal F, Kreuger JM. Effects of α-MSH on sleep, behavior and brain temperature: interactions with IL-1. Am J Physiol 1988; 255:R914-R922.
33. Martin SA, Malkinson TJ, Veale WL et al. Depletion of brain α-MSH alters prostaglandin and interleukin fever in rats. Brain Res 1990; 526.
34. Huang QH, Entwistle ML, Alvaro JD et al. Antipyretic role of endogenous melanocortins mediated by central melanocortin receptors during endotoxin-induced fever. J Neurosci 1997; 17:3343-3351.
35. Tatro JB. Endogenous antipyretics. Clin Infect Dis 2000; 31(Suppl)5:S190-201.
36. van der Poll T, Opal SM. Host-pathogen interactions in sepsis. Lancet Infect Dis 2008; 8:32-43.
37. Cinel I, Opal SM. Molecular biology of inflammation and sepsis: a primer. Crit Care Med 2009; 37:291-304.
38. Martin LW, Lipton JM. Acute phase response to endotoxin: rise in plasma alpha-MSH and effects of alpha-MSH injection. Am J Physiol 1990; 259:R768-772.
39. Delgado Hernandez R, Demitri MT, Carlin A et al. Inhibition of systemic inflammation by central action of the neuropeptide alpha-melanocyte-stimulating hormone. Neuroimmunomodulation 1999; 6:187-192.
40. Abou-Mohamed G, Papapetropoulos A, Ulrich D et al. HP-228, a novel synthetic peptide, inhibits the induction of nitric oxide synthase in vivo but not in vitro. J Pharmacol Exp Ther 1995; 275:584-591.
41. Lipton JM, Ceriani G, Macaluso A et al. Antiinflammatory effects of the neuropeptide alpha-MSH in acute, chronic and systemic inflammation. Ann N Y Acad Sci 1994; 741:137-148.
42. Chiao H, Foster S, Thomas R et al. Alpha-melanocyte-stimulating hormone reduces endotoxin-induced liver inflammation. J Clin Invest 1996; 97:2038-2044.
43. Pepys MB, Rogers SL, Evans DJ. Role of the acute phase response in the Shwartzman phenomenon. Clin Exp Immunol 1982; 47:289-295.
44. Scholzen TE, Sunderkotter C, Kalden DH et al. Alpha-melanocyte stimulating hormone prevents lipopolysaccharide-induced vasculitis by down-regulating endothelial cell adhesion molecule expression. Endocrinology 2003; 144:360-370.
45. Capsoni F, Ongari A, Colombo G et al. The synthetic melanocortin (CKPV)2 exerts broad anti-inflammatory effects in human neutrophils. Peptides 2007; 28:2016-2022.

46. Gatti S, Carlin A, Sordi A et al. Inhibitory effects of the peptide (CKPV)2 on endotoxin-induced host reactions. J Surg Res 2006; 131:209-214.
47. Ichiyama T, Zhao H, Catania A et al. Alpha-melanocyte-stimulating hormone inhibits NF-kappaB activation and IkappaBalpha degradation in human glioma cells and in experimental brain inflammation. Exp Neurol 1999; 157:359-365.
48. Haycock JW, Wagner M, Morandini R et al. Alpha-melanocyte-stimulating hormone inhibits NF-kappaB activation in human melanocytes and melanoma cells. J Invest Dermatol 1999; 113:560-566.
49. Manna SK, Aggarwal BB. Alpha-melanocyte-stimulating hormone inhibits the nuclear transcription factor NF-kappa B activation induced by various inflammatory agents. J Immunol 1998; 161:2873-2880.
50. Colombo G, Gatti S, Sordi A et al. Production and effects of alpha-melanocyte-stimulating hormone during acute lung injury. Shock 2007; 27:326-333.
51. Shen AS, Haslett C, Feldsien DC et al. The intensity of chronic lung inflammation and fibrosis after bleomycin is directly related to the severity of acute injury. Am Rev Respir Dis 1988; 137:564-571.
52. Matthay MA, Robriquet L, Fang X. Alveolar epithelium: role in lung fluid balance and acute lung injury. Proc Am Thorac Soc 2005; 2:206-213.
53. Guarini S, Schioth HB, Mioni C et al. MC(3) receptors are involved in the protective effect of melanocortins in myocardial ischemia/reperfusion-induced arrhythmias. Naunyn Schmiedebergs Arch Pharmacol 2002; 366:177-182.
54. Bazzani C, Mioni C, Ferrazza G et al. Involvement of the central nervous system in the protective effect of melanocortins in myocardial ischaemia/reperfusion injury. Resuscitation 2002; 52:109-115.
55. Bazzani C, Guarini S, Botticelli AR et al. Protective effect of melanocortin peptides in rat myocardial ischemia. J Pharmacol Exp Ther 2001; 297:1082-1087.
56. Huh SK, Lipton JM, Batjer HH. The protective effects of alpha-melanocyte stimulating hormone on canine brain stem ischemia. Neurosurgery 1997; 40:132-139; discussion 139-140.
57. Huang Q, Tatro JB. Alpha-melanocyte stimulating hormone suppresses intracerebral tumor necrosis factor-alpha and interleukin-1beta gene expression following transient cerebral ischemia in mice. Neurosci Lett 2002; 334:186-190.
58. Chiao H, Kohda Y, McLeroy P et al. Alpha-melanocyte-stimulating hormone protects against renal injury after ischemia in mice and rats. J Clin Invest 1997; 99:1165-1172.
59. Kwon TH, Frokiaer J, Han JS et al. Decreased abundance of major Na(+) transporters in kidneys of rats with ischemia-induced acute renal failure. Am J Physiol Renal Physiol 2000; 278:F925-939.
60. Deng J, Kohda Y, Chiao H et al. Interleukin-10 inhibits ischemic and cisplatin-induced acute renal injury. Kidney Int 2001; 60:2118-2128.
61. Jo SK, Yun SY, Chang KH et al. Alpha-MSH decreases apoptosis in ischaemic acute renal failure in rats: possible mechanism of this beneficial effect. Nephrol Dial Transplant 2001; 16:1583-1591.
62. Chiao H, Kohda Y, McLeroy P et al. Alpha-melanocyte-stimulating hormone inhibits renal injury in the absence of neutrophils. Kidney Int 1998; 54:765-774.
63. Hassoun HT, Zou L, Moore FA et al. Alpha-melanocyte-stimulating hormone protects against mesenteric ischemia-reperfusion injury. Am J Physiol Gastrointest Liver Physiol 2002; 282:G1059-1068.
64. Lipton JM, Catania A, Ichiyama T. Marshaling the anti-inflammatory influence of the neuroimmunomodulator alpha-MSH. News Physiol Sci 2000; 15:192-195.
65. Kwon TH, Frokiaer J, Fernandez-Llama P et al. Reduced abundance of aquaporins in rats with bilateral ischemia-induced acute renal failure: prevention by alpha-MSH. Am J Physiol 1999; 277:F413-427.
66. Pascual M, Swinford RD, Ingelfinger JR et al. Chronic rejection and chronic cyclosporin toxicity in renal allografts. Immunol Today 1998; 19:514-519.
67. Dallman MJ. Immunobiology of graft rejection. In: Ginns LC, Cosimi AB, Morris PJ, eds. Transplantation. Malden, MA: Blackwell Science, 1999;23-35.
68. Gatti S, Colombo G, Buffa R et al. Alpha-melanocyte-stimulating hormone protects the allograft in experimental heart transplantation. Transplantation 2002; 74:1678-1684.
69. Colombo G, Gatti S, Turcatti F et al. Gene expression profiling reveals multiple protective influences of the peptide {alpha}-melanocyte-stimulating hormone in experimental heart transplantation. J Immunol 2005; 175:3391-3401.
70. Colombo G, Sordi A, Lonati C et al. Treatment with alpha-melanocyte stimulating hormone preserves calcium regulatory proteins in rat heart allografts. Brain Behav Immun 2008; 22:817-823.

CHAPTER 10

Development of α-Melanocortin Analogs for Melanoma Prevention and Targeting

Zalfa A. Abdel-Malek*

Abstract

Melanocortins, particularly α-melanocortin (α-melanocyte stimulating hormone, α-MSH), were first identified as the physiological regulators of pigmentation in many vertebrate species. Their role in regulating human pigmentation was unequivocally demonstrated in the 1990s, with the cloning of the human melanocortin 1 receptor (*MC1R*) gene from human melanocytes and the demonstration that functional MC1R is expressed by these cells. α-Melanocyte stimulating hormone is a tridecapeptide, with the core sequence His[6]-Phe[7]-Arg[8]-Trp[9] shared with β- and γ-MSH and identified as essential for receptor activation and stimulation of pigmentation. The small size of α-MSH makes it an attractive molecule for drug design. There has been longstanding interest in the development of melanocortin analogs that target the MC1R expressed on normal melanocytes and melanoma cells. The aim has been to develop MC1R agonists that stimulate melanogenesis and confer photoprotection to human melanocytes and thus prevent skin cancer formation. Recent findings that the physiological α-MSH not only stimulates melanogenesis, but also reduces the extent of DNA damage caused by exposure to solar ultraviolet radiation have further rejuvenated the interest in developing synthetic MC1R agonists for skin cancer prevention. α-Melanocortin analogs have also been developed for imaging of melanoma tumors, localization of residual metastasis and specific delivery of radionuclides to eradicate melanoma tumors, sparing normal tissues. The main challenge is to develop specific MC1R agonists that will target melanocytes for skin cancer prevention, or for localization and treatment of metastatic melanoma.

Introduction

The first and perhaps best described physiological effect of melanocortins, particularly α-MSH, is stimulation of integumental pigmentation of many vertebrate species, including mammals.[1] Injection of mice that are wild type for *extension*, the genetic locus that codes for the MC1R, with α-MSH results in the development of black hairs due to stimulation of synthesis of eumelanin by follicular melanocytes.[2] On the other hand, mice harboring loss of function mutation in this gene (*e/e*; recessive yellow) fail to respond to physiological melanocortins with eumelanin synthesis and have a yellow coat color due to the predominance of pheomelanin, the red-yellow pigment.[3] In the 1960s, Lerner and McGuire[4] demonstrated that injection of human subjects with purified α-MSH and β-MSH increased skin darkening, particularly in sun-exposed anatomical sites. These early studies suggested that α-MSH affects human skin pigmentation, similar to its effects on follicular

*Zalfa A. Abdel-Malek—Department of Dermatology, University of Cincinnati, Cincinnati, Ohio 45267, USA. Email: abdelmza@email.uc.edu

Melanocortins: Multiple Actions and Therapeutic Potential, edited by Anna Catania.

melanocytes in mice. However, the observed increase in skin darkening of human subjects could not be definitely attributed to the direct effect of α-MSH on melanocytes, since it could be due to stimulation of production of autocrine or paracrine factor(s) that increase melanogenesis. It took almost three decades, until the 1990s, to prove unequivocally that cultured human melanocytes respond directly to α-MSH and ACTH with stimulation of melanogenesis and proliferation and that these effects are mediated by activation of the MC1R, which is expressed on the cell surface of melanocytes.[5-8] We showed that α-MSH and ACTH are equally potent and both are more potent than β-MSH, while γ-MSH is the least effective, in activating the MC1R expressed on human melanocytes.[9] That human epidermal melanocytes, as well as melanoma cells, express MC1R[10] generated interest in developing potent and stable α-melanocortin analogs to stimulate melanogenesis and to detect and target drug delivery to melanoma cells.

α-Melanocortin Analogs as Tanning Agents

The in vivo effect of melanocortins on human skin generated interest in developing α-MSH analogs for "sunless tanning". α-Melanocyte stimulating hormone is a tridecapeptide (Ac-Ser-Tyr-Ser-Met-Glu-His-Phe-Arg-Trp-Gly-Lys-Pro-Val-NH$_2$, with the core sequence His-Phe-Arg-trp shared with β- and γ-MSH and found to be sufficient for increasing pigmentation.[11] The small size of α-MSH has facilitated the design and development of analogs, many of which were agonists of the melanocortin receptors 1, 3, 4 and 5. It is common knowledge that increasing facultative pigmentation induced by sun exposure is photoprotective, since melanin, particularly eumelanin reduces the penetration of UV rays through the epidermal layers.[12,13] The first analog to be developed for this purpose was Ac-[Nle^4-D-Phe^7]-α-MSH (NDP-MSH), whereby Methionine in position 4 was replaced by Norleucine and L-Phe in position 7 was substituted by D-Phe.[14] This analog proved to be more potent and stable and with more prolonged effect than the physiological α-MSH in several bioassays, including frog and lizard bioassays and tyrosinase activity assay on mouse melanoma cells and cultured normal human melanocytes.[14-18]

The early results obtained by Lerner and McGuire were confirmed in 1991, when it was demonstrated that injection of human subjects with the NDP-MSH induced skin darkening, in addition to side effects, such as flushing and nausea.[19] The pigmentary effect of NDP-MSH was evident in individuals having skin phototype III or IV, according to the Fitzpatrick classification (those who tan and do not burn upon sun exposure) even in the absence of sun exposure and with application of sun screen and was maintained for a considerably long time.

Recently, the pigmentary effect of NDP-MSH was reported in individuals with skin Type I or II, who burn and have a poor tanning capacity.[20] The increase in pigmentation in response to NDP-MSH was due to stimulation of eumelanin synthesis without any effect on pheomelanin synthesis. This and the early study by Levine et al[19] relied on multiple injections of volunteers with NDP-MSH, which is not a practical method of delivery. To circumvent this, a time release patch was developed, which proved to be efficacious and reduced the undesirable effects of the analog by delivering it subcutaneously rather than systemically (reviewed by Hadley and Dorr).[21] The most recent human study with NDP-MSH showed that it reduced the extent of DNA photoproducts, as well as sunburn cells (i.e., apoptotic keratinocytes), that are induced by UV irradiation, indicating reduction of UV-induced DNA damage.[20]

Toxicological studies carried out with NDP-MSH demonstrated that it was not toxic or teratogenic to mice, rats or Yucatan miniature pigs (reviewed by Hadley and Dorr).[21] It did not increase the growth or metastasis of melanoma cells injected in mice, nor did it increase the growth of human melanoma tumors in SCID mice.[22,23] Furthermore, treatment of freshly isolated human melanoma tumor cells or melanoma cell lines with NDP-MSH did not increase their colony forming ability, suggesting lack of an effect of NDP-MSH on malignant transformation.[24]

The potency, stability and residual effect of NDP-MSH were due to stabilization of the β-turn structure involving the Phe^7 residue. Based on this, highly potent cyclic disulfide analogs of linear α-MSH were designed, such as Ac[Cys^4, Cys^{10}]-α-MSH.[25] Further computational studies led to the design of the cyclic lactam analog Ac-Nle^4 -c[Asp^5-His^6-D-Phe^7-Arg^8-Trp^9-Lys^{10}]-NH$_2$

(MT-II).[26] The fragment analog MT-II was developed as an attempt to deliver it transdermally. This analog has high potency at the human MC1R, MC3R and MC4R; it enhanced skin tanning, yet produced immediate penile erection in male volunteers. For that reason its pigmentary effect was no longer pursued. The stability and excellent biodistribution of NDP-MSH and MT-II made them very useful for examining agonist activities of melanocortin peptides. MT-II has been used to develop potent antagonists of the human melanocortin receptors. The best example is Ac-Nle[4]-c-[Asp[5]-His[6]-D-Nal(2')[7]-Arg[8]-Trp[9]-Lys[10]]-NH$_2$ (SHU-9119).[27] In contrast to its antagonistic activity at the MC3R and MC4R, this analog has high agonistic activity at the MC1R.

The pharmaceutical use of peptides is limited by their susceptibility to enzymatic degradation, which greatly compromises their bioavailability. To overcome this deficiency, peptoids that resemble the natural structure of peptides yet have less susceptibility for enzymatic degradation have been synthesized.[28] Peptoids are polymeric compounds composed of N-substituted glycine. When peptoids were modeled after the tetrapeptide His-Phe-Arg-Trp that is conserved in all melanocortins and account for their pigmentary effects, this resulted in compounds with reduced melanogenic activity but increased selectivity for each of the melanocortin receptors MC1R, MC3R, MC4R and MC5R.

α-Melanocortin Analogs Reduce UV-Induced DNA Damage

Our laboratory has made the important discovery that α-MSH confers photoprotection not only by increasing melanogenesis by human melanocytes, but also by reducing the burden of DNA damage caused by solar ultraviolet radiation (UV) (Fig. 1).[29] We have shown that treatment of UV-irradiated melanocytes with α-MSH reduced the generation of reactive oxygen species within minutes, as measured by decreased hydrogen peroxide generation and subsequently oxidative DNA damage, exemplified by less induction of 8-oxo-dG.[29,30] Furthermore, α-MSH inhibited oxidative damage by increasing the activity of catalase, as well as the levels of the antioxidant proteins catalase, hemeoxygenase-1 and ferritin. Moreover, α-MSH enhanced the repair of DNA photoproducts, evidenced by increased removal of cyclobutane pyrimidine dimers in α-MSH-pretreated, compared to untreated UV-irradiated melanocytes.[29] The effect of α-MSH on reduction of DNA photoproducts was also reported by Bohm et al.[31] and activation of nucleotide repair was confirmed more recently by Smith et al.[32] In our study, the above effects of α-MSH were observed before any measurable increase in eumelanin or total melanin content.[29] The timing of the above events and

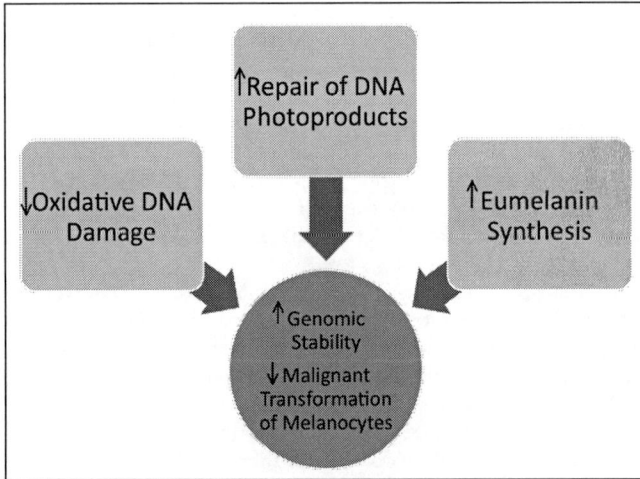

Figure 1. Mechanisms by which physiological α-MSH and synthetic MC1R agonists prevent malignant transformation of melanocytes to melanoma.

their occurrence in tyrosinase-negative albino melanocytes suggest that the effects of α-MSH on the DNA damage response to UV are independent of increased melanin content.[29]

Based on our results, we hypothesize that α-MSH has immediate effects on the UV response of human melanocytes, exemplified by reduced reactive oxygen species and oxidative DNA damage and enhanced repair of DNA photoproducts and latent effects, exemplified by stimulation of melanogenesis (Fig. 1). The former effects are critical for insuring genomic stability of melanocytes and prevention of mutagenesis and the latter are important for protection from subsequent UV exposures. The novel effects of α-MSH described above rejuvenated the interest in utilizing α-MSH-based analogs for skin cancer prevention, not merely for enhancing tanning, but also for stimulating mechanisms that reduce UV-induced DNA damage and thus prevent sun-induced skin cancer, including melanoma.

We have been interested in designing and testing small peptide analogs of α-MSH that are potent, long acting and lipophilic that can be applied topically for skin cancer prevention. We have reported the effects of a panel of N-capped tetrapeptide analogs, consisting of amino acids 6-9 of α-MSH, on human melanocytes and found two analogs, namely 5-phenylbutyryl (LK184) and n-pentadecanoyl-His-D-Phe-Arg-Trp-NH$_2$, to be significantly more potent than α-MSH and equally potent to the tridecapeptide analog NDP-MSH.[18,33,34] The former two analogs mimicked α-MSH in its effects on stimulation of pigmentation as well as reduction of generation of reactive oxygen species and enhancement of repair of DNA photoproducts (Fig. 1). The effects of these analogs were entirely mediated by binding to the MC1R, as they were absent in melanocytes that expressed loss-of-function MC1R and were blocked by the MC1R antagonist agouti signal protein. One of these analogs, n-phenylbutyryl-His-D-Phe-Arg-Trp-NH$_2$ was selective for MC1R and selectivity of the other analog is currently being determined.

More recently, we synthesized and tested smaller α-MSH analogs, tripeptides containing the 6-8 amino acid residues His-D-Phe-Arg that had N-capping or C-terminal modifications, or were Arginine mimetics. After testing a panel of 17 tripeptides, only 3 C-terminally modified analogs proved to be active on MC1R, evidenced by stimulating cAMP formation as well as tyrosinase activity in human melanocytes.[35] These tripeptides were less effective than α-MSH by 1 log unit, yet retained considerable activity at micromolar concentrations. The most potent of these C-terminally modified tripeptides mimicked α-MSH in reducing hydrogen peroxide generation and enhancing repair of DNA photoproducts by UV-irradiated human melanocytes (Fig. 1). The effects of this analog were mediated by binding MC1R since they were absent in melanocytes expressing loss of function MC1R. Generation of active tripeptide analogs of α-MSH is an important step towards the successful development of topically applied agents, due to the small size of these peptides. Improvement on the stability, lipophilicity and potency will help achieve this goal.

The *MC1R* gene is one of the most polymorphic pigmentary genes and is a major determinant of the diversity of human pigmentation. Additionally, the *MC1R* is recognized as a melanoma susceptibility gene, since some allelic variants, mainly R160W, R151C and D294H, that are strongly associated with red hair phenotype and poor tanning ability increase the risk for melanoma.[36-40] These variants are thought to have a heterozygous effect on melanoma risk and to increase the penetrance of the mutations in the melanoma locus CDKN2A.[38,39] Expression of these variants as heterozygotes reduces MC1R activity, thus are expected to compromise the ability of melanocytes to respond to physiological α-MSH with reduced DNA damage and repair of DNA photoproducts. We propose that treatment of melanocytes with these *MC1R* genotypes or mutations in *CDKN2A* with potent and stable melanocortin analogs should increase the activation of MC1R, thus augmenting the DNA damage response, as well as stimulating pigmentation, thus reducing the risk of melanoma.

α-Melanocortin Analogs for Melanoma Targeting

It is known that many melanoma tumors over express the MC1R, which enables them to respond to autocrine melanocortins for their autonomous growth.[10] For that, there has been long term interest in targeting MC1R with melanocortin peptides to diagnose melanoma, particularly metastases after resection of the primary tumor. Metastatic disease is the main cause of death of melanoma patients, hence the importance of detection for prognosis. Alpha-MSH analogs have been labeled with metals for potential medical uses. Many [111]In- and ^{18}F-labeled MC1R targeting peptides have been developed and primarily characterized as imaging agents.[41,42] The octapeptide [βAla[3], Nle[4], Asp[5], D-Phe[7]-Lys[10]]-α-MSH (MSH$_{oct}$) and NDP-MSH were conjugated to the metal chelator 1,4,7,10-tetrazocyclododecane 1,4,7,10-tetraacetic acid (DOTA) to allow for radiometal incorporation and labeled with [111]In.[41] DOTA-MSH$_{oct}$ bound the MC1R with high affinity, but its affinity was lower than that of DOTA-NDP-MSH. Both peptides exhibited high MC1R-mediated uptake by B16F1 tumors in tumor-bearing C57 mice, with DOTA-MSH$_{oct}$ having a poorer clearance from kidneys than DOTA-NDP-MSH, which showed poorer clearance from bone. Generally, ^{111}In-DOTA-MSH$_{oct}$ proved to have more favorable properties than ^{111}In-DOTA-NDP-MSH, suggesting that it might be a promising melanoma imaging agent.

For further improvement on DOTA-MSH$_{oct}$, a shorter linear α-MSH analog [Nle[4], Asp[5],D-Phe[7]]-α-MSH$_{4-11}$ (NAPamide) was synthesized and conjugated with DOTA on the C-terminal, rather than the N-terminal as in the case of the former analog.[43] DOTA-NAPamide had almost 7-fold higher binding affinity to MC1R and exhibited markedly higher uptake by B16F1 cells and less kidney uptake than DOTA-MSH$_{Oct}$. Another approach was undertaken to increase the tumor-to-kidney ratio of the melanocortin analog. This involved the synthesis of glycosylated derivatives of ^{111}In-labeled, DOTA-conjugated NAPamide. N-terminally positioned galactose in this analog slightly improved the tumor-to-kidney ratio, thus serving as a potential lead for novel MC1R targeting molecules.[44]

In one study, the biological properties of the cyclic pz-βAla-Nle-cyclo[Asp-His-D-Phe-Arg-Trp-Lys]-NH$_2$ a (Melanotan II) and linear pz-βAla-Nle-Asp-His-DPhe-Arg-Trp-Lys-NH$_2$, both labeled with *fac*-[[99m]Tc(CO)$_3$], were compared.[45] Cyclic constraint, as in Melanotan II resulted in increased affinity to MC1R, as well as greater potency, enzymatic stability and prolonged activity. The cyclic compound demonstrated higher levels of internalization and higher degree of cellular retention in B16F1 melanoma cells, compared to its linear counterpart.

Radiolabeled melanocortin analogs can be potentially used to target radiation to eradicate melanoma tumors. For that, DOTA-Re(Arg[11])CCMSH, a peptide cyclized by nonradioactive Re and contained an N-terminal DOTA chelator, was developed and radiolabeled with the beta-particle-emitter ^{177}Lu, or [212]Pb, the parent radionuclide of [212]Bi that yields an alpha and a beta particle upon decay.[46] The former resulted in 25-30% reduction in tumor size in melanoma tumor-bearing mice and a significant improvement in mean survival time with no evidence of radiation-related damage to the kidneys. The latter had the advantage of targeting melanoma tumor cells with minimal normal tissue exposures and dose-dependent therapeutic efficacy.

Conclusion

Numerous melanocortin analogs have been designed with the goal of utilizing them for increased tanning, or for screening or targeting melanoma tumors. The major challenges for the design of effective analogs are their potency, stability and importantly, selectivity for the MC1R. The issue of selectivity is of special importance, since many analogs can bind and activate MC1R, MC3R, MC4R and MC5R, resulting in additional effects other than the intended effects on pigmentation or melanoma targeting. In the skin, MC1R is expressed primarily on melanocytes[7] and MC1R and MC5R on sebocytes.[47,48] Keratinocytes and fibroblasts do not express melanocortin receptors, as determined by RT-PCR, as well as functional assays (receptor binding assay, coupling of the receptor to adenylate cyclase and increasing cAMP)[49] (our unpublished data). Overcoming these challenges should lead to the generation of highly efficacious analogs that can be utilized for skin cancer prevention or for localizing and treatment of metastatic melanoma.

Acknowledgements

This work was supported by R01 ES009110 from the National Institute from Environmental Health Sciences and R01CA114095 from the National Cancer Institute.

References

1. Sawyer TK, Hruby VJ, Hadley ME et al. α-Melanocyte stimulating hormone: Chemical nature and mechanism of action. Am Zool 1983; 23:529-540.
2. Levine N, Lemus-Wilson AL, Wood SH et al. Stimulation of follicular melanogenesis in the mouse by topical and injected melanotropins. J Invest Dermatol 1987; 89:269-273.
3. Tamate HB, Takeuchi T. Action of the e locus of mice in the response of phaeomelanic hair follicles to α-melanocyte-stimulating hormone in vitro. Science 1984; 224:1241-1242.
4. Lerner AB, McGuire JS. Effect of alpha- and beta-melanocyte stimulating hormones on the skin colour of man. Nature 1961; 189:176-179.
5. Mountjoy KG, Robbins LS, Mortrud MT et al. The cloning of a family of genes that encode the melanocortin receptors. Science 1992; 257:1248-1251.
6. Chhajlani V, Wikberg JES. Molecular cloning and expression of the human melanocyte stimulating hormone receptor cDNA. FEBS Lett 1992; 309:417-420.
7. Abdel-Malek Z, Swope VB, Suzuki I et al. Mitogenic and melanogenic stimulation of normal human melanocytes by melanotropic peptides. Proc Natl Acad Sci USA 1995; 92:1789-1793.
8. Hunt G, Donatien PD, Lunec J et al. Cultured human melanocytes respond to MSH peptides and ACTH. Pigment Cell Res 1994; 7:217-221.
9. Suzuki I, Cone R, Im S et al. Binding of melanotropic hormones to the melanocortin receptor MC1R on human melanocytes stimulates proliferation and melanogenesis. Endocrinology 1996; 137:1627-1633.
10. Ghanem GE, Comunale G, Libert A et al. Evidence for alpha-melanocyte stimulating hormone receptors on human malignant melanoma cells. Int J Cancer 1988; 41:248-255.
11. Hadley ME. Endocrinology. 4th ed. Upper Saddle River, NJ: Prentice-Hall, Inc., 1996.
12. Pathak MA, Fitzpatrick TB. The role of natural photoprotective agents in human skin. In: Fitzpatrick TB, Pathak MA, Haber LC et al, eds. Sunlight and Man. Tokyo: University of Tokyo Press, 1974; 725-750.
13. Kaidbey KH, Poh Agin P, Sayre RM et al. Photoprotection by melanin—a comparison of black and Caucasian skin. J Am Acad Dermatol 1979; 1:249-260.
14. Sawyer TK, Sanfilippo PJ, Hruby VJ et al. 4-Norleucine, 7-D-phenylalanine-α-melanocyte-stimulating hormone: A highly potent α-melanotropin with ultralong biological activity. Proc Natl Acad Sci USA 1980; 77:5754-5758.
15. Marwan MM, Abdel-Malek ZA, Kreutzfeld KL et al. Stimulation of S91 melanoma tyrosinase activity by superpotent α-melanotropins. Mol Cell Endocrinol 1985; 41:171-177.
16. Hadley ME, Abdel-Malek ZA, Kreutzfeld KL et al. [Nle⁺⁴, D-Phe⁺⁷]-α-MSH: A superpotent melanotropin that "irreversibly" activates melanoma tyrosinase. Endocr Res 1985; 11:157-170.
17. Abdel-Malek ZA, Kreutzfeld KL, Marwan MM et al. Prolonged stimulation of S91 melanoma tyrosinase by [Nle⁴, D-Phe⁷]-substituted α-melanotropins. Cancer Res 1985; 45:4735-4740.
18. Abdel-Malek ZA, Kadekaro AL, Kavanagh RJ et al. Melanoma prevention strategy based on using tetrapeptide alpha-MSH analogs that protect human melanocytes from UV-induced damage and cytotoxicity. FASEB J 2006; 20:1561-1563.
19. Levine N, Sheftel SN, Eytan T et al. Induction of skin tanning by the subcutaneous administration of a potent synthetic melanotropin. JAMA 1991; 266:2730-2736.
20. Barnetson RS, Ooi TK, Zhuang L et al. [Nle⁴-D-Phe⁷]-alpha-melanocyte-stimulating hormone significantly increased pigmentation and decreased UV damage in fair-skinned Caucasian volunteers. J Invest Dermatol 2006; 126(8):1869-1878.
21. Hadley ME, Dorr RT. Melanocortin peptide therapeutics: historical milestones, clinical studies and commercialization. Peptides 2006; 27(4):921-930.
22. Gehlsen KR, Hadley ME, Levine N et al. Effects of a melanotropic peptide on melanoma cell growth, metastasis and invasion. Pigment Cell Res 1992; 5:219-223.
23. Paine-Murrieta GD, Taylor CW, Curtis RA et al. Human tumor models in the severe combined immune deficient (scid) mouse. Cancer Chemother Pharmacol 1997; 40(3):209-214.
24. Jiang J, Sharma SD, Nakamura S et al. The melanotropic peptide, [Nle4,D-Phe7] alpha-MSH, stimulates human melanoma tyrosinase activity and inhibits cell proliferation. Pigment Cell Res 1995; 8(6):314-323.
25. Sawyer TK, Hruby VJ, Wilkes BC et al. Comparative biological activities of highly potent active-site analogues of α-melanotropin. J Med Chem 1982; 25:1022-1027.
26. Al-Obeidi F, Castrucci AM, Hadley ME et al. Potent and prolonged acting cyclic lactam analogues of alpha-melanotropin: design based on molecular dynamics. J Med Chem 1989; 32(12):2555-2561.
27. Hruby VJ, Lu D, Sharma SD et al. Cyclic lactam α-lelanotropin analogues of Ac-Nle⁺⁴-c[Asp⁺⁵,{UD}-Phe⁺⁷,Lys⁺¹⁰]-α-MSH(4-10)-NH₂ with bulky aromatic amino acids at position 7 show high antagonist potency and selectivity at specific melanocortin receptors. J Med Chem 1995; 38:3454-3461.

28. Holder JR, Bauzo RM, Xiang Z et al. Design and pharmacology of peptoids and peptide-peptoid hybrids based on the melanocortin agonists core tetrapeptide sequence. Bioorg Med Chem Lett 2003; 13(24):4505-4509.

29. Kadekaro AL, Kavanagh R, Kanto H et al. α-melanocortin and endothelin-1 activate anti-apoptotic pathways and reduce DNA damage in human melanocytes. Cancer Res 2005; 65:4292-4299.

30. Song X, Mosbi N, Yang J et al. Alpha-MSH activates immediate defense responses to UV-induced oxidative stress in human melanocytes. Pigment Cell Mel Res 2009, In press.

31. Bohm M, Wolff I, Scholzen TE et al. Alpha-melanocyte-stimulating hormone protects from ultraviolet radiation-induced apoptosis and DNA damage. J Biol Chem 2005; 280(7):5795-5802.

32. Smith AG, Luk N, Newton RA et al. Melanocortin-1 receptor signaling markedly induces the expression of the NR4A nuclear receptor subgroup in melanocytic cells. J Biol Chem 2008; 283(18):12564-12570.

33. Koikov LN, Ebetino FH, Solinsky MG et al. Analogs of sub-nanomolar hMC1R agonist LK-184 [Ph(CH$_2$)$_3$CO-His-DPhe-Arg-Trp-NH$_2$]. An additional binding site within the human melanocortin receptor 1? Bioorgan Med Chem Lett 2004; 14:3997-4000.

34. Todorovic A, Holder JR, Bauzo RM et al. N-terminal fatty acylated His-DPhe-Arg-Trp-NH$_2$ tetrapeptides: influence of fatty acid chain length on potency and selectivity at the mouse melanocortin receptors and human melanocytes. J Med Chem 2005; 48:3328-3336.

35. Abdel-Malek ZA, Ruwe AR, Kavanagh-Starner R et al. α-MSH tripeptide analogs activate the melanocortin 1 receptor and reduce UV-induced DNA damage in human melanocytes. Pigment Cell Mel Res 2009, In press.

36. Box NF, Wyeth JR, O'Gorman LE et al. Characterization of melanocyte stimulating hormone receptor variant alleles in twins with red hair. Hum Mol Genet 1997; 6:1891-1897.

37. Smith R, Healy E, Siddiqui S et al. Melanocortin 1 receptor variants in Irish population. J Invest Dermatol 1998; 111:119-122.

38. Palmer JS, Duffy DL, Box NF et al. Melanocortin-1 receptor polymorphisms and risk of melanoma: Is the association explained solely by pigmentation phenotype? Am J Hum Genet 2000; 66:176-186.

39. Kennedy C, ter Huurne J, Berkhout M et al. Melanocortin 1 receptor (MC1R) gene variants are associated with an increased risk for cutaneous melanoma which is largely independent of skin type and hair color. J Invest Dermatol 2001; 117:294-300.

40. van der Velden PA, Sandkuijl LA, Bergman W et al. Melanocortin-1 receptor variant R151C modifies melanoma risk in Dutch families with melanoma. Am J Hum Genet 2001; 69:774-779.

41. Froidevaux S, Calame-Christe M, Tanner H et al. A novel DOTA-alpha-melanocyte-stimulating hormone analog for metastatic melanoma diagnosis. J Nucl Med 2002; 43(12):1699-1706.

42. Cheng Z, Zhang L, Graves E et al. Small-animal PET of melanocortin 1 receptor expression using a 18F-labeled alpha-melanocyte-stimulating hormone analog. J Nucl Med 2007; 48(6):987-994.

43. Froidevaux S, Calame-Christe M, Schuhmacher J et al. A gallium-labeled DOTA-alpha-melanocyte-stimulating hormone analog for PET imaging of melanoma metastases. J Nucl Med 2004; 45(1):116-123.

44. Bapst JP, Calame M, Tanner H et al. Glycosylated DOTA-alpha-melanocyte-stimulating hormone analogues for melanoma targeting: Influence of the site of glycosylation on in vivo biodistribution. Bioconjug Chem 2009.

45. Raposinho PD, Xavier C, Correia JD et al. Melanoma targeting with alpha-melanocyte stimulating hormone analogs labeled with fac-[99mTc(CO)3]+: effect of cyclization on tumor-seeking properties. J Biol Inorg Chem 2008; 13(3):449-459.

46. Miao Y, Quinn TP. Peptide-targeted radionuclide therapy for melanoma. Crit Rev Oncol Hematol 2008; 67(3):213-228.

47. Bohm M, Schiller M, Stander S et al. Evidence for expression of melanocortin-1 receptor in human sebocytes in vitro and in situ. J Invest Dermatol 2002; 118(3):533-539.

48. Thiboutot D, Sivarajah A, Gilliland K et al. The melanocortin 5 receptor is expressed in human sebaceous glands and rat preputial cells. J Invest Dermatol 2000; 115(4):614-619.

49. Roberts DW, Newton RA, Beaumont KA et al. Quantitative analysis of MC1R gene expression in human skin cell cultures. Pigment Cell Res 2006; 19(1):76-89.

CHAPTER 11

MSH Radiopeptides for Targeting Melanoma Metastases

Alex N. Eberle,* Jean-Philippe Bapst, Martine Calame, Heidi Tanner and Sylvie Froidevaux

Abstract

Radiolabeled peptides have become important tools for preclinical cancer research and in nuclear oncology they serve as diagnostic and more recently also as therapeutic agents. Whereas the development of receptor-mediated targeting for therapy has been confined to some radiolabeled antibodies and somatostatin/SRIF analogs, recent research into radiolabeled α-melanocyte-stimulating hormone (α-MSH) and its receptor MC1R (over-)expressed by melanoma tumor cells has demonstrated that small metastatic melanoma lesions in experimental animals are specifically targeted by MSH radiopeptides. Thus MSH radiopharmaceuticals will eventually open a new avenue for the treatment of melanoma metastases in man, provided that the targeting efficiency can be further enhanced and nonspecific incorporation into nontarget organs, e.g., the kidneys, minimized. Some novel MSH lead compounds containing a glyco moiety, added negatively charged groups or a cyclic structure show very promising in vivo targeting characteristics.

Introduction

Ionizing radiation is one of the major means to kill tumor cells in patients suffering from cancer.[1,2] Although most patients undergoing radiation therapy are exposed to external beam radiation, internal radiotherapy based on targeting radioisotopes to the neoplastic tissue is receiving increased interest because targeting of radiolabeled peptides or antibodies to cancer cells can be made more specific than external radiation.[3,4] Because of their much lower molecular weight and hence their very low immunogenicity and excellent tumor penetration, radiopeptides have attracted steadily increasing interest in receptor-mediated tumor targeting during the past fifteen years. A variety of human tumors express or overexpress receptors for one or more of the many known regulatory neuropeptides or peptide hormones, thereby offering attractive targeting systems for tumor diagnosis and imaging.[5] The list of the different regulatory peptides for tumor targeting in preclinical development has now exceeded the number of thirty,[4,6,7] but routine application as diagnostics in the clinic is confined to a much smaller number[4] and internal radiotherapy is currently carried out with only a few selected radiopeptides.[8] The best example illustrating the rational of the strategy of receptor-mediated tumor targeting are radiolabeled analogs of somatostatin which are routinely used to image tumors expressing somatostatin receptors, thus demonstrating promise for internal radiotherapy in patients.[9,10]

The idea to apply radioactive peptides to receptor-mediated targeting of tumor cells dates back to the early 1970s, when in Robert Schwyzer's laboratory the first of several highly tritiated

*Corresponding Author: Alex N. Eberle—Laboratory of Endocrinology, Department of Biomedicine, University Hospital Basel and University Children's Hospital, University of Basel, Klingelbergstrasse 23, CH-4031 Basel, Switzerland. Email: alex-n.eberle@unibas.ch

Melanocortins: Multiple Actions and Therapeutic Potential, edited by Anna Catania.
©2010 Landes Bioscience and Springer Science+Business Media.

analogs of α-melanotropin (α-MSH) were prepared and later applied to in vitro and in vivo targeting experiments (reviewed by refs. 11,12). Although these radiopeptides became very useful for the identification and characterization of melanocortin receptors by binding experiments, autoradiography and crosslinking methods, in vivo targeting of melanoma in animal models was not successful: firstly, the analogs suffered from insufficient in vivo stability and secondly, the radiotoxicity of the tritium that had accumulated in the tumor was much too low to arrest tumor cell growth. On the other hand, these experiments demonstrated that radioactive peptides are readily taken up by tumor cells, an important advantage of peptides over antibodies for tumor targeting. In 1990 Bard et al showed in vitro and in vivo results with an ^{111}In-labeled analog of α-MSH with which melanoma tumors in experimental animals could be targeted.[13] This was the first report on a regulatory peptide carrying a chelating group for incorporation of radiometals.

α-MSH and many of its analogs have been studied extensively in the context of their melanogenic activity in melanocytes and melanoma cells as well as their binding to and regulation of melanocortin receptors (reviewed by refs. 11,14-16). Whereas human melanocytes generally express low numbers of melanocortin-1 receptor (MC1R)[17] and none of the other four MC receptor subtypes, melanoma cells frequently overexpress MC1R which is therefore regarded as useful marker for malignant melanoma.[18-22] These findings were the basis for our original studies on the in vivo targeting of melanoma with ^{111}In-labeled α-MSH containing DTPA (diethylenetriaminepentaacetic acid) as chelator for insertion of the radiometal.[23,24] In the past few years, our and other laboratories have developed short linear or cyclic α-MSH analogs containing the macrocyclic cyclen-type chelator DOTA (1,4,7,10-tetraazacyclododecane-1,4,7,10-tetraacetic acid). The characteristics of the most promising of these compounds with potential as melanoma targeting radiopharmaceutical will be presented in this chapter.

Radionuclides and Chelators for MSH Peptides

The general principle of tumor targeting with radiopeptides is outlined in Figure 1.[25] The radiopharmaceutical is applied systemically, in most cases intravenously, leading to accumulation in the target organ and also in nontarget tissues, mainly the kidneys, liver and spleen. Binding of the radiopeptide to its receptor induces receptor down-regulation and internalization of the receptor-ligand complex. The internalized receptor-ligand complexes are first found in endosomes and later part of the radioactivity may be seen in the nucleus and also in mitochondria. The selection of the radioisotopes depends on the purpose of the targeting: for diagnostic applications, isotopes emitting γ-radiation are necessary (e.g., ^{67}Ga, ^{99m}Tc, ^{111}In), or positron-emitters (e.g., ^{18}F, ^{64}Cu, ^{68}Ga, ^{124}I) which also produce γ-photons. For therapeutic application, short-range α-emitters (e.g., ^{211}At, ^{212}Pb, ^{213}Bi, ^{225}Ac) or β-emitters (e.g., ^{90}Y, ^{177}Lu, ^{67}Cu, ^{131}I, ^{188}Re) are selected or, alternatively, isotopes that emit Auger electrons (e.g., ^{99m}Tc, ^{111}In). The targeting characteristics of α-MSH radiopeptides have been tested with many of these radionuclides. DOTA turned out to be the most versatile chelator for radionuclide targeting of melanoma; it proved to be superior to nonmacrocyclic DTPA. Some other macrocyclic chelators have also been tested successfully with α-MSH analogs such as the cyclam-type chelator CBTE2A for ^{64}Cu labeling.[26] A different approach for the insertion of ^{99m}Tc or ^{188}Re into MSH peptides was developed without attachment of a dedicated chelator structure:[27] the side-chains of three Cys replacing specific residues in the MSH molecule together with an amino group can form an NS_3-type chelator after appropriate folding of the peptide. As a consequence of the complexation with the radiometal, the initially linear MSH peptide gets cyclized.[27] The ^{99m}Tc radiometal may also be attached to MSH peptides in form of *fac*[^{99m}Tc(CO)$_3$]$^+$ by complexing to a pyrazolyl chelator incorporated into MSH.[28]

MSH with High Potency for Melanoma Targeting

Radiopeptides for tumor targeting are only then an excellent alternative to radiolabeled antibodies when synthetic peptide analogs with excellent biostability and bioactivity are available to which suitable chemical groups for incorporation of a variety of different radioisotopes can be attached. Figure 2 list important requirements for MSH and other peptides that are used as

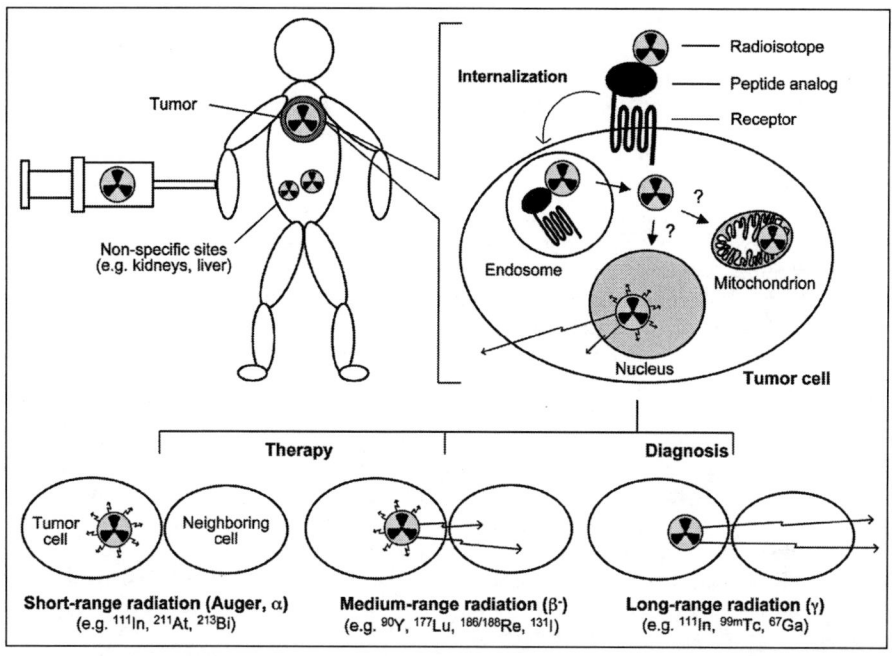

Figure 1. General principles of receptor-mediated targeting of tumor cells by radiopeptides labeled with diagnostic and therapeutic radioisotopes (for details see text; reproduced with permission from ref. 25).

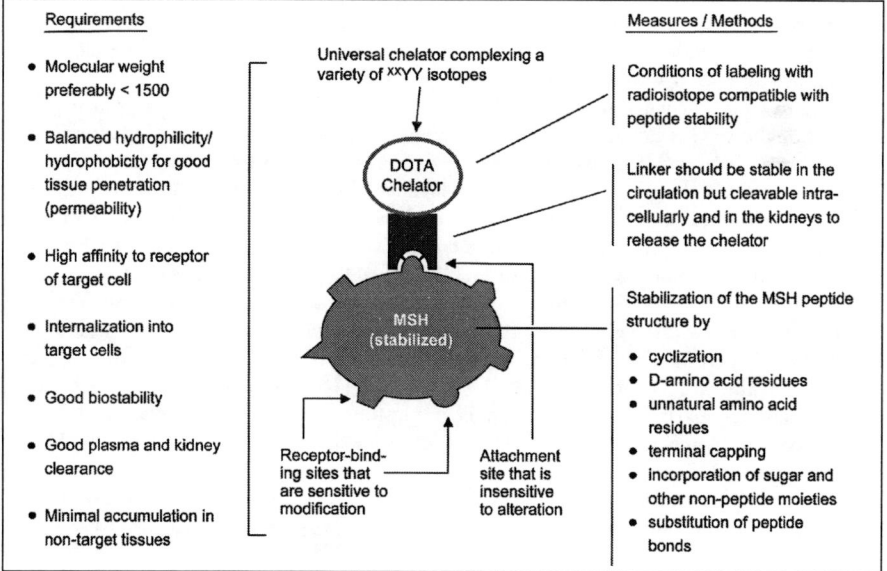

Figure 2. Important requirements for the design and development of MSH peptide radiopharmaceuticals include the limitation of the molecular weight of the peptide, a highest possible receptor affinity and internalization into target cells as well as excellent biostability, plasma clearance and low nonspecific tissue accumulation of the radiopeptide.

radiopharmaceuticals. Generally, screening and selection for high in vitro potency is not the sole indicator for obtaining good targeting characteristics. For example, when we prepared various MSH dimer peptides, they displayed excellent in vitro MC1R affinities and were amongst the most potent MSH ligands ever reported, but in vivo their nontarget organ accumulation (kidneys, liver and others) was dramatically increased as compared to monomeric MSH radiopeptides.[29] Thus, the rule to keep the molecular weight of the peptide to <1,500 was also true in this example and it is particularly important for rapid plasma and kidney clearance and to keep nontarget organ accumulation as low as possible. Other factors include good biostability which can be achieved by use of a D-Phe residue at position 7 of α-MSH and/or cyclization of the peptide as well as other structural modifications (e.g., capping of the N- and C-terminus), a well balanced hydrophilicity/hydrophobicity of the molecule (e.g., by insertion of sugar moieties) and a favorable distribution of positive and negative charges across the molecule.

The choice of the best suited chelator is an important factor,[30] but as most authors designing MSH radiopeptides have used DOTA, little experience with other chelators has been gathered for this class of peptide. Also, a systematic study on the way how the chelator should be linked to the MSH peptide and the ensuing influence on the in vivo characteristics has not yet been reported. From our own observation we assume that by introducing a cleavage site in the linker region specific for enzymes of the tubular system of the kidneys, the nonspecific accumulation in this organ may be reduced. In the search for general recommendations, Froidevaux et al found that the positive charge of a free lysine side-chain of α-MSH exerts an adverse effect on kidney retention.[31] This adverse effect can be eliminated when the DOTA chelator is attached directly on the lysine side-chain of the MSH analog or when the positive charge is neutralized by attaching, e.g., a small protecting group such as formyl.

In general, receptor binding and bioassays are the first screening methods for analyzing novel synthetic peptides, followed by receptor autoradiography using melanoma tissue sections to examine MC1R distribution in the tumor and to check for the suitability of the MSH radiopeptide for this type of application.[32] Receptor autoradiography is also important to assess the accumulation of MSH radiopeptides after in vivo biodistribution studies.[33] This latter method which has recently been complemented by PET analysis has become an important tool in the development of melanoma targeting systems. In addition the kinetics of cellular uptake of radiopeptides and the residence times of the radionuclide in the cell are also routinely examined.

Owing to its excellent receptor binding characteristics, DOTA-NDP-MSH was first MSH radiopeptide thoroughly examined in vitro and in vivo as it displayed good accumulation in the tumor.[34] Some of the nonspecific organ values, however, were relatively high which lead to the design and synthesis of fragments and fragment analogs of NDP-MSH with lower side-effects. As specified below, the first of these compounds was DOTA-MSH$_{oct}$ in which the DOTA chelator was placed at the N-terminus.[34] The second compound, DOTA-NAPamide,[33] contained the DOTA chelator on the side-chain of the lysine residue, i.e., at the C-terminus of the molecule. After labeling with ^{111}In or ^{67}Ga/^{68}Ga, high and specific melanoma uptake and relatively moderate or low kidney uptake was observed in mice. The amount of accumulated radioactivity in the kidneys observed with [^{67}Ga]DOTA-NAPamide was the lowest of all synthetic DOTA-α-MSH analogs studied at that time.[35-40] With both tracers, DOTA-MSH$_{oct}$ and DOTA-NAPamide, metastatic melanoma lesions could be detected by autoradiography following in vivo biodistribution (Fig. 3). A more recent development avoiding the presence of a chelator is the use of ^{18}F-containing MSH radiopeptides for PET analysis.[41]

As ^{99m}Tc and [188]Re cannot be complexed stably with DOTA-type chelators, Giblin et al studied Cys-containing α-MSH analogs with which these radioisotopes can be complexed internally by the peptide itself (see above).[27] The excellent biological potency and biostability of such cyclized MSH peptides initiated a series of studies with a large number of cyclic and linear analogs of this type, which turned out to be an interesting alternative to shorter linear peptides such as DOTA-NAPamide.[35-40] Comparison of the biodistribution data showed that the cyclic structures had the tendency of a slightly or markedly higher nonspecific accumulation,[42] in particular to the bone marrow. Nevertheless, other

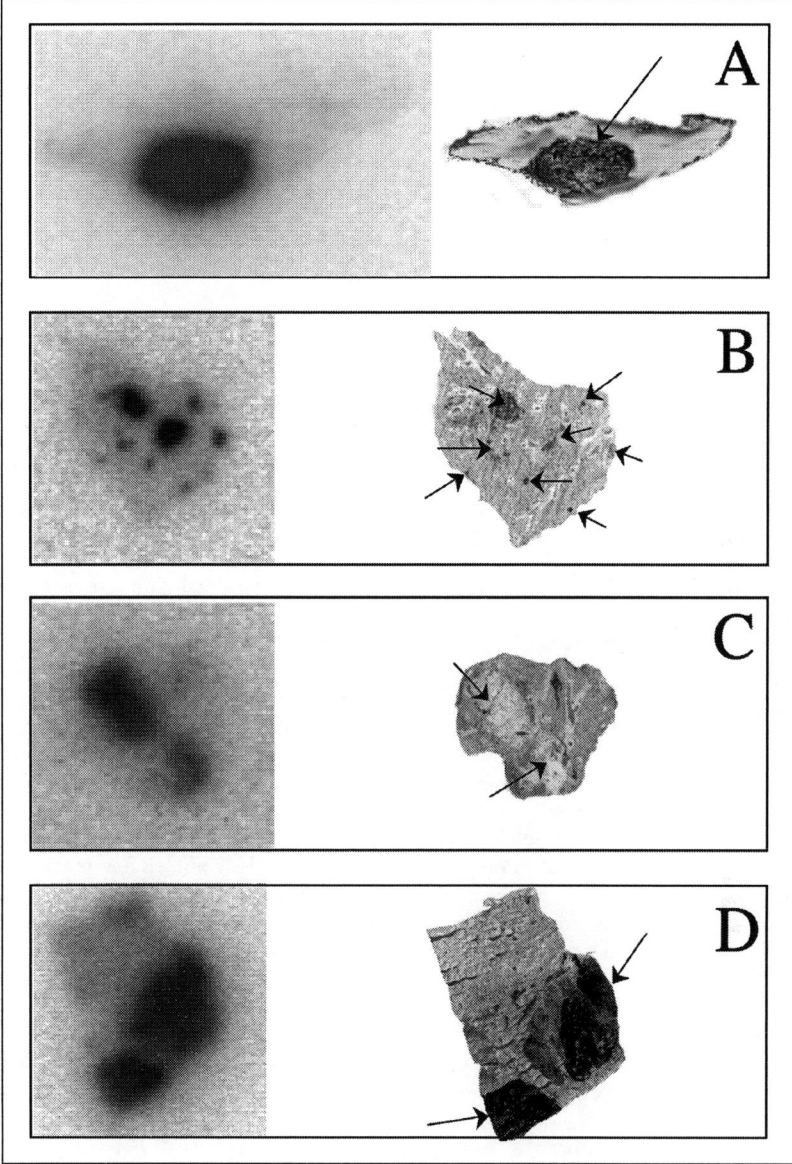

Figure 3. Autoradiographs of tissue sections from melanoma-bearing mice. [^{111}In]DOTA-MSH$_{oct}$ was injected to mice inoculated with B16F1 cells and tissues were collected 4 h postinjection. A-D, Autoradiographs (left panel) and scanner images (right panel) of a primary melanoma with surrounding skin tissue (A), lung with melanotic melanoma metastases (B), lung with amelanotic melanoma metastases (C), liver with melanotic melanoma metastases (D). Arrows indicate the melanoma lesions.

pharmacological criteria such as increased in vivo biostability or longer residence times in the tumor may perhaps compensate for the slight disadvantage of lower specificity.[43] This also applies to lactam bridge-cyclized analogs of the type of DOTA-NAPamide peptide.[44]

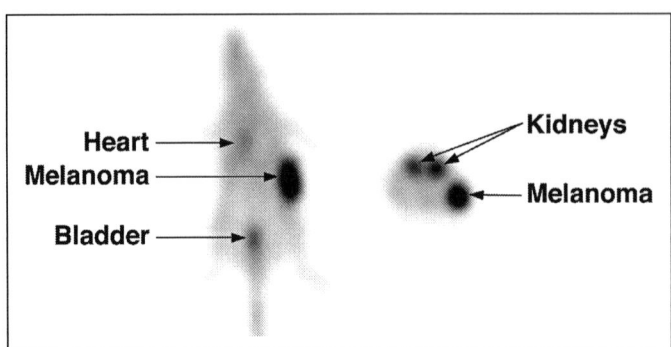

Figure 4. PET imaging of melanoma-bearing mice with [^{68}Ga]DOTA-NAPamide (scatter- and attenuation-corrected PET images of melanoma-bearing mice). [^{68}Ga]DOTA-NAPamide (50.1 GBq/μmol; 40 pmol) was injected into mice implanted in right flank with B16F1 melanoma and imaged at 0.5, 1, 2 and 3 h after injection (n = 2): coronal image (A) and transaxial image (B) of mice 0.5 h after injection. Only melanoma, kidneys, bladder and, to a lesser extent, heart are detectable. No further background reduction could be observed at later time points.

Nonspecific Targeting

The retention of considerable amounts of the injected dose by the kidneys limits the therapeutic efficacy of radiopeptides, as renal toxicity is a dose-limiting factor.[9,12] For the same reason diagnosis of tumors localized in the kidney region is strongly compromised. Renal accumulation is a general problem for all radiopeptides containing metal chelators such as DOTA or DTPA and is not confined to MSH analogs. In most of the published studies with DOTA-MSH radiopeptides, the uptake of radioactivity by the kidneys usually exceeded that of the tumor. DOTA-NAPamide showed tumor-to-kidney ratios >1, which means that with this radiopeptide more radioactivity was found in the tumor than the kidneys (Fig. 4). In order to reduce uptake by the kidneys further, various methods have been developed, such as infusion of basic amino acid cocktails,[45] which positively influenced excretion of MSH radiopeptides.[33] Other efforts should focus on the elucidation of the mechanism of retention of radiopeptides in the kidneys: It is now relatively well established that radiopeptides are reabsorbed by proximal tubules via luminal endocytosis after glomerular filtration. The peptides are then delivered to lysosomes where they are hydrolyzed to a final radioactive metabolite that cannot leave the lysosomes, leading to long-term sequestration of the radioisotope in the proximal tubular cells.[46] MSH radiopeptides exhibiting lower renal uptake per se would clearly represent a major step forward. However, as this is difficult to achieve before molecular details of the reuptake have been clarified, an alternative strategy is the development of MSH radiopeptides with markedly enhanced tumor uptake so that the dose of injected radiopeptide can be reduced, leading to lower kidney burden.

Relevant Lead Compounds

Figure 5 lists some of the most relevant lead compounds of MSH radiopeptides for melanoma targeting. Several additional compounds have appeared in the literature recently, but most of these have their roots in the structures shown here. In the last twenty years, NDP-MSH has become a kind of reference compound and it is usually the first ligand tested in any experimental system. As mentioned above, the targeting characteristics of DOTA-NDP-MSH are not optimal because of its higher accumulation in some nontarget tissues, e.g., the bone marrow, when compared to shorter peptides.[34] DOTA-MSH$_{oct}$ was the first lead compound with which excellent and specific accumulation in metastatic melanoma lesions could be demonstrated, with negligible accumulation in the bone marrow.[34] It is also the lead structure for a new derivative with phosphotyrosine yielding an excellent tumor-to-kidney ratio (unpublished data). With the DOTA-NAPamide molecule, kidney uptake could be further reduced, compared

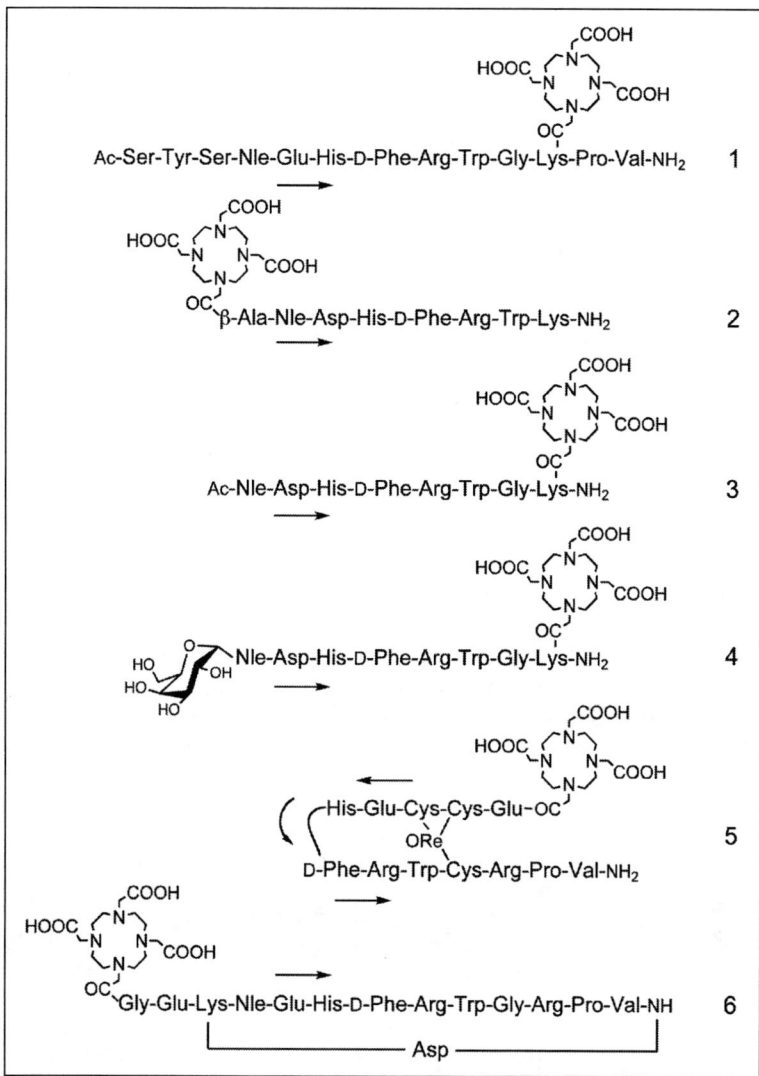

Figure 5. Lead structures for MSH radiopharmaceuticals. 1: [Nle⁴, D-Phe⁷, Lys(DOTA)¹¹]-α-MSH (DOTA-NDP-MSH); 2: DOTA-[β-Ala³, Nle⁴, Asp⁵, D-Phe⁷, Lys¹⁰]-α-MSH$_{3-10}$ (DOTA-MSH$_{oct}$); 3: [Nle⁴, Asp⁵, D-Phe⁷, Lys(DOTA)¹¹]-α-MSH$_{4-11}$ (DOTA-NAPamide); 4: Galactosyl-[Nle⁴, Asp⁵, D-Phe⁷, Lys(DOTA)¹¹]-α-MSH$_{4-11}$ (DOTA-Gal-NAPamide); 5: ReO-cyclized DOTA-[Glu², Cys³, Cys⁴, D-Phe⁷, Arg¹¹]-α-MSH$_{2-13}$ (DOTA-Re(Arg¹¹)CCMSH); 6: Lactam bridge-cyclized DOTA-[Gly¹, Glu², cyclo(Lys³, Nle⁴, D-Phe⁷, Arg¹¹, (Val-Asp)¹³)]-α-MSH (DOTA-CycMSH).

to that of DOTA-MSH$_{oct}$. Indeed, DOTA-NAPamide is one of the most potent MSH targeting molecules.[33] Addition of an N-terminal galactosyl residue to DOTA-NAPamide further enhances these positive characterstics so that DOTA-Gal-NAPamide exhibited even more favorable pharmacokinetic data.[47] Its high melanoma uptake and lower kidney retention and above all its improved tumor-to-kidney uptake ratio (Fig. 6), opens the door to the development of novel glycosylated radiolabeled α-MSH derivatives for melanoma targeting with further reduced nephrotoxicity. The literature on Re-cyclized lactam bridge-cyclized MSH

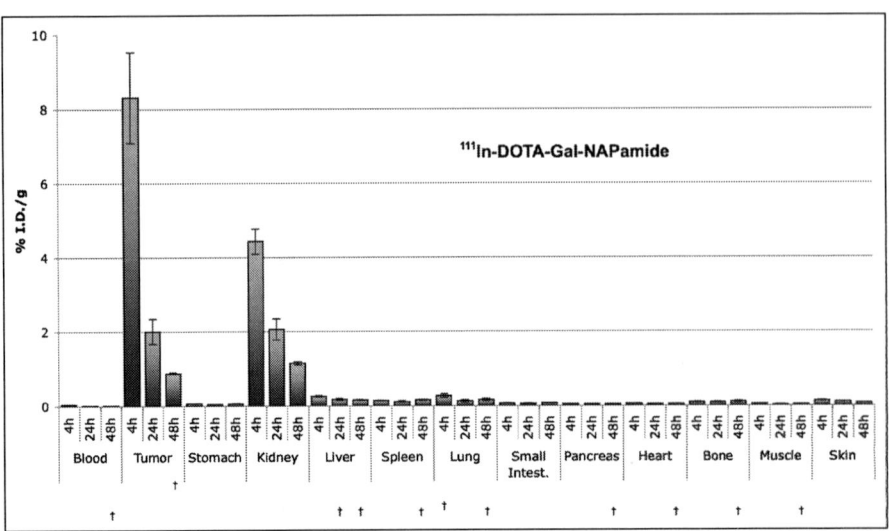

Figure 6. Tissue distribution of [¹¹¹In]DOTA-Gal-NAPamide at 4, 24 and 48 h postinjection. Results are expressed as % of injected dose per gram of tissue (%ID/g; means ± SEM; n = 4). †P < 0.05 vs [¹¹¹In]DOTA-NAPamide (reproduced with permission from ref. 47).

radiopeptides and the many different studies with therapeutic[37,39,40] and diagnostic[35,36,42,44,48-50] radionuclides with these peptides is impressive, leading to the expectation that a breakthrough to a clinical application may soon be reached (reviewed in ref. 43). Nonetheless, the targeting efficiency with these peptides so far does not show an advantage over linear peptides such as DOTA-Gal-NAPamide.

Conclusion

In the past few years, considerable progress in the design of more specific and stable α-MSH radiopeptides has been documented in the literature. The novel MSH compounds display comparable targeting characteristics in experimental melanoma models as achieved with the clinically used somatostatin radiopharmaceuticals in their experimental cancer models. A first breakthrough was DOTA-NAPamide which for a long time yielded the best tumor-to-kidney ratio when studied with in vivo biodistribution experiments. DOTA-Gal-NAPamide and a peptide containing a phosphorylated tyrosine residue further improved the targeting specificity of DOTA-NAPamide. For the rhenium-cyclized or lactam bridge-cyclized MSH analogs also marked progress has been reported. Yet, in view of the high tolerance of melanoma to ionizing radiation requiring a very high accumulation of radionuclide in tumor lesions and hence high doses of radiopharmaceutical, the rate of MSH-mediated tumor uptake and residence times of radionuclides in the tumor should first be enhanced further before clinical studies are started. We believe that it is less important to test too many different radionuclides with the same peptides and in the same experimental setting as there are more important open questions to solve at present: (1) the development of targeting systems with which the radionuclides are more rapidly and extensively internalized into tumor cells; (2) a better understanding of MC1R regulation in melanoma in vivo in order to find the most efficient targeting conditions; (3) the study of appearance of α-MSH antibodies in the circulation under specific pathophysiological conditions. Such antibodies could scavange MSH radiopharmaceuticals, thus reducing the efficiency of any therapy. Once these and other open questions are resolved, a clinical study with the then most appropriate MSH radiocompound may lead to a real breakthrough in clinical melanoma targeting.

References

1. Vikram B, Coleman CN, Deye JA. Current status and future potential of advanced technologies in radiation oncology. Part 1. Challenges and resources. Oncology (Williston Park) 2009; 23:279-83.
2. Vikram B, Coleman CN, Deye JA. Current status and future potential of advanced technologies in radiation oncology. Part 2. State of the science by anatomic site. Oncology (Williston Park) 2009; 23:380-5.
3. Harris M. Monoclonal antibodies as therapeutic agents for cancer. Lancet Oncol 2004; 5:292-302.
4. Eberle AN, Mild G, Froidevaux S. Receptor-mediated tumor targeting with radiopeptides. Part 1. General concepts and methods: applications to somatostatin receptor-expressing tumors. J Recept Signal Transduct 2004; 24:319-45.
5. Reubi JC. Neuropeptide receptors in health and disease: the molecular basis for in vivo imaging. J Nucl Med 1995; 36:1825-35.
6. Mariani G, Erba PA, Signore A. Receptor-mediated tumor targeting with radiolabeled peptides: there is more to it than somatostatin analogs. J Nucl Med 2006; 47:1904-6.
7. Britz-Cunningham SH, Adelstein SJ. Molecular targeting with radionuclides: state of science. J Nucl Med 2003; 44:1945-61.
8. Reubi JC, Mäcke HR, Krenning EP. Candidates for peptide receptor radiotherapy today and in the future. J Nucl Med 2005; 46(Suppl 1):67S-75S.
9. Froidevaux S, Eberle AN. Somatostatin analogs and radiopeptides in cancer therapy. Biopolymers 2002; 66:161-83.
10. Reubi JC. Somatostatin and other peptide receptors as tools for tumor diagnosis and treatment. Neuroendocrinology 2004; 80(Suppl 1):51-6.
11. Eberle AN. The melanotropins: chemistry, physiology and mechanisms of action. Basel: Karger; 1988.
12. Eberle AN, Froidevaux S. Radiolabeled α-melanocyte-stimulating hormone analogs for receptor-mediated targeting of melanoma: from tritium to indium. J Mol Recognit 2003; 16:248-54.
13. Bard DR, Knight CG, Page-Thomas DP. A chelating derivative of α-melanocyte stimulating hormone as a potential imaging agent for malignant melanoma. Br J Cancer 1990; 62:919-22.
14. Eberle AN. Proopiomelanocortin and the melanocortin peptides. In: Cone RD, ed. The Melanocortin Receptors. Totowa: Humana Press, 2000:3-67.
15. Eberle AN, Froidevaux S, Siegrist W. Melanocortins and melanoma. In: Cone RD, ed. The Melanocortin Receptors. Totowa: Humana Press, 2000:491-520.
16. Eves PC, MacNeil S, Haycock JW. α-Melanocyte-stimulating hormone, inflammation and human melanoma. Peptides 2006; 27:444-52.
17. De Luca M, Siegrist W, Bondanza S et al. α-Melanocyte stimulating hormone (α-MSH) stimulates normal human melanocyte growth by binding to high-affinity receptors. J Cell Sci 1993; 105:1079-84.
18. Siegrist W, Solca F, Stutz S et al. Characterization of receptors for α-melanocyte-stimulating hormone on human melanoma cells. Cancer Res 1989; 49:6352-58.
19. Ghanem GE, Comunale G, Libert A et al. Evidence for α-melanocyte-stimulating hormone (α-MSH) receptors on human malignant melanoma cells. Int J Cancer 1988; 41:248-55.
20. Siegrist W, Stutz S, Eberle AN. Homologous and heterologous regulation of α-melanocyte-stimulating hormone receptors in human and mouse melanoma cell lines. Cancer Res 1994; 54:2604-10.
21. Jiang J, Sharma SD, Fink JL et al. Melanotropic peptide receptors: membrane markers of human melanoma cells. Exp Dermatol 1996; 5:325-33.
22. Salazar-Onfray F, Lopez M, Lundqvist A et al. Tissue distribution and differential expression of melanocortin 1 receptor, a malignant melanoma marker. Br J Cancer 2002; 87:414-22.
23. Bagutti C, Stolz B, Albert R et al. [^{111}In]-DTPA-labeled analogues of α-MSH for the detection of MSH receptors in vitro and in vivo. Ann NY Acad Sci 1993; 680:445-7.
24. Bagutti C, Stolz B, Albert R et al. [^{111}In]-DTPA-labeled analogues of α-melanocyte-stimulating hormone for melanoma targeting: receptor binding in vitro and in vivo. Int J Cancer 1994; 58:749-55.
25. Eberle AN, Mild G. Receptor-mediated tumor targeting with radiopeptides. Part 1. General principles and methods. J Recept Signal Transduct 2009; 29:1-37.
26. Wei L, Butcher C, Miao Y et al. Synthesis and biologic evaluation of ^{64}Cu-labeled rhenium-cyclized α-MSH peptide analog using a cross-bridged cyclam chelator. J Nucl Med 2007; 48:64-72.
27. Giblin MF, Wang N, Hoffman TJ et al. Design and characterization of α-melanotropin peptide analogs cyclized through rhenium and technetium metal coordination. Proc Natl Acad Sci USA 1998; 95:12814-8.
28. Raposinho PD, Correia JD, Alves S et al. A ^{99m}Tc(CO)$_3$-labeled pyrazolyl-α-melanocyte-stimulating hormone analog conjugate for melanoma targeting. Nucl Med Biol 2008; 35:91-9.

29. Bapst JP, Froidevaux S, Calame M et al. Dimeric DOTA-α-melanocyte-stimulating hormone analogs: synthesis and in vivo characteristics of radiopeptides with high in vitro activity. J Recept Signal Transduct 2007; 27:383-409.

30. Heppeler A, Froidevaux S, Eberle AN et al. Receptor targeting for tumor localisation and therapy with radiopeptides. Curr Med Chem 2000; 7:971-94.

31. Froidevaux S, Calame-Christe M, Tanner H et al. Melanoma targeting with DOTA-α-melanocyte-stimulating hormone analogs: structural parameters affecting tumor uptake and kidney uptake. J Nucl Med 2005; 46:887-95.

32. Bagutti C, Oestreicher M, Siegrist W et al. α-MSH receptor autoradiography on mouse and human melanoma tissue sections and biopsies. J Recept Signal Transduct Res 1995; 15:427-42.

33. Froidevaux S, Calame-Christe M, Schuhmacher J et al. A gallium-labeled DOTA-α-melanocyte-stimulating hormone analog for PET imaging of melanoma metastases. J Nucl Med 2004; 45:116-23.

34. Froidevaux S, Calame-Christe M, Tanner H et al. A novel DOTA-α-melanocyte-stimulating hormone analog for metastatic melanoma diagnosis. J Nucl Med 2002; 43:1699-706.

35. Chen J, Cheng Z, Owen NK et al. Evaluation of an ^{111}In-DOTA-rhenium cyclized α-MSH analog: A novel cyclic-peptide analog with improved tumor-targeting properties. J Nucl Med 2001; 42:1847-55.

36. Cheng Z, Chen J, Miao Y et al. Modification of the structure of a metallopeptide: synthesis and biological evaluation of ^{111}In-labeled DOTA conjugated rhenium-cyclized α-MSH analogues. J Med Chem 2002; 45:3048-56.

37. Miao Y, Owen NK, Whitener D et al. In vivo evaluation of [188]Re-labeled α-melanocyte stimulating hormone peptide analogs for melanoma therapy. Int J Cancer 2002; 101:480-487.

38. Cheng Z, Chen J, Quinn TP et al. Radioiodination of rhenium cyclized α-melanocyte stimulating hormone resulting in enhanced radioactivity localization and retention in melanoma. Cancer Res 2004; 64:1411-18.

39. Miao Y, Hoffman TJ, Quinn TP. Tumor targeting properties of ^{90}Y and ^{177}Lu labeled α-melanocyte stimulating hormone peptide analogues in a murine melanoma model. Nucl Med Biol 2005; 32:485-93.

40. Miao Y, Fisher DR, Quinn TP. Reducing renal uptake of ^{90}Y and ^{177}Lu labeled α-melanocyte stimulating hormone peptide analogues. Nucl Med Biol 2006; 33:723-33.

41. Cheng Z, Zhang L, Graves E et al. Small animal PET of melanocortin 1 receptor expression using a ^{18}F-labeled α-melanocyte stimulating hormone analog. J Nucl Med 2007; 48:987-94.

42. Wei L, Zhang X, Gallazzi F et al. Melanoma imaging using [111]In-, [86]Y- and ^{68}Ga-labeled CHX-A''-Re(Arg[11]) CCMSH. Nucl Med Biol 2009; 36:345-54.

43. Miao Y, Quinn TP. Peptide-targeted radionuclide therapy for melanoma. Crit Rev Oncol Hematol 2008; 67:213-228.

44. Miao Y, Gallazzi F, Guo H et al. ^{111}In-labeled lactam bridge-cyclized α-melanocyte stimulating hormone peptide analogues for melanoma imaging. Bioconjug Chem 2008; 19:539-47.

45. Bernard BF, Krenning EP, Breeman WA et al. D-Lysine reduction of indium-111 octreotide and yttrium-90 octreotide renal uptake. J Nucl Med 1997; 24:761-9.

46. Behr TM, Goldenberg DM, Becker W. Reducing the renal uptake of radiolabeled antibody fragments and peptides for diagnosis and therapy: present status, future prospects and limitations. Eur J Nucl Med 1998; 25:201-12.

47. Bapst JP, Calame M, Tanner H et al. Glycosylated DOTA-α-melanocyte-stimulating hormone analogues for melanoma targeting: Influence of the site of glycosylation on in vivo biodistribution. Bioconjug Chem 2009; 20:984-93.

48. Cheng Z, Xiong Z, Subbarayan M et al. ^{64}Cu-labeled α-melanocyte stimulating hormone analog for microPET imaging of melanocortin-1 receptor expression. Bioconjug Chem 2007; 18:765-72.

49. Guo H, Shenoy N, Gershman BM et al. Metastatic melanoma imaging with an ^{111}In-labeled lactam bridge-cyclized α-melanocyte-stimulating hormone peptide. Nucl Med Biol 2009; 36:267-76.

50. Guo H, Yang J, Gallazzi F et al. Effect of DOTA position on melanoma targeting and pharmacokinetic properties of ^{111}In-labeled lactam bridge-cyclized α-melanocyte stimulating hormone peptide. Bioconjug Chem 2009; 20:2162-8.

CHAPTER 12

Applications of the Role of α-MSH in Ocular Immune Privilege

Andrew W. Taylor* and Darren Lee

Abstract

There is an important role for α-MSH and the melanocortin receptors in ocular immunity, development and health. This chapter will cover what is known about how α-MSH is part of the mechanisms of ocular immune privilege, about the expression of melanocortin receptors and the implications of these findings on the role of α-MSH in ocular physiology and its potential use to treat ocular pathologies.

Ocular Immune Privilege

It is greatly appreciated that the ocular microenvironment has an unique relationship with the immune system, in that immunity is highly regulated within the eye. It is considered to be an evolutionary adaptation to prevent excessive inflammatory responses that are often accompanied with collateral damage caused by vascular leakage, cell death and fibroses, which can permanently impair vision and cause blindness.[1] This immunoregulation is characterized by immunity failing to mount a response that would reject an allograft placed into the ocular microenvironment even if the immune response is primed.[2] Moreover, there is an induction of regulatory immunity to the foreign antigens.[3] This feature of ocular immunity defines immune privilege. The mechanisms of ocular immune privilege actively suppress the activation of effector T-cells, suppresses proinflammatory activation of macrophages and neutrophils and alters the presentation of antigen by antigen presenting cells to suppress inflammation and to promote regulatory T-cell activation.[4-7] The mediators of this immunosuppression are membrane bound proteins and soluble immunomodulating factors produced by parenchymal cells, neurons and immune cells within the ocular microenvironment.

The soluble immunomodulating factors within the ocular microenvironment are found primarily in aqueous humor, the fluid filling the anterior chamber of the eye. Aqueous humor suppresses inflammation mediated by macrophages stimulated with bacterial products.[8] In addition, aqueous humor treated macrophages and dendritic cells cannot function as antigen presenting cells that promote proinflammatory activity by T-cells.[9] Moreover, aqueous humor treatment of macrophages induces anti-inflammatory cytokine production and the presentation of antigen in a manner that promotes regulatory T-cell activation.[10,11] These findings suggest that resident ocular macrophages and dendritic cells are inhibited from mediating inflammation while they are still able to clear pathogens and damaged cells. When effector T-cells are treated with aqueous humor, the T-cells can no longer mediate hypersensitivity responses.[12] Aqueous humor changes the T-cell cytokine profile from interferon-gamma (IFN-γ), to transforming growth factor-beta (TGF-β).[11,13] This change is associated with the T-cells changing their functionality from inflam-

*Corresponding Author: Andrew W. Taylor—Schepens Eye Research Institute, 20 Staniford Street, Boston, Massachusetts 02114 USA. Email: andrew.taylor@schepens.harvard.edu

Melanocortins: Multiple Actions and Therapeutic Potential, edited by Anna Catania.
©2010 Landes Bioscience and Springer Science+Business Media.

matory to regulatory. The very ability of the ocular microenvironment to resist the activation of effector T-cells can be seen when effector T-cells are placed into the anterior chamber along with their specific antigen and antigen presenting cells.[12] Whereas, if this adoptive transfer of effector T-cells, antigen and antigen presenting cells were injected into the skin they would mediate a vigorous hypersensitivity response which does not occur when injected into the anterior chamber of the eye. Also, treatment of the effector T-cells with aqueous humor before injecting them with antigen and antigen presenting cells into the skin suppresses the expected inflammatory response.[12] Moreover, such aqueous humor treated T-cells function as regulatory T-cells and suppresses immunity.[13] Therefore, in aqueous humor there are constitutively expressed immunomodulating soluble factors that suppress the activation of inflammatory immunity while turning the immune response onto itself, further promoting immune privilege.

α-MSH in the Eye

Aqueous humor subjected to HPLC size separation revealed two fractions of immunomodulating activity.[14] The first fraction was found to be centered on 25 kDa associated with activated transforming growth factor-beta2 (TGF-β2). The second immunomodulating fraction was found to be the peptides contained in a fraction that was 2 kDa or less in molecular weight. It was in this low molecular weight fraction that the immunomodulating neuropeptides of aqueous humor were found. The first described immunomodulating neuropeptide in the eye was alpha-melanocyte stimulating hormone (α-MSH).[15] This thirteen amino acid long neuropeptide that is derived from sequential endoproteolytic cleavage and posttranslational modifications of pro-opiomelanocortin hormone (POMC) was originally described for its melanin-inducing activity in frogs.[16] In mammals it has become more evident that α-MSH has a more fundamental role in homeostasis of metabolism and immunity.[17-19]

The immunomodulating role of α-MSH is demonstrated by the suppression of endotoxin and proinflammatory cytokine (such as IL-1β and TNF-α) induced systemic inflammatory responses of animals injected with α-MSH.[20-27] At the cellular level, it is clear that α-MSH binds its melanocortin receptors on cells of innate immunity (macrophages, dendritic cells and neutrophils). The ability of these cells to generate reactive oxygen intermediates, nitric oxide, produce pro-inflammatory cytokines and to migrate are profoundly suppressed by α-MSH.[28-33] Endotoxin, IL-1β and TNF-α activated intracellular signaling pathways are blocked by α-MSH preventing the translocation of NF-kB from the cytoplasm to the nucleus.[34-41] This suppression is early in the signaling cascade and involves IRAK-M binding to IRAK-1.[42] In addition, α-MSH promotes production of anti-inflammatory cytokines like IL-10, its own production and up-regulates melanocortin receptor expression.[30,43-47] This action of α-MSH is not only anti-inflammatory, but it promotes a self-perpetuating anti-inflammatory autocrine loop.

In aqueous humor, α-MSH is constitutively present at a concentration of approximately 10^{-11} M.[15] Aqueous humor depleted of α-MSH can no longer modulate T-cell activity. The function that α-MSH plays in aqueous humor is to suppress IFN-γ production by effector T-cells. Also, it is through α-MSH that aqueous humor mediates a change in an antigen-specific T-cell response from proinflammatory to regulatory.[13,48] In this process, TGF-β2, also found in aqueous humor, helps enhance this activity of α-MSH induction of regulatory activity in T-cells.[48] The aqueous humor/α-MSH-induced regulatory T-cells express the expected regulatory T-cell marker of CD25 and are only CD4+ T-cells. These regulatory T-cells produce TGF-β, but not IL-4 or IL-10. It is possible to generate these T-cells in vitro by treating antigen-stimulated CD4+ T-cells with only α-MSH at its 10^{-11} M physiological concentration.[13,49,50] In adoptive transfer experiments it has been shown that these α-MSH-treated T-cells require restimulation with their specific antigen to activate their suppressive functionality, but they suppress the activation of neighboring T-cells that can be responding to other antigens.

The potential for α-MSH to induce regulatory T-cells in vivo was demonstrated by finding that melanocortin 5 receptor (MC5r) knocked-out mice naturally recovering from autoimmune uveitis lack the presence of retinal autoantigen-specific regulatory CD25+ CD4+ T-cells in their spleens, unlike wild type mice.[51,52] These results suggest that the natural recovery from autoimmune disease is not dependent on these regulatory T-cells, but that the induction of the regulatory T-cells through MC5r is a by-product of the recovery. A possible role for these regulatory T-cells is to prevent the expression of memory immunity to the autoantigens. When adoptively transferred, the regulatory T-cells from postrecovered wild type mice into post recovered MC5r mice prevent a rapid and severe uveitic response to a second immunization with retinal autoantigen.[51]

Melanocortin Receptors and the Eye

There are four melanocortin receptors for α-MSH that are differentially expressed throughout the body. In the eye, the melanocortin receptors MC3r, MC4r and MC5r are expressed in the inner neural retina layers with MC3r and MC4r localized to retinal ganglion cells, MC5r in the neural outer plexiform layers and the retinal pigment epithelial cells express MC1r and MC5r.[40,53] The expression of the melanocortin receptors in the eye are evolutionarily conserved and there is evidence that α-MSH, through its receptors, play an important role in retinal and neuronal development.[54-56] Neurite outgrowth from embryonic retinal explants can be stimulated with α-MSH treatment and there has been found a spatial and temporal expression of α-MSH in chick embryonic eye development with the retinal pigment epithelial cells as the source of α-MSH.[53,54] These indicate that with our previously described immunomodulating activity, α-MSH is also a neurotropic factor that may be necessary for development and survival of the retina.

Support of the dual role of α-MSH in the immune privileged eye is seen when we induce autoimmune disease in mice with MC5r knocked-out and when α-MSH is used as ocular therapy, which we will discuss in the next section.[51,57] As previously stated, the induction, tempo and resolution of autoimmune uveitis in the MC5r knock-out mice is no different from the wild type mouse. Also, while there is an induction of regulatory T-cells in the spleens of the wild type mice and not in the MC5r knock-out mice they are not necessary for the resolution of uveitis. One of the most striking differences is seen when comparing the histology of the post-uveitis retinas of the wild type and MC5r knock-out mice. The post-uveitic wild type mouse retina displays retinal folds and some granulomas formations, but is mostly intact with discernible retinal layers. In contrast, the retinas of post-EAU MC5r knock-out mice are severely damaged with losses in photoreceptors and disorganization of the retinal layers.[51,57] When a gene therapy approach was used to deliver α-MSH into the uveitic eyes of wild type mice and MC5r knock-out mice, only the uveitis of the wild type mouse was suppressed. The MC5r knock-out mice received no immunosuppressive benefit as observed in the wild type mice, but histological examination of the post-uveitis retina revealed less damage and some preservation of the retinal layers.[57] Such a benefit from α-MSH treatment may be due to it working through the other expressed melanocortin receptors in the eye. Such findings indicate the importance of the melanocortin system in the development, health, survival and immune privilege of the retina.

Application of α-MSH in Ocular Therapy

The immunomodulating activity and possible natural role in immune homeostasis of α-MSH has long suggested that it may be an effective and safe immunosuppressive therapy. There are multiple publications demonstrating the application of α-MSH either through peptide (cytokine-like) or gene therapy to suppress animal models of septic shock, contact hypersensitivity, allograft survival and multiple sclerosis.[23,24,27,31,35,43-45,57-66] Because of the intimate role of α-MSH in ocular immune privilege, the potential of delivering α-MSH into an inflamed or wounded eye to reimpose ocular immunosuppression has been an intriguing possibility. Several rodent models of ocular pathology have been tested and treated with α-MSH to see if it is possible to prevent, suppress and restore ocular immune privilege. Experimental autoimmune uveitis (EAU) and endotoxin induced uveitis (EIU) are rodent models for endogenous uveitis in humans, which in the USA 2 million persons are afflicted. Persistent and reoccurring uveitis leads to visual impairment and possible blindness. The current treatments are limited to steroids, which because of serious side effects limits their use. The potential of using an immunomodulating neuropeptide like α-MSH that has the additional possibility of (re)imposing immune privilege or immune tolerance is an exciting possibility of a new therapeutic approach.

The mouse model of EAU is an antigen specific, CD4$^+$ T-cell dependent, uveitis, in which mice are immunized to break tolerance and activate effector T-cells specific to the retinal antigens such as interphotoreceptor retinoid-binding protein (IRBP) and retinal soluble antigen (SAg).[67] The resulting inflammation of the retina is easily monitored and scored. The uveitis, unlike in many humans, is limited in that it lasts from 30 to 90 days depending on the strain of mouse when it spontaneously resolves. Analyzing how mouse uveitis spontaneously resolves led to finding the presence of MC5r-dependent regulatory T-cells in the spleens of EAU-recovered mice, which we discussed in the last two sections.[51,52] The methods of delivering α-MSH into mice with EAU have included systemic injections of α-MSH peptide and conjunctival injection of an α-MSH expression plasmid. If α-MSH is systemically injected when the uveitis is at its maximum, the treatment accelerates the recovery.[68] When α-MSH is injected at the start of uveitis it can delay the onset of the disease and when an α-MSH encoded plasmid is injected into the conjunctiva of mouse eyes at the onset of inflammation it suppresses the severity and hastens the resolution of the autoimmune disease.[57] The mechanism of immunosuppression mediated by these α-MSH therapies are not completely understood, but it is likely a combination of α-MSH antagonizing proinflammatory cytokines and chemokines and its induction of regulatory and immunosuppressive activity in immune cells. Whether these α-MSH therapies alone are sufficient to reestablish immune privilege is to be seen.

The EIU model of uveitis in rats is induced by the injection of bacterial endotoxin, lipopolysaccharide, which results in ocular inflammation within hours of the injection and is fully resolved by 48 hours.[69] This model of uveitis involves a stepwise change in the expression of intraocular inflammatory cytokines and chemokines.[69] These are followed by a breakdown in the blood ocular barrier and infiltration of immune cells. Around 24 hours, intraocular immunosuppressive molecules begin to be re-expressed, inflammation subsides and immune privilege is restored. It is viewed that in EIU, immune privilege is able to naturally reassert itself in response to the induction of innate immune mediated intraocular inflammation. A systemic injection of α-MSH peptide effectively inhibits the ocular inflammation and suppresses infiltration of cells into the ocular microenvironment.[63,64] The mechanism by which α-MSH can suppress EIU is through suppression of cyclooxygenase 2 production by macrophages within the ocular microenvironment.[64] The effect of α-MSH treatment is the suppression of the early events of EIU; therefore, preventing the subsequent infiltration of immune cells and production of proinflammatory cytokines and chemokines in the eye.[63] A similar anti-inflammatory efficacy was seen when α-MSH was systemically injected or topically applied to the eye of rabbits with surgical trauma to the cornea.[70]

The potential benefits of α-MSH therapy are not limited to only ocular inflammatory disease. There is a potential of α-MSH therapy to be effective in treating other ocular pathologies. Intravitreal injection of α-MSH analogs retard photoreceptor loss in RCS rat, which is a model of retinal dystrophy.[71] This may be working through the melanocortin receptors inducing some undefined neurotropic activity. It has also been demonstrated that topical application of α-MSH is effective in lowering the intraocular pressure in normal tension rabbits for up to six hours by stimulating PGE2 and prostacyclin levels in iris and ciliary body cells.[72] This finding suggests a potential for α-MSH therapy to be an effective antiglaucoma drug.

There is also the potential of using α-MSH in more unconventional therapies that involve manipulating immune cells ex vivo to generate antigen-specific regulatory T-cells. It is possible in a mouse model to generate ocular autoantigen specific T-cells that when restimulated and treated with α-MSH they become antigen-specific regulatory T-cells capable of suppressing EAU.[48] The only requirement of antigen specificity for these regulatory T-cells is that they are specific for any retinal autoantigen, not necessarily the target autoantigen.[13,48,50] Adoptive transfer of similarly generated α-MSH regulatory T-cells specific to retinal autoantigens into mice with neonatal retinal allografts suppressed graft rejection and promoted retinal tissue development.[65] This activity of the α-MSH generated regulatory T-cells tells us that these regulatory T-cells need to see their antigen to activate their immunosuppressive activity in vivo and the regulatory T-cells can create a supportive environment that promotes tissue survival and development. Therefore, a potential exists to take advantage of this feature of α-MSH generated regulatory T-cells and use the regulatory T-cells to suppress inflammation by generating α-MSH regulatory T-cells to any antigen expressed within the target tissue. It may even be possible to suppress autoimmunity by using an antigen that is purposely introduced into the tissue to activate the regulatory T-cells. This would be a benefit of using the α-MSH generated regulatory T-cells in autoimmune diseases where it is unclear as to what is the target antigen.

Conclusion

The role of α-MSH in mediating the expression of ocular immune privilege has further added to our understanding of α-MSH in the maintenance of immune homeostasis. The mechanisms of α-MSH modulation of immunity have suggested new therapeutic approaches to inflammatory and autoimmune diseases. Whether it is necessary to find ways that single out the immunomodulating activity of α-MSH from α-MSH's role in skin pigmentation and metabolic homeostasis is to be determined. The characterization of α-MSH in ocular immunity defines its importance and its place in the evolutionary adaptation of the ocular microenvironment to highly regulate immunity for the purpose of preserving vision.

References

1. Taylor AW. Ocular immune privilege. Eye 2009. Epub ahead of print (Epub ahead of print).
2. Medawar P. Immunity to homologous grafted skin. III. the fate of skin homografts transplanted to the brain to subcutaneous tissue and to the anterior chamber of the eye. Br J Exp Path 1948; 29:58-69.
3. Streilein JW. Ocular immune privilege: therapeutic opportunities from an experiment of nature. Nat Rev Immunol 2003; 3(11):879-889.
4. Taylor A. A review of the influence of aqueous humor on immunity. Ocul Immunol Inflamm 2003; 11(4):231-241.
5. Niederkorn JY. The immune privilege of corneal grafts. J Leukoc Biol 2003; 74(2):167-171.
6. Streilein JW, Masli S, Takeuchi M et al. The eye's view of antigen presentation. Hum Immunol 2002; 63(6):435-443.
7. Ferguson TA, Griffith TS. The role of Fas ligand and TNF-related apoptosis-inducing ligand (TRAIL) in the ocular immune response. Chemical Immunology and Allergy 2007; 92:140-154.
8. Taylor AW, Yee DG, Streilein JW. Suppression of nitric oxide generated by inflammatory macrophages by calcitonin gene-related peptide in aqueous humor. Invest Ophthalmol Vis Sci 1998; 39(8):1372-1378.
9. Taylor AW, Streilein JW, Cousins SW. Alpha-melanocyte-stimulating hormone suppresses antigen-stimulated T-cell production of gamma-interferon. Neuroimmunomodulation 1994; 1(3):188-194.
10. Lin HH, Faunce DE, Stacey M et al. The macrophage F4/80 receptor is required for the induction of antigen-specific efferent regulatory T-cells in peripheral tolerance. J Exp Med 2005; 201(10):1615-1625.
11. Taylor AW, Alard P, Yee DG et al. Aqueous humor induces transforming growth factor-beta (TGF-beta)-producing regulatory T-cells. Curr Eye Res 1997; 16(9):900-908.
12. Cousins SW, Trattler WB, Streilein JW. Immune privilege and suppression of immunogenic inflammation in the anterior chamber of the eye. Curr Eye Res 1991; 10(4):287-297.
13. Nishida T, Taylor AW. Specific aqueous humor factors induce activation of regulatory T-cells. Invest Ophthalmol Vis Sci 1999; 40(10):2268-2274.
14. Granstein R, Staszewski R, Knisely T et al. Aqueous humor contains transforming growth factor-β and a small (<3500 daltons) inhibitor of thymocyte proliferation. Journal of Immunology 1990; 144:3021-3027.
15. Taylor AW, Streilein JW, Cousins SW. Identification of alpha-melanocyte stimulating hormone as a potential immunosuppressive factor in aqueous humor. Curr Eye Res 1992; 11(12):1199-1206.
16. Lee TH, Lerner AB, Buettner-Janusch V. The isolation and structure of α- and β-melanocyte-stimulating hormones from monkey pituitary glands. Journal of Biological Chemistry 1961; 236:1390-1394.
17. Tung YC, Piper SJ, Yeung D et al. A comparative study of the central effects of specific POMC-derived melanocortin peptides on food intake and body weight in Pomc null mice. Endocrinology 2006.
18. Guijarro A, Laviano A, Meguid MM. Hypothalamic integration of immune function and metabolism. Prog Brain Res 2006; 153:367-405.
19. Lipton JM, Catania A. Anti-inflammatory actions of the neuroimmunomodulator alpha-MSH. Immunology Today 1997; 18(3):140-145.

20. Holdeman M, Khorram O, Samson WK et al. Fever-specific changes in central MSH and CRF concentrations. Am J Physiol 1985; 248:R125-R129.
21. Martin LW, Catania A, Hiltz ME et al. Neuropeptide alpha-MSH antagonizes IL-6- and TNF-induced fever. Peptides 1991; 12:297-299.
22. Martin LW, Lipton JM. Acute phase response to endotoxin: rise in plasma alpha-MSH and effects of alpha-MSH injection. Am J Physiol 1990; 259(4 Pt 2):R768-772.
23. Watanabe T, Hiltz ME, Catania A et al. Inhibition of IL-1b-induced periferal inflammation by peripheral and central administration of analogs of the neuropeptide α-MSH. Brain Res Bull 1993; 32:311-314.
24. Hiltz ME, Catania A, Lipton JM. Alpha-MSH peptides inhibit acute inflammation induced in mice by rIL-1 beta, rIL-6, rTNF-alpha and endogenous pyrogen but not that caused by LTB4, PAF and rIL-8. Cytokine 1992; 4(4):320-328.
25. Shih ST, Khorram O, Lipton JM et al. Central administration of alpha-MSH antiserum augments fever in the rabbit. Am J Physiol 1986; 250(5 Pt 2):R803-806.
26. Shih ST, Lipton JM. Intravenous alpha-MSH reduces fever in the squirrel monkey. Peptides 1985; 6(4):685-687.
27. Chiao H, Foster S, Thomas R et al. Alpha-melanocyte-stimulating hormone reduces endotoxin-induced liver inflammation. J Clin Invest 1996; 97(9):2038-2044.
28. Cannon JG, Tatro JB, Reichlin S et al. Alpha melanocyte stimulating hormone inhibits immunostimulatory and inflammatory actions of interleukin 1. J Immunol 1986; 137(7):2232-2236.
29. Catania A, Rajora N, Capsoni F et al. The neuropeptide alpha-MSH has specific receptors on neutrophils and reduces chemotaxis in vitro. Peptides 1996; 17(4):675-679.
30. Star RA, Rajora N, Huang J et al. Evidence of autocrine modulation of macrophage nitric oxide synthase by alpha-melanocyte-stimulating hormone. Proc Natl Acad Sci USA 1995; 92(17):8016-8020.
31. Rajora N, Boccoli G, Burns D et al. Alpha-MSH modulates local and circulating tumor necrosis factor-alpha in experimental brain inflammation. J Neurosci 1997; 17(6):2181-2186.
32. Mason MJ, Van Epps D. Modulation of IL-1, tumor necrosis factor and C5a-mediated murine neutrophil migration by alpha-melanocyte-stimulating hormone. J Immunol 1989; 142(5):1646-1651.
33. Manna SK, Sarkar A, Sreenivasan Y. Alpha-melanocyte-stimulating hormone down-regulates CXC receptors through activation of neutrophil elastase. Eur J Immunol 2006; 36(3):754-769.
34. Brzoska T, Kalden DH, Scholzen T et al. Molecular basis of the alpha-MSH/IL-1 antagonism. Ann N Y Acad Sci 1999; 885:230-238.
35. Ichiyama T, Sakai T, Catania A et al. Inhibition of peripheral NF-kappaB activation by central action of alpha-melanocyte-stimulating hormone. J Neuroimmunol 1999; 99(2):211-217.
36. Mandrika I, Muceniece R, Wikberg JE. Effects of melanocortin peptides on lipopolysaccharide/interferon-gamma-induced NF-kappaB DNA binding and nitric oxide production in macrophage-like RAW 264.7 cells: evidence for dual mechanisms of action. Biochemical Pharmacology 2001; 61(5):613-621.
37. Luger TA. Neuromediators—a crucial component of the skin immune system. Journal of Dermatological Science 2002; 30(2):87-93.
38. Sarkar A, Sreenivasan Y, Manna SK. Alpha-Melanocyte-stimulating hormone induces cell death in mast cells: involvement of NF-kappaB. FEBS Lett 2003; 549(1-3):87-93.
39. Teare KA, Pearson RG, Shakesheff KM et al. Alpha-MSH inhibits inflammatory signalling in Schwann cells. Neuroreport 2004; 15(3):493-498.
40. Cui HS, Hayasaka S, Zhang XY et al. Effect of alpha-melanocyte-stimulating hormone on interleukin 8 and monocyte chemotactic protein 1 expression in a human retinal pigment epithelial cell line. Ophthalmic Res 2005; 37(5):279-288.
41. Li D, Taylor AW. Diminishment of alpha-MSH anti-inflammatory activity in MC1r siRNA-transfected RAW264.7 macrophages. J Leukoc Biol 2008; 84(1):191-198.
42. Taylor AW. The immunomodulating neuropeptide alpha-melanocyte stimulating hormone (α-MSH) suppresses LPS-stimulated TLR4 with IRAK-M in macrophages. J Neuroimmunol 2005; 162:43-50.
43. Grabbe S, Bhardwaj RS, Mahnke K et al. Alpha-Melanocyte-stimulating hormone induces hapten-specific tolerance in mice. J Immunol 1996; 156(2):473-478.
44. Luger TA, Kalden D, Scholzen TE et al. Alpha-melanocyte-stimulating hormone as a mediator of tolerance induction. Pathobiology 1999; 67(5-6):318-321.
45. Raap U, Brzoska T, Sohl S et al. Alpha-melanocyte-stimulating hormone inhibits allergic airway inflammation. J Immunol 2003; 171(1):353-359.
46. Lam CW, Perretti M, Getting SJ. Melanocortin receptor signaling in RAW264.7 macrophage cell line. Peptides 2006; 27(2):404-412.
47. Taherzadeh S, Sharma S, Chhajlani V et al. alpha-MSH and its receptors in regulation of tumor necrosis factor-alpha production by human monocyte/macrophages. Am J Physiol 1999; 276(5 Pt 2):R1289-1294.
48. Taylor A, Namba K. In vitro induction of CD25+ CD4+ regulatory T-cells by the neuropeptide alpha-melanocyte stimulating hormone (alpha-MSH). Immunol Cell Biol 2001; 79(4):358-367.

49. Namba K, Kitaichi N, Nishida T et al. Induction of regulatory T-cells by the immunomodulating cytokines alpha-melanocyte-stimulating hormone and transforming growth factor-beta2. J Leukoc Biol 2002; 72(5):946-952.
50. Taylor AW. Modulation of regulatory T-cell immunity by the neuropeptide alpha-melanocyte stimulating hormone. Cell Mol Biol (Noisy-le-grand) 2003; 49(2):143-149.
51. Taylor AW, Kitaichi N, Biros D. Melanocortin 5 receptor and ocular immunity. Cell Mol Biol 2006; 52:141-147.
52. Kitaichi N, Namba K, Taylor AW. Inducible immune regulation following autoimmune disease in the immune-privileged eye. J Leukoc Biol 2005; 77(4):496-502.
53. Lindqvist N, Napankangas U, Lindblom J et al. Proopiomelanocortin and melanocortin receptors in the adult rat retino-tectal system and their regulation after optic nerve transection. Eur J Pharmacol 2003; 482(1-3):85-94.
54. Teshigawara K, Takahashi S, Boswell T et al. Identification of avian alpha-melanocyte-stimulating hormone in the eye: temporal and spatial regulation of expression in the developing chicken. J Endocrinol 2001; 168(3):527-537.
55. Ringholm A, Fredriksson R, Poliakova N et al. One melanocortin 4 and two melanocortin 5 receptors from zebrafish show remarkable conservation in structure and pharmacology. J Neurochem 2002; 82(1):6-18.
56. Cerda-Reverter JM, Ling MK, Schioth HB et al. Molecular cloning, characterization and brain mapping of the melanocortin 5 receptor in the goldfish. J Neurochem 2003; 87(6):1354-1367.
57. Lee DJ, Biros DJ, Taylor AW. Injection of an alpha-melanocyte stimulating hormone expression plasmid is effective in suppressing experimental autoimmune uveitis. Int Immunopharmacol 2009: In press.
58. Lee TH, Jawan B, Chou WY et al. Alpha-melanocyte-stimulating hormone gene therapy reverses carbon tetrachloride induced liver fibrosis in mice. The Journal of Gene Medicine 2006; 8(6):764-772.
59. Taylor AW, Kitaichi N. The diminishment of experimental autoimmune encephalomyelitis (EAE) by neuropeptide alpha-melanocyte stimulating hormone (alpha-MSH) therapy. Brain, Behavior and Immunity 2008; 22(5):639-646.
60. Wang CH, Jawan B, Lee TH et al. Single injection of naked plasmid encoding alpha-melanocyte-stimulating hormone protects against thioacetamide-induced acute liver failure in mice. Biochem Biophys Res Commun 2004; 322(1):153-161.
61. Ceriani G, Diaz J, Murphree S et al. The neuropeptide alpha-melanocyte-stimulating hormone inhibits experimental arthritis in rats. Neuroimmunomodulation 1994; 1(1):28-32.
62. Delgado Hernandez R, Demitri MT, Carlin A et al. Inhibition of systemic inflammation by central action of the neuropeptide alpha-melanocyte-stimulating hormone. Neuroimmunomodulation 1999; 6(3):187-192.
63. Nishida T, Miyata S, Itoh Y et al. Anti-inflammatory effects of alpha-melanocyte-stimulating hormone against rat endotoxin-induced uveitis and the time course of inflammatory agents in aqueous humor. Int Immunopharmacol 2004; 4(8):1059-1066.
64. Shiratori K, Ohgami K, Ilieva IB et al. Inhibition of endotoxin-induced uveitis and potentiation of cyclooxygenase-2 protein expression by alpha-melanocyte-stimulating hormone. Invest Ophthalmol Vis Sci 2004; 45(1):159-164.
65. Ng TF, Kitaichi N, Taylor AW. In vitro generated autoimmune regulatory T-cells enhance intravitreous allogeneic retinal graft survival. Invest Ophthalmol Vis Sci 2007; 48(11):5112-5117.
66. Gatti S, Colombo G, Buffa R et al. alpha-Melanocyte-stimulating hormone protects the allograft in experimental heart transplantation. Transplantation 2002; 74(12):1678-1684.
67. Caspi R, Roberge F, Chan C et al. A new model of autoimmune disease, experimental autoimmune uveoretinitis induced in mice with two different retinal antigens. Journal of Immunology 1988; 140:1490-1495.
68. Taylor AW, Yee DG, Nishida T et al. Neuropeptide regulation of immunity. The immunosuppressive activity of alpha-melanocyte-stimulating hormone (alpha-MSH). Ann NY Acad Sci 2000; 917:239-247.
69. Ohta K, Yamagami S, Taylor AW et al. IL-6 antagonizes TGF-beta and abolishes immune privilege in eyes with endotoxin-induced uveitis. Invest Ophthalmol Vis Sci 2000; 41(9):2591-2599.
70. Naveh N, Marshall J. Melanocortins are comparable to corticosteroids as inhibitors of traumatic ocular inflammation in rabbits. Graefes Arch Clin Exp Ophthalmol 2001; 239(11):840-844.
71. Naveh N. Melanocortins applied intravitreally delay retinal dystrophy in Royal College of Surgeons rats. Graefes Arch Clin Exp Ophthalmol 2003; 241(12):1044-1050.
72. Naveh N, Kaplan-Messas A, Marshall J. Mechanism related to reduction of intraocular pressure by melanocortins in rabbits. Br J Ophthalmol 2000; 84(12):1411-1414.

Index